J. Grote und C. Stick

Tissue Reactions in Response
to Hypoxia and Ischemia

Akademie der Wissenschaften und der Literatur
Mathematisch-naturwissenschaftliche Klasse

Funktionsanalyse biologischer Systeme

25 (1996)

Redaktion: Gerhard Thews

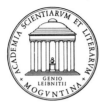

Akademie der Wissenschaften und der Literatur · Mainz · 1996

Tissue Reactions in Response to Hypoxia and Ischemia

7. Westerländer Gespräch
Erwin Riesch-Symposium
Westerland, 24 to 27 September 1992

Edited by J. Grote and C. Stick

With 69 Figures and 18 Tables

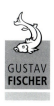

Gustav Fischer Verlag · Stuttgart · Jena · Lübeck · Ulm · 1996

Gefördert durch das Ministerium für Bildung, Wissenschaft und Weiterbildung
des Landes Rheinland-Pfalz, Mainz

Redaktion: Prof. Dr. Dr. Gerhard Thews, Akademie der Wissenschaften und der Literatur
Geschwister-Scholl-Str. 2, 55131 Mainz

Die Deutsche Bibliothek - CIP Einheitsaufnahme

Tissue reactions in response to hypoxia and ischemia : with 18
tables / 7. Westerländer Gespräch. Erwin-Riesch-Symposium,
Westerland, 24 to 27 September 1992. Ed. by J. Grote and C.
Stick. - Jena ; Lübeck : G. Fischer, 1996
  (Funktionsanalyse biologischer Systeme ; 25)
  ISBN 3-437-25148-1
NE: Grote, Jürgen [Hrsg.]; Westerländer Gespräch <7, 1992>; GT

©1996 by Akademie der Wissenschaften und der Literatur, Mainz.
Alle Rechte einschließlich des Rechts zur Vervielfältigung, zur Einspeisung in elektronische
Systeme sowie der Übersetzung vorbehalten. Jede Verwertung außerhalb der engen Grenzen
des Urheberrechtsgesetzes ist ohne ausdrückliche Genehmigung der Akademie und des Verlages unzulässig und strafbar.
Satz: Computersatz Karola Kammerdiener, Nieder-Olm
Druck: Strauss Offsetdruck GmbH, Mörlenbach
Gedruckt auf säurefreiem, chlorfrei gebleichtem Papier

ISBN 3-437-25148-1

Contents

List of speakers	7
Preface	9
G. HEUSCH, R. SCHULZ: Characterization of short-term hibernating myocardium	11
J.D. SCHIPKE, G. ARNOLD: Can ventricular function be down-regulated?	23
T. NOLL, H.M. PIPER: Mitochondrial contribution to energy metabolism in the hypoxic myocardial cell	33
R. MEYER, U. POHL, S.Y. WANG, B. REUFELS, O. ZIMMERMANN: The influence of $MgCl_2$ and Mg-Aspartate on membrane currents, cytoplasmic Ca^{2+} concentration and contraction of cardiac myocytes	43
L. NEYSES, A. BLAUFUSS, C. KUBISCH, B. WOLLNIK, A. MAASS, S. OBERDORF, C. GROHE, H. VETTER: Use of antisense oligonucleotides for selective inhibition of gene expression in adult cardiomyocytes	53
F. VETTERLEIN, P. N. TRAN, G. SCHMIDT: Effects of diltiazem on cellular redox-state and capillary perfusion in the hypoperfused myocardium of the anesthetized rat	63
G. SIEGEL, F. SCHNALKE, R. HETZER: Hyperpolarization, relaxation, and ionic concentrations in hypoxic human coronary arteries	69
E. SCHLICKER, B. MALINOWSKA: Six histamine H_1, H_2 or H_3 receptor-mediated effects in the cardiovascular system of pithed rats	83
M. HECKER, A.T. BARA, F. NESTLER, I. PÖRSTI, R. BUSSE: On the mechanism of the coronary dilator response to ACE inhibitors	91
A.R. PRIES, P. GAEHTGENS: Endothelium-dependent regulation of arteriolar tone in skeletal muscle *in vivo*	103
M. WAHL, L. SCHILLING, A. PARSONS: Nitric oxide (NO) acting as an endothelial and parenchymal vasodilating factor in cerebral arteries	113
M. WEHLER, J. GROTE: Effects of endothelium-derived nitric oxide on cerebral cortical blood flow during normoxia and hypoxia in rats	121
U. GÖBEL, H. THEILEN, W. KUSCHINSKY: Completness of brain capillary perfusion	131
A. HAGENDORFF, C. DETTMERS, M. MANZ, B. LÜDERITZ, A. HARTMANN, J. GROTE: Regional cerebral and myocardial blood flow during ventricular pacing in rats	137

A. WINKLER, F. STAUB, J. PETERS, O. KEMPSKI, A. BAETHMANN: Glial swelling and glial acidosis induced by arachidonic acid 145

M.D. MENGER, P. VAJKOCZY, C. BEGER, K. MESSMER: The study of the microcirculation of islets of Langerhans: An *in vivo* microscopic approach 153

O. AEDTNER, A. GRILLHÖSL, E. MANECK, R. GÖTZ, W. MOLL: Arterial blood flow velocity and elasticity in the fetal guinea pig 161

U. PEIPER, J. DEE, S. KLABUNDE, K. SCHUMACHER: Smooth muscle contraction kinetics in relation to membrane depolarization and sarcoplasmatic calcium concentration 169

G. GROS, H.-W. MÜLLER-DETHARD, W. BRUNS, W. ZINGEL: Carbonic anhydrase III regulation under chronic hypoxia and creatine depletion . . . 177

J. FANDREY, H.F. BUNN: Quantitation of erythropoietin messenger RNA in organs of the rat 193

K.-U. ECKARDT, A. KURTZ: Protein kinase C is a modulator of erythropoietin formation 201

W. JELKMANN, J. FANDREY, M. WOLFF, S. FREDE, H. PAGEL: Mechanism of action of thyroid hormones (T_3/T_4) on erythropoietin production 209

H. PAGEL, A. ENGEL: The increased production of erythropoietin by antidiuretic hormone is not mediated by vasoconstriction 219

U. RAUEN, W. LAUCHART, H.D. BECKER, H. DE GROOT: Energy-dependent injury to hepatic endothelial cells in organ preservation solutions 227

G. GRONOW, O. JUNG, M. MALYUSZ: Modulation of oxygen deprivation-induced cellular dysfunction by glycine and alanine 235

A. BRATTSTRÖM, E. APPENRODT, M. SONNTAG, H. LISTING, A. BRATTSTRÖM JR, R. MILLER, W. DEJONG, E. SIMEONOVA, L. PHAROW: Modulation of the baroreflex by central neuropeptides is due to the route of administration 245

J. LÜDEMANN, H. BRAUER, A. GENS, J. EXNER, S. WUSSOW, D. ROSSKOPF, W. SIFFERT, A. HONIG: Cardiorespiratory reactions to hyperoxia in young caucasian men with different platelet Na^+/H^+-antiporter activity 257

U. ZWIENER, R. BAUER, H. WITTE, W. BUCHENAU, D. HOYER: A feedforward control of vital compensation of hypoxic-acidotic effects in piglets . 265

H. HELLER, K.-D. SCHUSTER, B.O. GÖBEL: Influence of blood transfusion on fractionation of stable oxygen isotopes under the condition of severe anemia 273

E. SCHUBERT, W. LAUBE, A. PATZAK: Power spectral analysis of the heart period duration under conditions of rest and load 281

List of speakers

BRATTSTRÖM, A., Prof. Dr., Knoll Deutschland GmbH, Medizin, Minden
ECKARDT, K.-U., Priv.Doz. Dr., Abteilung Nephrologie, Universitätsklinikum Rudolf Virchow Berlin
FANDREY, J., Priv.Doz. Dr., Physiologisches Institut I der Universität Bonn
GRONOW, G., Priv.Doz. Dr., Physiologisches Institut der Universität zu Kiel
GROS, G., Prof. Dr., Zentrum Physiologie, Abteilung Vegetative Physiologie der Medizinischen Hochschule Hannover
HAGENDORFF, A., Dr., Medizinische Klinik und Poliklinik der Universität Bonn mit den Schwerpunkten Kardiologie und Pneumologie
HECKER, M., Priv.Doz. Dr., Zentrum der Physiologie, Klinikum der Johann Wolfgang Goethe-Universität Frankfurt
HELLER, H., Dr., Physiologisches Institut I der Universität Bonn
HEUSCH, G., Prof. Dr., Abteilung für Pathophysiologie, Zentrum für Innere Medizin, Universitätsklinikum Essen
JELKMANN, W., Prof. Dr., Institut für Physiologie, Medizinische Universität zu Lübeck
KUSCHINSKY, W., Prof. Dr., I. Physiologisches Institut der Universität Heidelberg
LÜDEMANN, J., Dr., Institut für Physiologie der Universität Greifswald
MENGER, M.D., Prof. Dr., Institut für Klinisch-Experimentelle Chirurgie, Universität des Saarlandes, Homburg/Saar
MEYER, R., Priv.Doz. Dr., Physiologisches Institut II der Universität Bonn
MOLL, W., Prof. Dr., Institut für Physiologie der Universität Regensburg
NEYSES, L., Priv.Doz. Dr., Medizinische Klinik der Universität Würzburg
PAGEL, H., Dr., Institut für Physiologie, Medizinische Universität zu Lübeck
PEIPER, U., Prof. Dr., Universitäts-Krankenhaus Eppendorf, Physiologisches Institut, Abteilung für Vegetative Physiologie
PIPER, H.M., Prof. Dr., Physiologisches Institut der Universität Gießen
PRIES, A.R., Prof. Dr., Institut für Physiologie der Freien Universität Berlin

RAUEN, U., Dr., Institut für Physiologische Chemie, Universitätsklinikum Essen

SCHIPKE, J. D., Priv.Doz. Dr., Institut für experimentelle Chirurgie der Universität Düsseldorf

SCHLICKER, E., Prof. Dr., Institut für Pharmakologie und Toxikologie der Universität Bonn

SCHUBERT, E., Prof. Dr., Institut für Physiologie, Medizinische Fakultät (Charite) der Humboldt-Universität zu Berlin

SIEGEL, G., Prof. Dr., Institut für Physiologie der Freien Universität Berlin

VETTERLEIN, F., Prof. Dr., Zentrum Pharmakologie und Toxikologie, Abteilung Neuropharmakologie, Universität Göttingen

WAHL, M., Prof. Dr., Physiologisches Institut der Universität München

WEHLER, M., Dr., Physiologisches Institut I der Universität Bonn

WINKLER, A., Dr., Institut für Chirurgische Forschung der Universität München, Klinikum Großhadern

ZWIENER, U., Prof. Dr. Dr., Institut für Pathophysiologie des Klinikums der Friedrich-Schiller-Universität, Jena

Preface

It is with great gratitude that we would like to dedicate the proceedings of the 7th Westerland Conference (Westerländer Gespräch) to the memory of Professor Dr. med. Erich Witzleb (1924 - 1991). Being engaged in experimental as well as in clinical research since 1956 Erich Witzleb organized several interdisciplinary conferences on the physiology and pathophysiology of the circulatory and respiratory system. From the very beginning the aim of the meetings was to bring together experts to discuss recent results from research fields of mutual interest. The symposia were held in Bad Oeynhausen, where Erich Witzleb was head of the Department of Physiology at the Gollwitzer-Meier-Institute from 1959 to 1970. It is obvious from the proceedings, published by Springer between 1957 and 1964 and by Thieme in 1968, that the seven Bad Oeynhausen Conferences (Bad Oeynhausener Gespräche) permitted a comprehensive review of the principal results of clinical and experimental investigations relevant to the topics of the symposia.

In 1970 Erich Witzleb accepted the offer of the University of Kiel to take the chair of the Department of Applied Physiology (Institut für angewandte Physiologie und medizinische Klimatologie). He moved to Kiel where he worked with great success over a period of more than two decades as a distinguished teacher and scientist.

The tradition of the Bad Oeynhausen Conferences was continued in Westerland on the island Sylt, where a branch of the Department of Applied Physiology is located. The first Westerland Conference was held in 1981. Since then every two years scientists from different clinical departments as well as from departments of physiology, biochemistry, molecular biology and pharmacology meet each other in Westerland for a stimulating exchange of their recent results of clinical, experimental or theoretical studies on tissue respiration and metabolism or the regulation of blood flow.

This volume contains the papers presented at the 7th Westerland Conference held in September 1992. The contributions discussed under the topic: Tissue Reactions in Response to Hypoxia and Ischemia, report on experimental and clinical studies.

The editors would like to express their gratitude to the Erwin Riesch-Stiftung, Lorch, for supporting the conference and to the Akademie der Wissenschaften und der Literatur, Mainz, for publishing these proceedings.

Jürgen Grote, Carsten Stick, Gerhard Thews

Characterization of short-term hibernating myocardium

G. Heusch and R. Schulz

Abteilung für Pathophysiologie, Zentrum für Innere Medizin, Universität Essen

Transition from a supply-demand imbalance to a state of perfusion-contraction matching

Upon acute coronary artery occlusion contractile function in the ischemic region rapidly ceases. Within a few cardiac cycles systolic segment shortening and systolic wall thickening are reduced (hypokinesis), later abolished (akinesis) and within 30 s to 2 min replaced by paradoxic systolic segment lengthening and systolic wall thinning (dyskinesis, bulging) [25,30,31]. The mechanisms underlying the rapid loss of contractile function in ischemic myocardium are less clear. Of particular interest in this context is the temporal course of changes in high-energy phosphates as compared to changes in contractile function. ATP is the ultimate energy source of the contractile machinery. While in a number of studies the decrease in myocardial ATP-content developed too slowly to account for the rapid reduction in contractile function [3,8,11], in a recent study a decrease in the subendocardial ATP-content occurred within the first 15 beats following the onset of myocardial ischemia [1]. While this recent finding would support the hypothesis that the decrease in the ATP-content might be responsible for the early ischemic decrease in contractile function, a compelling argument against the loss of ATP as the mediator of acute ischemic contractile failure, as noted by Katz, is that the result of ATP loss should be rigor of the myofibril rather than the observed *loss* of wall tension [12]. This obvious contradiction could be partially resolved by the fact that a small decrease in the intracellular ATP-content may not necessarily act as an energy restriction, but may act through modulation of excitation-contraction coupling [14] or activation of ion channels such as the ATP-dependent potassium channel [18,19,22]. Activation of ATP-dependent potassium channels shortens the action potential, thereby reducing the intracellular calcium concentration and finally decreasing contractile function. Alternatively, energy turnover rather than steady-state high-energy phosphate concentrations may be important to the ischemia-induced dysfunction. A decrease in the free energy change of ATP-hydrolysis parallels the decline of ventricular function in isolated rat hearts [11]. Also, a decreased rephosphorylation rate of cytosolic ADP from creatine phosphate (CP) [2], which serves as an intracellular energy reservoir, and is reduced very rapidly during ischemia [8], has been proposed to be involved in the early contractile failure. Other mechanisms which have been proposed include the development of intracellular acidosis [10], accumulation of inorganic phosphate [13] or impairment of sarcoplasmic calcium transport kinetics, which again may be pH- or ATP-dependent [14,17].

After 2-3 min of ischemia, there is a consistent relation between the reduced regional myocardial blood flow and reduced function [6,7,32]. These studies demonstrate that during steady-state ischemia reductions in regional myocardial blood flow, i.e. the supply of oxygen, are associated with appropriate reductions in regional myocardial function, i.e. the major determinant of the demand for oxygen. The initial transient state of myocardial ischemia which may be characterized as a supply-demand imbalance has been termed "relative ischemia", whereas the ensuing steady-state condition, characterized by proportionally reduced regional blood flow and function, was termed "absolute ischemia" by Gallagher et al. [7] and later "perfusion-contraction-matching" by Ross [24]. Both these concepts apply to a situation where some residual blood flow occurs via the stenotic coronary artery or via collaterals. It appears fair and attractive to view the transition from a short-lasting supply-demand imbalance to a steady-state balance of regional myocardial blood flow and function as an adaptative process. The ischemic myocardium may through reduction of its contractile function reduce energy expenditure by the contractile machinery, thereby adjusting to the reduced energy available, and protecting itself from the development of irreversible damage, and finally prolonging its viability.

The "hibernating" myocardium

With severe myocardial ischemia resulting from complete coronary occlusion, irreversible damage starts to develop after 20 min; the infarct develops as a transmural wavefront from the most ischemic subendocardial to the less ischemic subepicardial layers [23]. However, with more moderate non-transmural ischemia, regional myocardial blood flow and systolic wall thickening may be reduced by about 40 % for 5 hours without evidence of irreversible damage and gradual, but complete recovery of function over 1 week after reperfusion [16]. In a previous study from our laboratory, a reduction in regional myocardial work by as much as 70 % was tolerated for 90 min without the development of myocardial infarction [27].

Thus, a balance between supply and demand may not only exist during very early steady-state ischemia but for prolonged periods of time. Rahimtoola provided clinical evidence for such prolonged depression of regional myocardial function in ischemic myocardium which was reversible upon reperfusion [21] and termed this situation myocardial "hibernation" [15].

Recent experimental studies have revealed some metabolic features of such adaptation to prolonged moderate ischemia. During 3 hours of coronary stenosis in pigs, regional subendocardial blood flow was reduced by 50 % and remained stable throughout the ischemic period. Regional myocardial oxygen consumption was also reduced immediately after coronary inflow reduction and remained stable at this reduced level. Coronary venous pH and lactate extraction were significantly reduced and coronary venous Pco_2 increased immediately after coronary inflow reduction, but these parameters gradually returned towards control values during continued ischemia [4]. Likewise, within the first 60-90 min of moderate ischemia in anesthetized, open-chest pigs, subendocardial blood flow, systolic wall thickening and regional myocardial oxygen consumption remained stable at a reduced level. However, myocardial CP-content was significantly decreased at 5 min of ischemia, but gradually recovered to near control values over the ischemic period [20,27]. These recent studies are consistent with the idea that there is only a transient phase of an energetic supply-demand imbalance during early myocardial ischemia. The ensuing reduction in regional myocardial function induces a decrease of energy-demand and allows stabilization at a new level characterized by an energetic balance, as indicated by recovery of metabolic markers. As suggested previously [8], CP or the ratio of CP : ATP may be a particularly well suited marker of the balance between energy demand and energy supply.

Inotropic challenge of the "hibernating" myocardium

Myocardium subjected to 5 min of moderate ischemia retains its responsiveness to adrenoceptor activation using dobutamine [28]. This response to an inotropic challenge indicates that the mechanisms responsible for the decreased contractile function can be overridden. Additionally, the response to an inotropic challenge demonstrates that energy is available in the ischemic myocardium to support the response to inotropic activation. Since at least some metabolic features tend to improve during prolonged moderate ischemia, such inotropic responsiveness may persist or even improve in the "hibernating" myocardium. Thus, an inotropic reserve may be characteristic of viable myocardium successfully adapted to ischemia and therefore could be of diagnostic value to identify such areas. The objective of our studies performed in the last few years was to follow the time course of the inotropic responsiveness of myocardium subjected to moderate ischemia and to determine its aerobic and anaerobic metabolic correlates.

For these studies anesthetized swine were used, in which the left anterior descending (LAD) coronary artery was cannulated and perfused at constant flow (for details see: [28]). Regional myocardial blood flow was measured using radioactive tracer microspheres and the thickness of the anterior wall was continuously measured using sonomicrometry. For calculation of regional contractile performance a work index was used [28]. In brief, wall thickening was multiplied by the instantaneous left ventricular pressure; this product was then integrated throughout ventricular systole. Thus, dimensional change against a load during systole was used as an estimate of regional myocardial work. This measurement is useful in view of the ventricular asynchrony observed during regional ischemia and inotropic activation [9]. Regional myocardial oxygen and lactate consumption (cannulation of a local cardiac vein) as well as high-energy phosphates and glycogen content (transmural biopsies, bioluminescence technique) were measured. Following the instrumentation and a set of control measurements, coronary inflow was reduced to achieve a 55 % - 70 % reduction in the regional myocardial work index of the anterior wall.

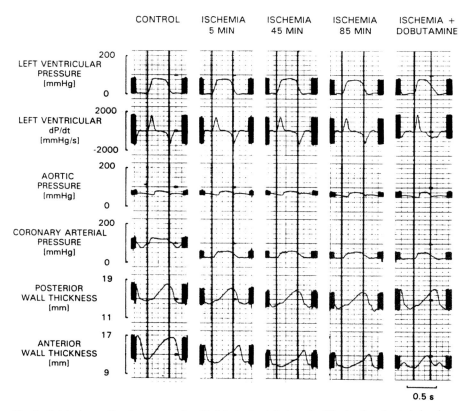

Fig. 1: Original recording from one study with dobutamine infusion after 90 min of moderate ischemia, showing left ventricular pressure, LV dP/dt, aortic pressure, coronary artery pressure, coronary blood flow and wall thickness of the anterior wall.
After control measurements coronary arterial pressure was reduced to decrease regional myocardial function by 70%. There was a tendency for a further decrease in function between 5 and 85 min of moderate ischemia. Infusion of dobutamine after 90 min of ischemia resulted in an increase in regional myocardial function.
(From [27] by permission of the American Heart Association).

At different time points during 85 min of coronary hypoperfusion, dobutamine was infused into the hypoperfused artery as an inotropic challenge. After 5 min of ischemia, transmural blood flow to the anterior wall was reduced from 0.61 ± 0.11 to 0.33 ± 0.08 ml/min/g, with no further change occurring between 5 and 85 min of ischemia and the subsequent infusion of dobutamine. This short-term inotropic stimulation increased positive LVdP/dt and decreased negative LVdP/dt. The work index was reduced by 54 % after 5 min of moderate ischemia with a tendency for a further decrease between 5 and 85 min of ischemia (Fig. 2). Infusion of dobutamine after 85 min of ischemia resulted in an increase in the work index by 61 %

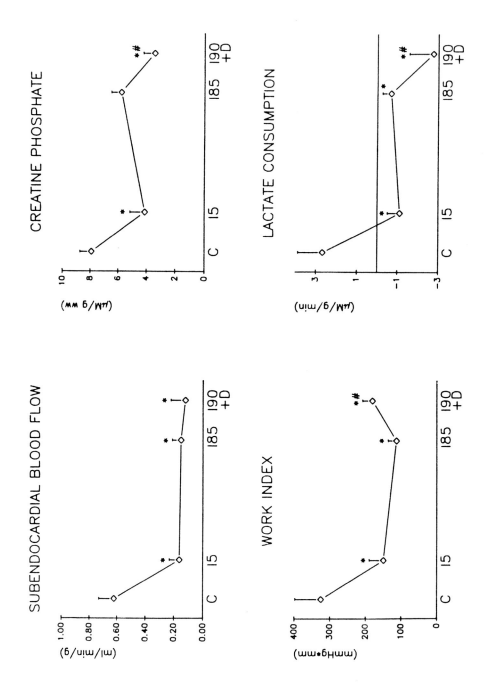

(Fig. 2). At 5 min of ischemia regional myocardial oxygen consumption was decreased by 38 %, CP-content fell by 48 % (Fig. 2) and lactate consumption was reversed to net lactate production (Fig. 2). Prolonging the ischemia to 85 min had no additional effect on regional myocardial oxygen consumption or the myocardial ATP-content. Myocardial lactate production tended to be attenuated (Fig. 2) and the CP-content returned to near control values (Fig. 2). Infusion of dobutamine again caused increased lactate production and the CP-content decreased (Fig. 2); the ATP-content and regional myocardial oxygen consumption were unaffected [27].

These results once again indicate that regional contractile function is decreased in response to moderate ischemia thereby allowing for partial normalization of metabolism. Despite this decrease in baseline function, the hypoperfused myocardium retains its responsiveness to an inotropic challenge by dobutamine. Thus, adrenoceptors are still accessible, excitation-contraction coupling can be stimulated and the myofibrils respond appropriately with increased work. This increase in work implies increased energy utilization. Since lactate production was once more increased by the inotropic challenge, an anaerobic energy production is suggested. This is further supported by failure of regional myocardial oxygen consumption to increase. The fact that CP fell with the enhanced regional function indicates that this energy reservoir was utilized more rapidly than it was being replenished. Thus, inotropic challenge once again can upset the balance between regional myocardial blood flow and regional myocardial function in moderately ischemic myocardium.

Fig. 2: A = Regional work performed by the anterior myocardium during moderate myocardial ischemia and the subsequent intracoronary dobutamine (+DOB) infusion. The work index was reduced at 5 min of ischemia with a tendency for a further decrease during ongoing ischemia. Infusion of dobutamine after 85 min of ischemia resulted in an increase of the work index.
2: B = Subendocardial blood flow of the anterior myocardium during moderate myocardial ischemia and the subsequent intracoronary dobutamine (+DOB) infusion. Subendocardial blood flow was reduced at 5 min of ischemia and did not change further during ongoing ischemia or the subsequent infusion of dobutamine.
2: C = Creatine phosphate (CP) concentration of the anterior myocardium during moderate myocardial ischemia and the subsequent intracoronary dobutamine (+DOB) infusion. Five min of ischemia resulted in a decrease in CP content. During ongoing ischemia CP content increased; at 85 min of ischemia CP had returned to near the control value. Infusion of dobutamine again caused a decrease in CP content.
2D: Lactate consumption (V_{Lac}) of the anterior myocardium during moderate myocardial ischemia and the subsequent intracoronary dobutamine (+DOB) infusion. Five min of ischemia resulted in a net lactate production which, however, was attenuated when ischemia was prolonged to 85 min. Infusion of dobutamine after 85 min of ischemia again caused a marked increase in lactate production.
Data from [27]

Prolonged inotropic stimulation and precipitation of myocardial infarction

More prolonged inotropic stimulation may not only impair metabolic recovery, but disrupt the state of hibernation and precipitate infarction. To study the impact of prolonged inotropic stimulation on hibernating myocardium, coronary inflow was reduced to decrease the regional myocardial work index by 70 % at 5 min of ischemia in 12 swine. Dobutamine was then infused for an additional 85 min. The work index increased at 5 min of dobutamine infusion from 73 ± 35 mmHg·mm to 139 ± 34 mmHg·mm ($p<0.05$ vs. 5 min of ischemia). However, this increase was only transient and after 85 min of dobutamine infusion, the work index was decreased below the initial ischemic value (42 ± 34 mmHg·mm). At 5 min of ischemia, CP-content was reduced from 8.80 ± 1.97 to 6.21 ± 3.87 $\mu M \cdot g^{-1}$ wet wt, and myocardial ATP-content was slightly decreased from 4.75 ± 0.92 to 4.12 ± 1.29 $mM \cdot g^{-1}$ wet wt (both NS). After 5 min of dobutamine infusion, further reductions in the CP-content to 3.11 ± 0.76 $mM \cdot g^{-1}$ wet wt and ATP to 3.14 ± 0.81 $mM \cdot g^{-1}$ wet wt were observed (both $p<0.05$). During the remainder of the continuous dobutamine infusion, the CP-content remained unchanged, while the ATP-content further decreased significantly to 1.68 ± 0.96 $mM \cdot g^{-1}$ wet wt. The ß-adrenoceptor density of the LAD-perfused myocardium was 36.5 ± 5.8 fmol ICYP·mg^{-1} protein under control conditions and was unchanged during ischemia and the subsequent dobutamine infusion. Following 2 hrs of reperfusion, infarct size (TTC-staining) was 26.3 ± 7.5 % of the area at risk. These results demonstrate that prolonged inotropic stimulation can disrupt the adaptation process of moderately ischemic myocardium, disrupt the state of hibernation and finally precipitate myocardial infarction [29].

Short-term vs. long-term myocardial "hibernation"

Myocardial hibernation in the clinical setting is a situation of contractile dysfunction in patients with coronary artery disease which exists for months or years, but is fully reversible upon reperfusion. Such long-term hibernation, in contrast to the short-term hibernation studied in animal models so far, is accompanied by morphological alterations of the ischemic myocardium. In biopsies taken during coronary bypass grafting from patients with reversible contractile dysfunction, desorganisation of sarcomer filaments and loss of the sarcoplasmic reticulum were demonstrated [5]. Thus, although the myocardium remains viable during prolonged periods of hypoperfusion, morphological alterations nevertheless occur and may explain why contractile function recovers only slowly during reperfusion.

Conclusions and perspectives

It is currently unclear, for how long and to what levels of blood flow the ischemic myocardium can successfully adapt. However, it is clear that the clinical identification of such viable, hibernating myocardium using imaging techniques is of utmost importance for the selection of patients to undergo reperfusion procedures. NMR-spectroscopy [33] to analyze myocardial high- energy phosphates and PET techniques [26] to analyze anaerobic glycolysis appear to be particularly suited to distinguish reversibly injured, hibernating from irreversibly injured, necrotic myocardium both of which may exhibit hypokinesis. Also, recruitment of an inotropic reserve may be taken as evidence of hibernating myocardium. However, prolonged inotropic stimulation will certainly deplete the remaining energy reservoirs and once again upset the balance of supply and demand in the hibernating myocardium, thereby jeopardizing its successful adaptation to the reduction in blood flow. It also needs to be emphasized that with complete coronary occlusion and in the absence of collateral blood flow myocardial infarction will inevitably occur. Only in the presence of some residual blood flow, can a reduction in metabolic demand delay infarct development.

References

1. ARAI, A. E., G. A. PANTELY, W. J. THOMA, C. G. ANSELONE & J. D. BRISTOW (1992): Energy metabolism and contractile function after 15 beats of moderate myocardial ischemia. Circ. Res. 70: 1137-1145.
2. BITTL, J. A., J. A. BALSCHI & J. S. INGWALL (1987): Contractile failure and high-energy phosphate turnover during hypoxia: 31P-NMR surface coil studies in living rat. Circ. Res. 60: 871-878.
3. BRAASCH, W., S. GUDBJARNASON, P. S. PURI, K. G. RAVENS & R. J. BING (1968): Early changes in energy metabolism in the myocardium following acute coronary artery occlusion in anesthetized dogs. Circ. Res. 23: 429-438.

4. FEDELE, F. A., H. GEWIRTZ, R. J. CAPONE, B. SHARAF & A. S. MOST (1988): Metabolic response to prolonged reduction of myocardial blood flow distal to a severe coronary artery stenosis. Circulation 78: 729-735.
5. FLAMENG, W., R. SUY, F. SCHWARZ, M. BORGERS, J. PIESSENS, F. THONE, H. VAN ERMEN & H. DE GEEST (1981): Ultrastructural correlates of left ventricular contraction abnormalities in patients with chronic ischemic heart disease: Determinants of reversible segmental asynergy postrevascularization surgery. Am. Heart J. 102: 846-857.
6. GALLAGHER, K. P., M. MATSUZAKI, J. A. KOZIOL, W. S. KEMPER & J. ROSS JR. (1984): Regional myocardial perfusion and wall thickening during ischemia in conscious dogs. Am. J. Physiol. 247: H727-H738.
7. GALLAGHER, K. P., M. MATSUZAKI, G. OSAKADA, W. S. KEMPER & J. ROSS JR. (1983): Effect of exercise on the relationship between myocardial blood flow and systolic wall thickening in dogs with acute coronary stenosis. Circ. Res. 52: 716-729.
8. GUTH, B. D., J. F. MARTIN, G. HEUSCH & J. ROSS JR. (1987): Regional myocardial blood flow, function and metabolism using phosphorus- 31 nuclear magnetic resonance spectroscopy during ischemia and reperfusion. J. Am. Coll. Cardiol. 10: 673-681.
9. GUTH, B. D., R. SCHULZ, AND G. HEUSCH (1990): Evaluation of parameters for the assessment of regional myocardial contractile function during asynchronous left ventricular contraction. Basic Res. Cardiol. 85: 550-562.
10. JACOBUS, W. E., I. H. PORES, S. K. LUCAS, M. L. WEISFELDT & J. T. FLAHERTY (1982): Intracellular acidosis and contractility in normal and ischemic hearts examined by 31p NMR. J. Mol. Cell. Cardiol. 14: 13-20.
11. KAMMERMEIER, H., P. SCHMIDT & E. JÜNGLING (1982): Free energy change of ATP-hydrolysis: a causal factor of early hypoxic failure of the myocardium? J. Mol. Cell. Cardiol. 14: 267-277.
12. KATZ, A. M. (1973): Effects of ischemia on the contractile processes of heart muscle. Am. J. Cardiol. 32: 456-460.
13. KUSUOKA, H., M. L. WEISFELDT, J. L. ZWEIER, W. E. JACOBUS & E. MARBAN (1986): Mechanism of early contractile failure during hypoxia in intact ferret heart: Evidence for modulation of maximal Ca-activated force by inorganic phosphate. Circ. Res. 59: 270-282.
14. KÜBLER, W. & A. M. KATZ (197): Mechanism of early "pump" failure of the ischemic heart: possible role of adenosine triphosphate depletion and inorganic phosphate accumulation. Am. J. Cardiol. 40: 467-471.
15. LUNDE, H., T. HEDNER, O. SAMUELSSON, J. LÖTVALL, L. ANDREN, L. LINDHOLM, & B.-E. WIHOLM (1994): Dyspnoea, asthma, and bronchospasm in relation to treatment with angiotensin converting enzyme inhibitors. Br. Med. J. 308: 18-21.
16. MATSUZAKI, M., K. P. GALLAGHER, W. S. KEMPER, F. WHITE & J. ROSS JR. (1983): Sustained regional dysfunction produced by prolonged coronary stenosis: gradual recovery after reperfusion. Circulation 68: 170-182.
17. NAYLER, W. G., P. A. POOLE-WILSON & A. WILLIAMS (1979): Hypoxia and calcium. J. Mol. Cell. Cardiol. 11: 683-706.
18. NICHOLS, C. G., C. RIPOLL & W. J. LEDERER (1991): ATP-sensitive potassium channel modulation of guinea pig ventricular action potential and contraction. Circ. Res. 68: 280-287.
19. NOMA, A. (1983): ATP- regulated K+ channels in cardiac muscle. Nature 305: 147-148.

20. PANTELY, G. A., S. A. MALONE, W. S. RHEN, C. G. ANSELONE, A. ARAI, J. BRISTOW & J. D. BRISTOW (1990): Regeneration of myocardial phosphocreatine in pigs despite continued moderate ischemia. Circ. Res. 67: 1481-1493.
21. RAHIMTOOLA, S. H. (1989): A perspective on the three large multicenter randomized clinical trials of coronary bypass surgery for chronic stable angina. Circulation 72 Suppl.V: V-123-V-135.
22. REFFELMANN, T. & H. KAMMERMEIER (1992): Energetics and function of hypoxic isolated rat hearts as influenced by modulation of the K+-ATP-channel-system. Pfluegers Arch. 420 (Suppl 1): R105.
23. REIMER, K. A., J. E. LOWE, M. M. RASMUSSEN & R. B. JENNINGS (1977): The wavefront phenomenon of ischemic cell death. 1. Myocardial infarct size vs duration of coronary occlusion in dogs. Circulation 56: 786-794.
24. ROSS JR., J. (1991): Myocardial perfusion-contraction matching. Implications for coronary heart disease and hibernation. Circulation 83: 1076-1083.
25. SASAYAMA, S., D. FRANKLIN, J. ROSS JR., W. S. KEMPER & D. MCKOWN (1976): Dynamic changes in left ventricular wall thickness and their use in analyzing cardiac function in the conscious dog. Am. J. Cardiol. 38: 870-879.
26. SCHELBERT, H. R. (1991): Positron emission tomography for the assessment of myocardial viability. Circulation 84 (Suppl I): I-122-I-131.
27. SCHULZ, R., B. D. GUTH, K. PIEPER, C. MARTIN & G. HEUSCH (1992): Recruitment of an inotropic reserve in moderately ischemic myocardium at the expense of metabolic recovery: a model of short-term hibernation. Circ. Res. 70: 1282-1295.
28. SCHULZ, R., S. MIYAZAKI, M. MILLER, E. THAULOW, G. HEUSCH, J. ROSS JR. & B. D. GUTH (1989): Consequences of regional inotropic stimulation of ischemic myocardium on regional myocardial blood flow and function in anesthetized swine. Circ. Res. 64: 1116-1126.
29. SCHULZ, R., J. ROSE, C. MARTIN, O. E. BRODDE & G. HEUSCH (1993): Development of short-term myocardial hibernation: its limitation by the severity of ischemia and inotropic stimulation. Circulation 88: 684-695.
30. THEROUX, P., D. FRANKLIN, J. ROSS JR. & W. S. KEMPER (1974): Regional myocardial function during acute coronary artery occlusion and its modification by pharmacological agents in the dog. Circ. Res. 35: 896-908.
31. THEROUX, P., J. ROSS JR., D. FRANKLIN, W. S. KEMPER & S. SASAYAMA (1976): Regional myocardial function in the conscious dog during acute coronary occlusion and responses to morphine, propranolol, nitroglycerin, and lidocaine. Circulation 53: 302-314.
32. VATNER, S. F. (1980): Correlation between acute reductions in myocardial blood flow and function in conscious dogs. Circ. Res. 47: 201-207.
33. WEISS, R. G., P. A. BOTTOMLEY, C. J. HARDY & G. GERSTENBLITH (1990): Regional myocardial metabolism of high-energy phosphates during isometric exercise in patients with coronary artery disease. N. Engl. J. Med. 323: 1593-1600.

Can ventricular function be down-regulated?

J.D. Schipke and G. Arnold

Institut für Experimentelle Chirurgie der Universität Düsseldorf

Introduction

It is well accepted that during physiologic conditions, cardiac function and oxygen supply match. Moreover, function can only be increased, if oxygen supply can increase and, in turn, function will decrease, if oxygen supply is reduced. In the present paper, this paradigm of balanced oxygen demand and supply will be challenged on the basis of the more recent literature and on the basis of own investigations.

Down-Regulation

Myocardial function and coronary blood flow are tightly coupled. Due to the autoregulation, coronary blood flow remains constant within the physiologic range of perfusion pressure. Thus, ventricular function is not affected if coronary perfusion pressure is moderately reduced, and is not impaired unless the perfusion pressure falls below a critical value. These previous statements are displayed in Fig. 1 where regional function, expressed in terms of wall thickening is plotted against coronary arterial pressure [1]. Within the autoregulatory range, reductions in coronary arterial pressure are not associated with reductions in regional function. Once a critical pressure is reached, decreases in coronary arterial pressure and hence, oxygen supply, are paralleled by decreases in regional function.

This condition is known as myocardial ischemia which is almost generally believed to reflect a mismatch between oxygen supply and oxygen demand, and to result in necrosis in case it persists. In the following, this view will be challenged for particular myocardial states.

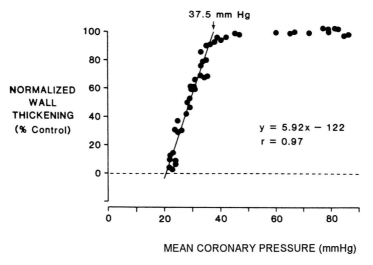

Fig. 1: Dependency of regional ventricular function (normalized wall thickening) on mean coronary arterial pressure. (Canty, 1988)

Down-Regulation in Isolated Hearts

Jacobus and coworkers [2] showed from their experiments on isolated rat hearts that reducing coronary flow, and likewise oxygen supply, down to about 50 % of normal, did not result in the common signs of ischemia (Fig. 2). Because the flow reductions were paralleled by decreases in ventricular function, expressed in terms of developed pressure (DP), the authors suggested a mechanism that specifically reduces ventricular function and thus, reduces, oxygen demand. They termed this mechanism 'down-regulation' of function.

The biochemical background of such a phenomenon remains unclear. It is known, however, that the occlusion of a coronary artery results in reduced intracellular phosphocreatine and increased inorganic phosphate. Thus, depletion of high energy phosphates could induce the decreased ventricular function during reduced coronary blood flow.

In our own experiments on isolated, blood-perfused canine hearts, the perfusion pressure was systematically varied [3]. Ventricular function was assessed in terms of peak isovolumic left ventricular pressure, and the intracellular content of high energy phosphates was assessed with the help of NMR-spectroscopy. In Fig. 3, three ranges of coronary arterial pressure

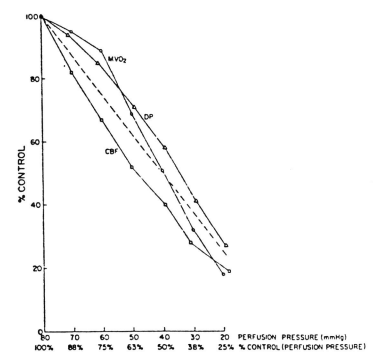

Fig. 2: Effect of reduction in perfusion pressure on coronary flow (CBF), developed pressure (DP) and myocardial oxygen consumption ($M\dot{V}O_2$) in buffer-perfused rat hearts. (Jacobus et al., 1982)

can be differentiated: a range in which decreased perfusion pressure had no effect on either ventricular function or high energy phosphates. This range is most probably identical to the autoregulatory range. Further reductions in arterial pressure were associated with reductions in ventricular function, whereas high energy phosphates remained unchanged (second range). If coronary arterial pressure was further reduced, both function and phosphorous metabolism declined and did not reach steady state (third range).

The major finding of our experiments was that for perfusion pressures between about 25 and 50 mmHg, i.e., in a range below autoregulation, ventricular function was impaired without exhibiting the common signs of myocardial ischemia, that means, phosphocreatine was not depleted and inorganic phosphate did not accumulate, suggesting a down-regulated ventricular function at equilibrium phosphorous metabolism. It was an additional characteristic of the second range that ventricular function remained constant throughout the 15 min duration of the experimental step.

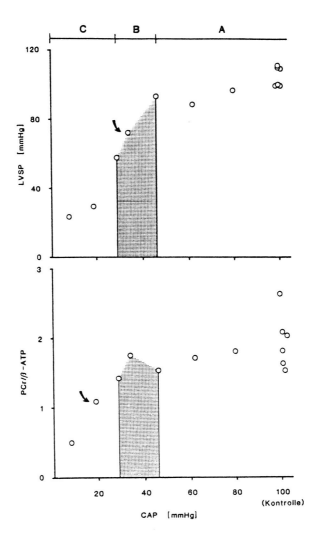

Fig. 3: Effects of reduction in coronary arterial pressure (CAP) on left ventricular peak systolic pressure (LVSP, top) and the tissue concentrations of phosphocreatine (PCr/β-ATP, bottom). The shaded area represents a range, where ventricular function was already impaired whereas the ratio of PCr over β-ATP was unchanged.

Moreover, ventricular function quickly achieved its initial value after physiologic perfusion was reinstated, whereas function remained considerably depressed during reperfusion following decreases in perfusion pressure to very low values.

Can ventricular function be down-regulated?

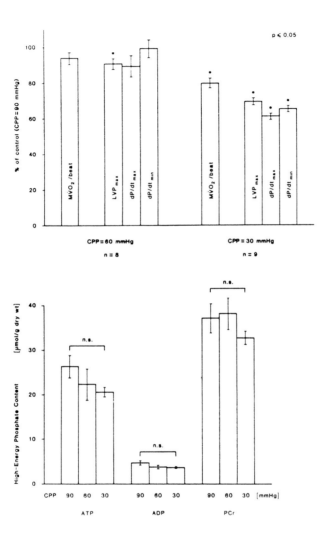

Fig. 4: Effects of reduction of the coronary perfusion pressure (CPP) from 90 to 60 and 30 mmHg on myocardial oxygen consumption (MVO_2) and left ventricular function (top), and on the intracellular concentrations of ATP, ADP and phosphocreatine (bottom). At both levels of reduced oxygen supply, function remained stable and the content in high energy phosphates was only insignificantly reduced.

In more recent investigations on isolated, saline-perfused rabbit hearts, coronary arterial pressure was reduced from 90 to 60 and 30 mmHg [4]

(Fig. 4). Both oxygen consumption and ventricular function stepwise decreased and achieved always steady state conditions within the observation period supporting the view that no mismatch had occurred between the reduced oxygen supply and the reduced function. Because the intracellular content of high energy phosphates showed no major alterations, these results support our view of a new low-level equilibrium.

An additional aspect of down-regulation of function was investigated on isolated ferret hearts [5]. After reducing the perfusion pressure down to values that did not yet affect the intracellular concentration of high energy phosphates, the authors observed a decrease in the phasic concentration of free, intracellular Ca^{++}, i.e. in the Ca^{++} transients. The authors infer from the down-regulated Ca^{++} transients that there exists a protective mechanism, which minimizes the myocardial energy requirements during a period of reduced coronary flow.

In Situ Down-Regulation

In investigations on isolated piglet hearts, Downing and Chen [6] extended the state of reduced oxygen supply to 2 h. They decreased the perfusion pressure so that the oxygen supply was reduced to 20 % of control. After decrease of ventricular function, intracellular phosphocreatine content remained unchanged whereas the ATP content was reduced to 75 %. Because a new equilibrium was achieved during the observation period, the authors conclude that the myocardium employs an intrinsic property to adapt its function to the reduced oxygen supply. They interpret their observation as a result of a mechanism that protects the myocardium towards irreversible ischemic damage. The results show that the phenomenon is not only short lasting and that it exists already in juvenile animals.

When investigating the effects of hypoxia on cardiac function in adult anaethetized rats, Bittl and coworkers [7] could demonstrate a decreased turnover of high energy compounds that might be responsible for contractile failure during hypoxia. Their findings support the concept that the myocardium, to a certain extent, employs mechanisms to down-regulate its mechanical activitiy in order to avoid the consequences of ischemia.

Comparable conclusions can be drawn from a paper by Gallagher and coworkers [8] who observed in conscious exercising dogs, following restriction in coronary blood flow, a myocardial dysfunction which, in turn, reduced the oxygen demand in the involved myocardial region until a new equilibrium was reached between oxygen supply and demand.

In experiments on anesthetized pigs, coronary blood flow was decreased during 1 h to about 30 % of control [9]. Likewise, regional function was reduced to about 30 %. Compared with control, ATP and phosphocreatine concentrations of the myocardium were decreased during early ischemia. In the course of the experiments, ATP concentration continued to decrease, while the PCr concentration slowly recovered. At the end of the experiments, oxygen consumption was increased by electrically pacing the hearts. The fact that the PCr concentration decreased during this intervention, shows that the myocardial cells could utilize the normalized PCr stores. The authors conclude from their findings that the down-regulatory process is not a passive adaptation but an active process.

Trigger of Down-Regulation

No particular trigger is identified, so far, to initiate down-regulation. Both the intracellular concentrations and the turnover of high energy phosphate compounds are discussed, as well as the Ca^{++} transients. Recently, also the activity of ATP-depending K^+ channels was made responsible for initiating the down-regulation of function [10]. From the observation that myocardial function quickly recovers upon successful reperfusion, Rutishauser and colleagues [11] conclude that restoration of the intravasal pressure might be responsible for the functional recovery via an 'erectile' effect. In turn, decrease of the intravasal pressure could be another candidate for initiating down-regulation.

Hibernation

Some authors used the term hibernation for the particular myocardial state that results from a down-regulation of function. Rahimtoola first defined the hibernating myocardium as abnormal left ventricular function due to chronic, painless, resting, persistent, *severe* myocardial 'ischemia' which was reversible [12] but later considered hibernating myocardium as a result of mild to moderate ischemia [13]. By others, hibernating myocardium was characterized by akinetic/dyskinetic segments, reduced perfusion, and yet active metabolism [14,15].

Such myocardial segments have been shown to recover following surgical revascularization. A number of clinical groups have demonstrated that hibernating myocardium in patients quickly regained normal function during reperfusion, i.e. after successful revascularization.

Summary

On the basis on the literature and on our own experiments, we challenge the common concept that myocardial ischemia is an allornothing process. As long as the extent of myocardial ischemia is mild to moderate, it can be longlasting because the reduced metabolism matches the down-regulated function. It is unclear, however, whether down-regulation represents an active process. As possible triggers for such down-regulation, concentration and/or turnover of high-energy phosphates, Ca^{++} transients, ATP-dependent K^+ channels, and the loss of intravasal pressure are discussed. As the result of a down-regulatory process, there exists no mismatch between supply and demand, no cellular damage will occur, and the cells will remain viable. We suggest that this state does not reflect ischemia in its more classical sense but should be termed hibernation. After reperfusion, the myocardial state will return to normal, i.e. the state will be physiologic with its function being normal.

References

1. CANTY, J.M. (1988): Coronary pressure-function and steady-state pressure-flow relations during autoregulation in the unanesthetized dog. Circ. Res. 63, 821-836.
2. JACOBUS, W.E., I.H. PORES, S.K. LUCAS, C.H. KALIMAN, M.L. WEISFELDT & J.T. FLAHERTY (1982): The role of intracellular pH in the control of normal and ischemic myocardial contractility: A 31P nuclear magnetic resonance and mass spectrometry study. New York: Alan R. Liss, 537-565.
3. SCHIPKE, J.D., Y. HARASAWA, D. BURKHOFF, V.P. CHACKO, K. SAGAWA & W.E. JACOBUS (1989): Decreased LV function secondary to decreased coronary arterial pressure (CAP) is not due to reduced high-energy phosphate content. Faseb J. 3(3), A249.
4. SUNDERDIEK, U., I. BERGFELD, M. SCHWENEN, G. ARNOLD & J. D. SCHIPKE (1992): Myocardial function and energy balance during reduced myocardial perfusion. Eur. Heart J. 13, 43.
5. MARBAN, E., M. KITAKAZE, V.P. CHACKO & M.M. PIKE (1988): Ca2+ transients in perfused hearts revealed by gated 19F NMR spectroscopy. Circ. Res. 63, 673-678.

6. DOWNING, S.E. & V. CHEN (1990): Myocardial hibernation in the ischemic neonatal heart. Circ. Res. 66, 763-772.
7. BITTL, J.A., J.A. BALSCHI, & J.S. INGWALL (1987): Contractile failure and high-energy phosphate turnover during hypoxia: 31P-NMR surface coil studies in living rat. Circ. Res. 60, 871-878.
8. GALLAGHER, K.P., M. MATSUZAKI, G. OSAKADA, W.S. KEMPER & J. ROSS Jr. (1983): Effect of exercise on the relationship between myocardial blood flow and systolic wall thickening in dogs with acute coronary stenosis. Circ. Res. 52, 716-729.
9. ARAI, E.A., A. PANTELY, C.G. ANSELONE, J. BRISTOW & J.D. BRISTOW (1991): Active downregulation of myocardial energy requirements during prolonged moderate ischemia in swine. Circ. Res. 69, 1458-1469.
10. REFFELMANN, T. & H. KAMMERMEIER (1992): Energetics and function of hypoxic isolated rat hearts as influenced by modulation of the K+ATP-channel-system. Eur. Heart J. 13, 105.
11. MELCHIOR, J., P.A. DORIOT, P. CHATELANI, B. MEIER, P. URBAN, L. FINCI & W. RUTISHAUSER (1987): Improvement of left ventricular contraction and relaxation synchronism after recanalization of chronic total coronary occlusion by angioplasty. J. Am. Coll Cardiol. 9, 763-768.
12. RAHIMTOOLA, S.H. (1985): A perspective on the three large multicenter randomized clinical trials of coronary bypass surgery for chronic stable 0angina. Circulation 72 Suppl.V, 123-135.
13. RAHIMTOOLA, S.H. (1989): The hibernating myocardium. Am. Heart J. 117: 111-121.
14. BASHOUR, T.T. (1986): Of myocardial life, hibernation, and death. Am. Heart J. 112, 427-428.
15. BRAUNWALD, E. & J.D. RUTHERFORD (1986): Reversible ischemic left ventricular dysfunction: evidence for the "hibernating myocardium". J. Am. Coll Cardiol. 8, 1467-1470.

Mitochondrial contribution to energy metabolism in the hypoxic myocardial cell

T. Noll and H. M. Piper

Physiologisches Institut I, Universität Düsseldorf

Introduction

It has been demonstrated in studies by Rouslin and collaborators [1, 2] that in ischemic and autolysing heart muscle mitochondrial ATP hydrolysis contributes to energy depletion. The mitochondrial site of ATP hydrolysis was identified to be the oligomycin-sensitive F_1,F_0 -proton ATPase. This mechanism is of great potential therapeutic interest since an inhibition of this energy wasting effect might be used to improve myocardial protection against ischemic injury.

The presumed mechanism of the activation of mitochondrial ATP hydrolysis is the following [1, 2]: When blood flow to cardiac muscle is interrupted, there is a rapid depletion of tissue oxygen and consequent cessation of mitochondrial electron flow. Dissipation of the mitochondrial transmembrane electrochemical gradient activates mitochondrial ATPase hydrolytic activity, as well known from studies in isolated mitochondria. Even though the possibility of this mechanism is well established, it is not yet proven to which extent the whole mechanism contributes to energy loss in the oxygen depleted myocardial cell. In the cited studies [1, 2], the decline of high-energy phosphates and the stimulation of glycolysis were taken to indicate an aerobic-anaerobic metabolic transition within the tissue preparations. It is not established, however, that these signs of an aerobic-anaerobic metabolic transition occur only in response to the *cessation* of mitochondrial electron flow and the consequent dissipation of the mitochondrial electrochemical gradient.

The present study was undertaken to investigate whether hypoxic states of the heart muscle cell are possible in which it shows the signs of an aerobic-anaerobic metabolic transition and yet retains a polarized state of its mitochondria. The model system used were isolated ventricular cardiomyocytes from the rat heart in a homogeneous suspension in which the oxygen tension was continuously monitored and factors other than oxygen and substrate limitation, influencing cells in ischemic tissue, were excluded. To prevent a masking of ATP hydrolytic processes in the cellular energetic balance by great activity of glycolytic energy production [2], the cells were incubated in the absence of exogenous glucose. The two main conditions under investigation were, first, the reduction of the ambient Po_2 to one-thousandfold below its normal arterial level ($Po_2 \leq 0.1$ mmHg) and, second, the additional chemical blockade of any residual electron flux through the mitochondrial respiratory chain. The signs of the aerobic-anaerobic metabolic transition, ATP decay and increased lactate production, were monitored under these conditions. The contribution of the mitochondrial F_1,F_0-proton ATPase to the cellular energetic changes was determined by comparing incubations in the presence and absence of the specific inhibitor oligomycin.

The results of this study demonstrate that deep hypoxia can cause a full aerobic-anaerobic metabolic transition in the myocardial cell and yet leave its mitochondria polarized.

Methods and Materials

1. Incubation of isolated cells in the oxystat system

Ventricular myocytes were isolated from Wistar rats (200-250g) as described previously [3]. The cell material consisted of 72 ± 3 % rod shaped cells (n = 21 cell preparations). Suspensions of isolated cardiomyocytes were incubated at defined Po_2 levels from 150 to 0.2 mmHg and at Po_2 0.1 mmHg. A modified substrate-free Tyrode's solution was used as incubation medium (composition in mM: 140.0 NaCl, 5.0 KCl, 1.0 $CaCl_2$, 1.2 $MgSO_4$, 30.0 N-2-hydroxyethylpiperazine-N'-ethanesulphonic acid; pH 7.4, 37 °C). The cell density of the suspension was 2 mg/ml. As specified in the experimental protocols, the following metabolic inhibitors were added to cardiomyocytes when $Po_2 \leq 0.1$ mmHg was established: oligomycin, 20 μM; NaCN, 5 mM.

Experiments were carried out at 37 °C in the oxystat system [4, 5]. In this system cellular energy metabolism can be studied at any preselected Po_2 under steady state conditions. The cells are stirred in suspension (350 rpm) to provide homogeneous and direct access of oxygen to the surfaces of the individual cells. The oxygen uptake of the cells is monitored constantly. In the experiments described metabolic inhibitors were not added to the cell suspension unless oxygen consumption fell below the limit of detection. This procedure assured that the inhibitors were not added to cells which were still sufficiently respiring. During incubations the pH remained in the range of 7.3 - 7.4 in all experiments.

2. Analytical methods
For the analysis of acid soluble metabolites, samples of the cell suspension were taken up directly into 0.6 M $HClO_4$. The neutralized extracts were analyzed for lactate according to [3], creatine phosphate (CrP) according to [6], ATP and ADP according to [7]. In order to determine total lactate production, samples of the effluent from the oxystat incubation chamber were also analyzed for lactate. In all samples withdrawn from the cell suspension protein was determined, using bovine serum albumin as standard [8].

Statistical discriminations were performed with the non-paired Student's t-test, $p < 0.05$ was regarded as significant. Given are mean values ± SD.

3. Materials
Bovine serum albumin, oligomycin and NaCN were obtained from Sigma (Deisenhofen, Germany). All other chemicals used were of analytical quality.

Results

1. Effect of variations of the Po_2 on the energetic state
In the Po_2 range between 5 and 150 mmHg, the rates of oxygen consumption were nearly constant at 30 nmol O_2/min/mg protein. Below 5 mmHg, the oxygen consumption of cardiomyocytes declined and approached half-maximal rates at approximately 1 mmHg. When cell suspensions were depleted from oxygen below 0.1 mmHg, oxygen consumption

fell below the limit of detection. The lowest level of oxygen established by the oxygen consumption of cardiomyocytes contained in the oxystat incubation vessel is, therefore, specified as "≤ 0.1 mmHg".

Lactate production did not significantly increase unless the Po_2 had dropped below 0.2 mmHg. Compared to the small lactate production seen also at 150 mmHg, it was tenfold increased at ≤ 0.1 mmHg. The average rates during the first 20 min under the indicated condition were (n = 4) at 150 mmHg (≤ 0.1 mmHg; ≤ 0.1 mmHg and addition of 20 μM oligomycin after 1 min): 0.9 ± 0.6 nmol lactate/min/mg protein (10.9 ± 1.2; 10.4 ± 1.2 nmol lactate/min/mg protein). Lack of a difference of hypoxic lactate production in absence and presence of oligomycin demonstrates that these rates are maximal.

At 150 mmHg, the cardiomyocytes contained 17.8 ± 0.2 nmol ATP/mg protein (n = 21 cell preparations). After 60 min incubation in presence of 5 mM glucose, contents of high-energy phosphates were virtually the same: 17.2 ± 0.7 nmol ATP/mg protein (n = 4 cell preparations). Since it has been shown that in these preparations hypercontracted cells are nearly devoid of high-energy phosphates [3], the values can be corrected for the percentage of rod-shaped cells (72 %, see above). The initial contents then correspond, on average, to 25 nmol ATP/mg protein.

2. The effect of oligomycin on hypoxic energetic state

Upon establishing a Po_2 ≤ 0.1 mmHg, ATP contents declined (Fig. 1), with a delay of 10 min during which two thirds of CrP were degraded. Levels of ATP below 20 % were reached at times later than 30 min. When oligomycin was added upon establishment of hypoxic conditions, the decline of ATP contents started earlier than in the absence of oligomycin. When compared 15 min after oligomycin addition, the ATP reserve of the cardiomyocytes amounted to 50 % of that found in non-treated cells, at the same time ADP had accumulated to a greater extent in oligomycin-treated cells. The accelerating effect of oligomycin on ATP depletion showed that net ATP synthesis is catalysed at the F_1,F_0-proton ATPase in hypoxic cardiomyocytes.

3. The effect of cyanide on the hypoxic energetic state

Since deep hypoxia alone did not cause mitochondrial depolarization, experiments were carried out in which the effect of hypoxia on

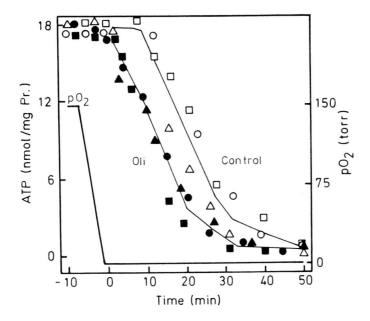

Fig. 1: ATP depletion of hypoxic cardiomyocytes in absence and presence of oligomycin. Oligomycin (Oli, 20 µM) was added at time zero, i.e. 1 min after a $Po_2 \leq 0.1$ mmHg (torr) was reached. Open symbols: experiments in the absence of Oli; closed symbols: experiments in the presence of Oli. Data of 3 experiments of separate cell preparations.

mitochondrial polarization was combined with the effect of specific inhibition by cyanide which blocks the reduction of molecular O_2 at the site of cytochome oxidase. Cyanide was added upon establishment of $Po_2 \leq 0.1$ mmHg.

In presence of cyanide, the hypoxic breakdown of high-energy phosphates was greatly accelerated, leading to a loss of ATP greater 90 % within the first 10 min of action (Fig. 2). Oligomycin given immediately prior to the blocker, slowed down energy depletion to a rate comparable to the one observed in hypoxic cardiomyocytes treated with oligomycin alone. These results demonstrate that an effective respiratory blockade in hypoxic cardiomyocyte can cause mitochondrial depolarization and activation of net ATP hydrolysis at the site of the F_1,F_0-proton ATPase.

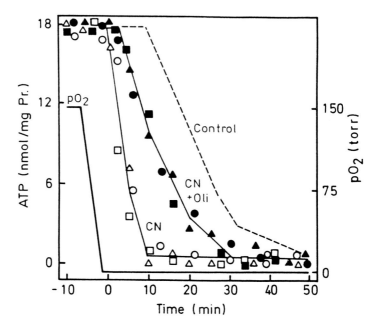

Fig. 2: Effect of NaCN (CN, 5 mM) oligomycin (Oli, 20 µM) on ATP depletion of hypoxic cardiomyocytes. Oli and CN were added at time zero, i.e. 1 min after a $Po_2 \leq 0.1$ mmHg (torr) was reached. Open symbols: experiments in the absence of Oli; closed symbols: experiments in the presence of Oli. Broken line (Control indicates ATP depletion in the absence of inhibitors (see Fig. 1). Data of 3 experiments of separate cell preparations.

Discussion

The central result of this study is that an one-thousandfold reduction of the extracellular oxygen tension below the normal arterial level, i.e. $Po_2 \leq 0.1$ mmHg, is compatible with mitochondrial polarization in ventricular myocardial cells even though it leads to an aerobic-anaerobic metabolic transition with the signs of a maximal stimulation of glycolysis and progressive decline of the cellular contents of high-energy phosphates. This has the implication that activation of glycolysis and the development of an energetic deficit per se cannot be taken to indicate mitochondrial depolarization and therefore, possibly, activation of mitochondrial ATPase hydrolytic activity.

In cardiomyocytes incubated at a $Po_2 \leq 0.1$ mmHg oligomycin did not decelerate but accelerate the decline of cellular ATP content. The results show that at this very low level of ambient oxygen net synthesis of ATP still occurred. Since oligomycin is a specific inhibitor of mitochondrial ATP synthesis of hydrolysis at the F_1,F_0-proton ATPase [9] and this complex catalyses net ATP synthesis only in polarized mitochondria [10], it can be concluded that the mitochondrial membranes were not depolarized in these hypoxic cells. As demonstrated by LaNoue et al. [11] it needs only a partial depolarization to shift mitochondrial net synthesis of ATP to net hydrolysis of ATP.

The results of the present study do not provide direct evidence that at oxygen still serves as electron acceptor since at these low oxygen levels oxygen consumption was not detectable. It is indicated, however, that preservation of a polarized mitochondrial state at these extremely low Po_2 levels depends on flux of electrons through at least parts of the electron chain since it could be abolished by the specific blocker of electron flux cyanide. In presence of cyanide the decline of ATP was greatly accelerated, beyond the rate observed in the presence of oligomycin. This acceleration demonstrates activation of mitochondrial ATPase hydrolytic activity and, therefore, also mitochondrial depolarization. The effects of cyanide on the hypoxic cardiomyocytes are comparable to the effect of an uncoupler. This similarity suggests that in the presence of the respiratory blocker the electrochemical gradient across the mitochondrial inner membrane is rapidly reduced, causing then the activation of ATP hydrolysis.

It is demonstrated by this study that hypoxic states of the heart muscle cell are possible in which it exhibits the signs of aerobic-anaerobic metabolic transition and yet retains a low level of mitochondrial ATP synthesis, which indicates a polarized state of its mitochondria. It has the implication that deep hypoxia does not have to cause mitochondrial ATP hydrolysis. The results are in accordance with the finding that in hepatocytes, too, deep hypoxia can lead to an aerobic-anaerobic metabolic transition and yet permit retention of a nearly normal proton electrochemical gradient [12]. The results on hepatocytes suggested that a distinct decrease of ion permeability of anoxic mitochondria in the living cell accounted for preservation of the proton electrochemical gradient, and not ATP-hydrolysis.

In human pathology, regional ischemia is the most frequent natural case of myocardial oxygen deficiency. To a variable degree collateral flow can prevent very deep levels of hypoxia. The distribution of residual flow and, thereby, of residual oxygenation is known to be inhomogeneous in regionally ischemic myocardium. It is interesting to speculate whether small differences in the degree of hypoxia [13] represent a cause for the micro-inhomogeneity of ischemic tissue injury, in that small local differences in the Po_2 at very low levels may prevent activation of mitochondrial ATP hydrolysis in one cell but not in the adjacent one.

The results of the present study are of relevance also for the experimental use of blockers and uncouplers of mitochondrial respiration with the intention to imitate the conditions of hypoxia or ischemia (often called "chemical anoxia" or "chemical ischemia"). This study and previous observations by Haworth et al. [14] demonstrate that in "chemical anoxia" one must expect a substantial contribution of mitochondrial ATP hydrolysis to the progression of energy depletion. Mitochondrial depolarization causes large changes in the subcellular distribution of metabolites and ions. From the results of the present study it seems likely that these changes occur in "chemical anoxia" more rapidly than in a natural course of progressive oxygen depletion. At present it must remain an open question whether the more drastic effects of blockers of mitochondrial electron transport compared to deep hypoxia alone are due to their ability to abolish residual small amounts of electron flux (which are not detectable with present methods) or to other additional effects of these agents (as hypothesized by Aw et al. [15]).

Acknowledgement

This study was supported by the Deutsche Forschungsgemeinschaft grant C6, SFB 242.

References

1. ROUSLIN, W., J.L. ERICKSON & R.J. SOLARO (1986): Effects of oligomycin and acidosis on rates of ATP depletion in ischemic heart muscle. Am. J. Physiol. 250, H503-H508.
2. ROUSLIN, W., C.W. BROGE & I.L. GRUPP (1990): ATP depletion and functional loss during ischemia in slow and fast heart-rate hearts. Am. J. Physiol. 259, H1759-H1766.
3. PIPER, H.M., I. PROBST, P. SCHWARTZ, J.F. HÜTTER & P.G. SPIECKERMANN (1982): Culturing of calcium stable adult cardiac myocytes. J. Mol. Cell. Cardio. 14, 397-412.
4. NOLL, T., H. DE GROOT & P. WISSEMANN (1986): A computer-supported oxystat system maintaining steady-state O_2 partial pressures and simultaneously monitoring O_2 uptake in biological systems. Biochem. J. 236, 765-769.
5. MERTENS, S., T. NOLL, R. SPAHR, A. KRÜTZFELDT & H.M. PIPER (1990): The energetic response of coronary endothelial cells to hypoxia. Am. J. Physiol. 258, H689-H694.

6. GUTMAN, I. & A.W. WAHLEFELD (1974): L(+)-Lactat. In: BERGMEYER, H.U. (ed.) Methoden der enzymatischen Analyse, pp. 1510-1514, Weinheim: Verlag Chemie.
7. JÜNGLING, E. & H. KAMMERMEIER (1980): Rapid assay of adenine nucleotides or creatine compounds in extracts of cardiac tissue by paired-ion reverse-phase high performance liquid chromatography. Anal. Biochem. 102, 358-361.
8. LOWRY, O.H., N.J. ROSEBROUGH. A.L. FARR & R.J. RANDALL (1951): Protein measurement with the folin phenol reagent. J. Biol. Chem. 193, 265-275.
9. LARDY, H.A. (1981): Antibiotic inhibitors of mitochondrial energy transfer. In: ERECINSKA, M. & D.F. WILSON (eds.) Inhibitors of Mitochondrial Function, pp. 187-198, Oxford: Pergamon Press.
10. SCHWERZMANN, K. & P. PEDERSEN (1986): Regulation of the mitochondrial ATP Synthase/ATPase complex. Arch. Biochem. Biophys. 250, 1-18.
11. LANOUE, K.F., F.M.H. JEFFRIES & G.K. RADDA (1986): Kinetic control of mitochondrial ATP synthesis. Biochemistry 25, 7667-7675.
12. ANDERSSON, B.S., T.Y. AW & D.P. JONES (1987): Mitochondrial transmembrane potential and pH gradient during anoxia. Am. J. Physiol. 252, C349-C355.
13. STEENBERGEN, C., DELEEUW, C. BARLOW, B. CHANCE & J.R. WILLIAMSON (1977): Heterogeneity of the hypoxic state in perfused rat heart. Circ. Res. 41, 606-615.
14. HAWORTH, R.A., D.R. HUNTER & H.A. BERKHOFF (1981): Contracture in isolated adult rat heart cells: Role of Ca^{2+}, ATP and compartmentation. Circ. Res. 49, 1119-1128.
15. AW, T.Y., B.S. ANDERSSON & D.P. JONES (1987): Suppression of mitochondrial respiratory function after short-term anoxia. Am. J. Physiol. 252, C362-C368.

The influence of $MgCl_2$ and Mg-Aspartate on membrane currents, cytoplasmic Ca^{2+}-concentration and contraction of cardiac myocytes

R. Meyer, U. Pohl, S.Y. Wang, B. Reufels and O. Zimmermann

Department of Physiology, University of Bonn

Introduction

The contraction of heart muscle is induced by the calcium-inward current, I_{Ca}, during the action potential. This inward current triggers a Ca^{2+}-release from the sarcoplasmic reticulum, SR. The amount of Ca^{2+}-released from the SR depends on the amplitude of I_{Ca} and on the Ca^{2+}-load of the SR. As the height of contraction is proportional to the cytoplasmic calcium concentration, $[Ca^{2+}]_i$, both Ca^{2+}-load of the SR and the amplitude of the I_{Ca} determine the height of contraction of heart muscle [11].

Increasing the external Ca^{2+}-concentration, $[Ca^{2+}]_o$, increases both the amplitude of I_{Caa} and the Ca^{2+}-load of the SR, thus $[Ca^{2+}]_o$ has a positive ionotropic effect on the contraction of heart muscle [6]. The positive inotropic effect of $[Ca^{2+}]_o$ is antagonized by the external Mg^{2+}-concentration, $[Mg^{2+}]_o$, (Ca/Mg-Antagonism [10]). The mechanism, by which $[Ca^{2+}]_o$ brings about its positive inotropic effect, has been investigated in detail, whereas the reasons for the negative inotropic influence of $[Mg^{2+}]_o$ have not been characterized to such an extent. It has been shown several times that the size of the I_{Ca} depends on $[Mg^{2+}]_o$, increasing $[Mg^{2+}]_o$ causes a decrease in the amplitude of I_{Ca} [recent works 1, 8, 13]. This decrease in I_{Ca} will lead to a decrease in Ca^{2+}-release from the SR thus causing a weaker force of contraction. In most investigations Mg-ions were applied as $MgCl_2$ or $MgSO_4$ salts. Very little is known about the influence of the Mg-(DL)-hydrogenaspartate salt, Mg-Asp, which is a widely used Mg-salt in clinical application. Therefore, it was the aim of this study to investigate the effects of Mg-Asp on membrane currents, intracellular calcium concentration, $[Ca^{2+}]_i$, and the amplitude of shortening of isolated guinea pig heart muscle cells.

Methods

All measurements were carried out on isolated ventricular myocytes of the guinea pig in permanently perfused experimental chambers at 36 °C. As control solution served Tyrode's solution (in mM): NaCl 135, KCl 4, $CaCl_2$ 1.8, $MgCl_2$ 1, Glucose 10, HEPES 2; BSA 1 mg/ml. If Mg-(DL)-hydrogenaspartate was tested, all Mg^{2+} present was added in this form.

Contractions were recorded optically as unloaded shortening with a pair photodiodes mounted in the ray tracing of an inverted microscope, Zeiss IM 35 [9]. For primary magnification a 100 X objective was utilized (aperture 1,25). The cells were partly attached to the ground of the experimental chamber by laminin. They were stimulated externally at 1 Hz by biphasic pulses. Contractions are expressed in relative values compared to contractions measured in a solution without Mg^{2+}.

Membrane currents were recorded with patch electrodes (resistances 2 - 5 M; filling solution in mM: KCl 140, HEPES 10, EGTA 0.5 titrated with about 7 mM NaOH to pH 7.2) in whole cell recording mode by means of a List EPC7 amplifier. For L-channel-Ca^{2+}-current recording Na^+-current, I_{Na}, was always inactivated by an appropriate preclamp. I_{Ca} amplitude was calculated as the difference current between the current minimum and the current after 200 ms.

Intracellular Ca^{2+} was measured as fura-2 fluorescence in externally stimulated cells [5]. The cells were loaded with fura-2/AM by incubation in control solution containing 0,5 µM fura-2/AM for 15 min at 36 °C. After incubation the external fura-2/AM was washed away and the cells were allowed to rest for 20 min to obtain full deestrification of fura-2/AM. Fura-2 signals were recorded with a Zeiss-system (fast fluorescence photometry, FFP), a microspectrofluorimeter consisting of an inverted microscope (Axiovert 135) equipped with epifluorescence xenon-lamp illumination. In the epifluorescence pathway a fast rotating filter wheel and a shutter was installed (sampling rate up to 200 Hz, we utilized 50 Hz, excitation wavelenght 340 and 380 nm). Signals were detected with a photomultiplier tube, mounted on the third outlet of the binoculartube. All measurements were carried out with the Ultrafluar 100 X, 1.3 aperture objective.

Calibration was carried out with rectangular glass capillaries of 50 μm height [4]. These capillaries were filled with a solution of an ionic composition comparable to the cytoplasm (in mM: KCl 135, NaCl 10, $MgCl_2$ 1, HEPES 10, EGTA 10 with graded Ca^{2+}-concentrations pCa, 9, 8, 7, 6, 5, 4, 3). The measured values were fitted with the calibration function [5] to construct a full calibration curve. A calibration curve was valid only for experiments, which have been carried out with identical settings on the microspectrofluorimeter.

Results

Contractions recorded from single cells have a good signal to noise ratio and differences of less than 10 % in amplitude can be resolved (Fig. 1A). They remain stable during experiments of more than 40 min, in which various ionic concentrations are tested (Fig. 1A). In the beginning of each experiment a Tyrode's solution without Mg^{2+} is applied. Contraction amplitude in this solution is used as relative value for the normalization of all contractions. Switching to normal Tyrode's solution with 1 mM $MgCl_2$ decreased the amplitude of shortening by about 14 %. A further increase in the external Mg^{2+}-concentration, $[Mg^{2+}]_o$, to 5 mM led to a decrease of the contraction amplitude to 53 %. Exchanging the 5 mM $MgCl_2$ for 5 mM Mg-Asp restored the contraction to 98 % of the situation without Mg^{2+}. Obviously there is a difference between the two Mg-salts, which gets clearer, if the whole dose/response curve for Mg^{2+}/contraction is regarded. In the case of $MgCl_2$ the amplitude of shortening decreases steadily over the whole concentration range, it reaches its 50 % value around 5 mM and approaches its minimum above 30 mM. The curve for $MgCl_2$ is nearly superimposible to one recorded in $MgSO_4$ (not shown). In the case of Mg-Asp a negative inotropic effect is obtained only above 5 mM (Fig. 1 B). The dose/response curve of Mg-Asp has its 50 % value between 15 and 20 mM and approaches the curve of $MgCl_2$ above 20 mM. The difference between $MgCl_2$ and Mg-Asp is maximal at 5 mM, therefore both salts were applied in this concentration subsequently to the same cells (Fig. 1 A). If the concentration of aspartic acid is increased alone, without changing the Mg^{2+}-concentration, a positive inotropic effect is visible (not shown). All effects on contraction are completely reversible, but the washout time for Mg-(DL)-aspartate as well as aspartic acid is longer than for $MgCl_2$.

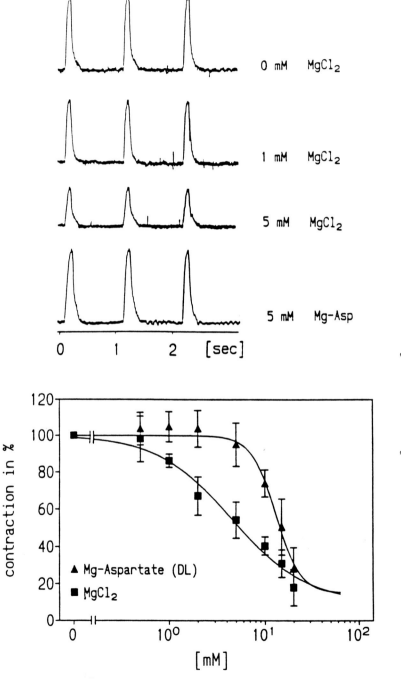

Fig. 1: A = Records of shortening at different $[Mg^{2+}]_0$. The actual $[Mg^{2+}]_0$ is marked beside each trace, Mg-Asp means Mg-(DL)-hydrogen aspartate. Shortening amplitude at 0 mM was always regarded as 100%.
Fig. 1: B = Dose/response curves of Mg/contraction. Shortening amplitude is plotted in linear scale, the $[Mg^{2+}]_0$ in logarithmic scale.

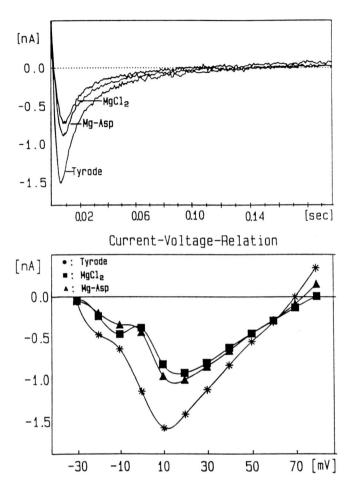

Fig. 2: **A** = Current records obtained from the same cell in three different external solutions a) Tyrode: Control solution; b) $MgCl_2$: 5 mM $MgCl_2$; c) Mg-Asp: 5 mM Mg-(DL)-hydrogenaspartate $[Mg^{2+}]_0$. The currents were elicited by a clamp pulse to 10 mV at a stimulation frequency of 0.2 Hz.
B = Current-voltage-relation of the experiment shown in 2 A. The amplitude of the inward current is plotted versus the potential of the test clamp.

A comparison of the two Mg-salts with respect to their influence on the L-channel-Ca^{2+}-current seems to be most interesting at a concentration of 5 mM, where the difference in contraction amplitude is maximal. L-channel Ca^{2+}-currents were recorded with 13 voltage clamp pulses applied at a frequency of 0.2 Hz. Each pulse consisted of a constant preclamp of 200 ms duration to inactivate the sodium inward current (from -80 mV to around -

40 mV) and a test clamp of 500 ms duration to varying potentials between -30 and 80 mV graded in steps of 10 mV. In the beginning of the test clamp the I_{Ca} is the dominating current component. It reaches its maximum during the first 10 ms and inactivates slowly within the following 100 - 200 ms (Fig. 2 A).

The current flowing at the end of the 500 ms lasting test clamp is mainly K^+-current. The biggest inward current amplitude is reached at a test potential of 0 - 10 mV. At negative test potentials the current amplitude increases with growing membrane depolarizations, in the positive potential range additional depolarization decreases the current amplitude. This behavior leads to a bell-shaped current/voltage-relation with its minimum around 10 mV (Fig. 2 B). In a series of experiments both Mg^{2+}-salts were applied one after another on the same cells. In the beginning of the experiment I_{Ca} was recorded in control solution containing 1 mM $MgCl_2$, then I_{Ca} was measured in solutions with elevated Mg^{2+} and at the end current was recorded in control solution again. Cells with more than 10 % current "run down" [1] during the experiment were rejected, i.e. the control currents recorded at the end of the experiment had to reach at least 90 % of those monitored at the beginning. Raising the $[Mg^{2+}]_o$ from 1 to 5 mM attenuates the amplitude of the inward current as shown in the original current records (Fig. 2A) no matter whether the anion is chloride or aspartate. The current voltage relation for the two Mg-salts is also very similar. Both salts decrease the current and shift the maximum of the current voltage relation to more positive potentials (Fig. 2 B).

The shift of the maximum of the current voltage relation gets more obvious when it is demonstrated as a shift in the steady state activation curve (not shown). The small shift in the reversal potential, which is present in the example shown in Fig. 2 B, is not a typical Mg^{2+}-effect. In the average of 10 cells from different animals carried out at 5 mM Mg^{2+} the the peak of the current/voltage relation was reduced to 77,4 % ± 7.2 by 5 mM $MgCl_2$ and to 77,8 % ± 5.3 by 5 mM Mg-Asp. 5 mM $MgCl_2$ shifted the activation curve by 6 mV ± 2.9 in positive potential direction and 5 mM Mg-Asp induced a shift of 4,7 mV ± 1.9 (n = 11), a difference being small, but significant ($p < 0.05$).

As the difference in the contractile behaviour is obviously not due to differences in the I_{Ca} it might be induced by differences in the $[Ca^{2+}]_i$. Therefore we measured $[Ca^{2+}]_i$ in externally stimulated cells. At a stimulation frequency of 1 Hz the diastolic $[Ca^{2+}]_i$ in normal Tyrode's was between 150 and 200 nM. After the stimulus the $[Ca^{2+}]_i$ rises within 100 ms from 173 ±

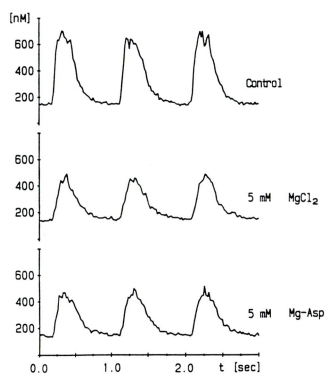

Fig. 3: $[Ca^{2+}]_i$-transients recorded subsequently at the same cell in three different external solutions.

54 nM to a peak value of 801 ± 328 nM (n = 6), 500 ms after the stimulus the $[Ca^{2+}]_i$ has decreased nearly to its control level (Fig. 3). After perfusion with 5 mM $MgCl_2$ the diastolic $[Ca^{2+}]_i$ remained unchanged (165 ± 37 nM), but the amplitude of the $[Ca^{2+}]_i$-transients has been depressed from 628 ± 297 to 434 ± 120 nM, i.e. a reduction to 69 % of control amplitude. This is a significant decrease at a level of $p < 0.1$. After exchanging the $MgCl_2$ containing solution against one with 5 mM Mg-Asp the amplitude of the $[Ca^{2+}]_i$-transients remained practically unchanged (446 ± 126 nM;) as well as the diastolic $[Ca^{2+}]_i$ (163 ± 39 nM; Fig. 3), i.e. a specific influence of aspartate on $[Ca^{2+}]_i$ is not visible in this experiment. The effect of raising the external Mg^{2+} was fully reversible.

Discussion

The influence of $MgCl_2$ on excitation-contraction coupling can be explained by the effect of Mg^{2+} on the cell membrane of the heart muscle cells. Negative surface charges on the outer surface of the membrane attract cations from the external bulk solution, resulting in an enrichment of cations close to the cell surface. These cations surround the cell completely and partly compensate the negative surface charges by screening or binding. These effects deminish the electric field in the membrane and thereby shift the gating of the channels to more positive potentials. Divalent cations are far more effective in shifting the gating kinetics of channels than monovalent cations. Therefore the external Ca^{2+}-concentration, $[Ca^{2+}]_o$, is an important factor for the activation and inacitvation curves of sodium and calcium current. External Ca^{2+} is concentrated directly over the cell membrane and varyiing the $[Ca^{2+}]_o$ shifts the gating curves for I_{Na} [3] and I_{Ca} [12] along the voltage axis. In addition to Ca^{2+} Mg^{2+} is also enriched over the cell membrane. Both compete for the same binding sites.

Thus Ca^{2+} and Mg^{2+} have similar effects on the voltage dependence of Ca^{2+} channel gating. Rising the $[Mg^{2+}]_o$ leads to an increased screening and binding by Mg^{2+} at the external surface of the membrane. This displaces Ca^{2+} from the external membrane surface and thus from the mouth of the Ca^{2+} channel, resulting in a reduced driving force for Ca^{2+} and thus a diminished I_{Ca}-amplitude. In addition to the substitution of Ca^{2+} by Mg^{2+} at the external membrane surface direct interaction of Mg^{2+} with the Ca^{2+}-channel has also been discussed as another reason for the influence of Mg^{2+} on the I_{Ca} [2,7]. In both cases Mg^{2+} develops its effect on I_{Ca} from the external side of the cell membrane.

The decreased I_{Ca} will also induce the release of less Ca^{2+} from the sarcoplasmic reticulum and will supply less Ca^{2+} for its refilling. These two effects will cause smaller $[Ca^{2+}]_i$-transients, like the ones measured in this investigation. As $[Ca^{2+}]_i$-transients and the amplitude of contraction are usually in proportion, smaller transients are expected to elicit smaller contractions. This is true for the experiments with $MgCl_2$. In these experiments the three parameters current, $[Ca^{2+}]_i$, and contraction are all in close proportion. The reduction of the current to about 75 % induced by raising the $[Mg^{2+}]_o$ from 1 mM to 5 mM matches well with the $[Ca^{2+}]_i$-transients, which were deminished to about 69 %.

For comparison with these data the shortening has to be normalized to the 1 mM $MgCl_2$ value, which served as control in the current and $[Ca^{2+}]_i$-

transient measurements. In this case shortening amplitude in 5 mM $MgCl_2$ is reduced to about 79 % of control level. Thus the three parameters of electromechanical coupling are supressed to less than 80 % of control level by the increase of $[Mg^{2+}]_O$. Therefore the effects of $MgCl_2$ can all be attributed to the substitution of Ca^{2+} by Mg^{2+} on the external surface of the membrane.

The exchange of $MgCl_2$ against Mg-Asp did not change I_{Ca} and $[Ca^{2+}]_i$-transients but the amplitude of shortening was increased distinctly. As the influence of Mg^{2+} on the I_{Ca} is independent of the salt, Mg^{2+} seems to be concentrated near the cell surface in a comparable amount. Consequently this leads to an appropriate decrease in the $[Ca^{2+}]_i$-transients. Aspartate seems to have only little or no influence on the Ca^{2+}-exchange mechanisms controlling excitation contraction coupling. Therefore the positive inotropic effect of aspartate has to be attributed to other reactions of the contraction mechanism, possibly the energy metabolism. If Mg-Asp had the same effect in vivo as in our experiments, it would be an ideal antiarrhythmic substance, because it reduces the Ca^{2+}-load of the heart muscle cell without decreasing the amplitude of contraction. This means it could help depressing dangerous effects of high Ca^{2+}-load like early and delayed afterdepolarizations without changing the contractile performance of the heart.

References

1. BELLES, B., C.O. MALECOT, J. HESCHLER & W. TRAUTWEIN (1988): "Run-down" of the Ca current during long whole-cell recordings in guinea pig heart cells: role of phosphorylation and intracellular calcium. Pflügers Arch. 411, 353-360.
2. DICHTL, A. & W. VIERLING (1992): Inhibition of calcium inward current by magnesium in heart ventricular muscle. Europ. J. Pharmacol. 204, 243-248.
3. FRANKENHAEUSER, B. & A.L. HODGKIN (1957): The action of calcium on the electrical properties of squid axons. J. Physiol 137, 218-244.
4. GOLLNICK, F., R. MEYER & W. STOCKEM (1991): Visualization and measurement of calcium transients in *Amoeba proteus* by fura-2 fluorescence. Europ. J. Cell Biol. 55, 262-271.
5. GRYNKIEWICZ, G., M. POENIE & R.Y. TSIEN (1985): A new generation of Ca^{2+}-indicators with greatly improved fluorescence properties. J. Biol. Chem. 260, 3440-3450.
6. KATZ, A.M. (1992): Physiology of the heart. 2. Edition, Raven Press, New York.
7. LANSMAN, J.B., P. HESS & R.W. TSIEN (1986): Blockade of current through single calcium channels by Cd^{2+}, Mg^{2+}, and Ca^{2+}. Voltage and concentration dependence of calcium entry into the pore. J. Gen. Physiol. 88, 321-347.

8. MEYER, R., S.Y. WANG & U. POHL (1992): Magnesium, Kalium und Calcium in der Herzelektrophysiologie. In: VETTER, H. & L NEYSES (eds.) Elektrolyte im Blickpunkt - Neue Ansätze in der Pathophysiologie und Behandlung kardiovaskulärer Erkrankungen, Thieme Verlag Stuttgart, New York, 68-77.
9. MEYER, R., J. WIEMER, J. DEMBSKI & H.-G. HAAS (1987): Photoelectric recording of mechanical responses of cardiac myocytes. Pflügers Arch. 408, 390-394.
10. VIERLING, W., F. EBNER & M. REITER (1978): The opposite effects of magnesium and calcium on the contraction of guinea-pig ventricular myocardium in dependence on the sodium concentration. Naunyn-Schmiedeb. Arch. Pharmacol. 303, 111-119.
11. WIER, W.G. (1990): Cytoplasmic [Ca^{2+}] in mammalian ventricle: Dynamic control by cellular processes. Ann. Rev. Physiol. 52, 467-485.
12. WILSON, D.L., K. MORIMOTO, Y. TSUDA & A.M. BROWN (1983): Interaction between calcium ions and surface charge as it relates to calcium currents. J. Membrane Biol. 72, 117-130.
13. WU, J. & S.L. LIPSIUS (1990): Effects of extracellular Mg^{2+} on T- and L-type Ca^{2+} currents in single atrial myocytes. Am. J. Physiol. 259, H1842-H1850.

Use of antisense oligonucleotides for selective inhibition of gene expression in adult cardiomyocytes

L. Neyses, A. Blaufuß, C. Kubisch, B. Wollnik, A. Maass, S. Oberdorf, C. Grohé and H. Vetter

Medizinische Poliklinik der Universität Bonn

Introduction

Traditional tools for studying the function of single genes have been inhibitors that act on the level of the gene product, i.e. proteins. Examples are the use of ouabain to inhibit the sarcolemmal Na^+/K^+- ATPase or the inhibition of the sarcoplasmic calcium release channel by ryanodine [reviewed in 1]. The application of molecular biological techniques to eukaryotic organisms has considerably widened our options for targeting single genes to investigate their function.

Once a gene is isolated and cloned (either as c-DNA or as genomic DNA), the two main choices to study gene regulation are selective overexpression or inhibition of genes [2]. Overexpression is either possible in the whole organism using a transgenic animal approach or by in vitro cell culture. In the latter case, genes are transferred into the cells by a process called transfection for which precipitation of circular plasmid DNA onto crystals of calciumphosphate, liposomes, electroporation, or various other methods are used.

On the other hand, selective inhibition of gene expression can be achieved by creating animals carrying a gene that interrupts the gene of interest by a process coined homologous recombination [5]. On the cell culture level, cells can be transfected by vectors carrying DNA that is transcribed in the reverse direction (with respect to the natural gene) thus creating RNA with a sequence complementary to the natural RNA of the targeted gene. The resulting double stranded RNA is rapidly degraded by

RNAse inhibiting the translation of the message into corresponding protein [reviewed in 6].

The major drawback of the transgenic approaches is their high cost in terms of time and money, whereas transfection of genes for either over-expression or antisense inhibition requires that the cells of interest be largely resistant to the agents used for transfection in order to survive the treatment used for the transfection procedure. Furthermore, gene constructs have to be created.

Recently, a new technique has received great attention, the use of antisense oligonucleotides for targeted inhibition of single genes. The initial report observed the inhibition of viral sequences in cells infected with the Rous sarcoma virus [reviewed in 7,8]; this technique has rapidly been extended to the eukaryotic cell's own mRNA sequences. In this approach, antisense oligonucleotides are synthesized and incubated with the cells. Most cells take up these molecules, probably via a DNA-surface receptor [9] that has been incompletely characterized (some modified oligonucleotides, e.g. methylphosphonates, diffuse through the cell membrane [7,10]). The oligonucleotide then forms a hybrid double strand with the homologous mRNA. The RNA of the hybrid is degraded by (the ubiquitous) RNAse H (H for hybrid) [11].

Recently, first successes in experimental antisense therapy have been reported [12]. An antisense oligonucleotide (modified as the phosphorothioate analogue because of better in vivo stability) complementary to the mRNA of the transcription factor c *myb* inhibited restenosis after balloon angioplasty in rat carotid arteries [12].

Because of our interest in cardiac hypertrophy, we have used this technique to investigate potential mechanisms of endo-/ paracrine induction of hypertrophic cardiac growth. Furthermore, we have recently begun to study the role of the sarcolemmal Ca^{2+}-pumping ATPase in the cardiac contraction cycle. In particular, we asked whether the relaxation delay that is one of the prominent features of the contractile cycle in the hypertrophied heart [13] could be due to reduced function of the Ca^{2+}-pump of the sarcolemma.

Methods

An unmodified antisense oligodeoxyribonucleotide to the first 5 base triplets of the Egr-1 coding region was synthesized using the sequence for rat Egr-1 (NGFI-A) [14]. The ATG codon suggested by Sukhatme [15] was taken as the start site; originally, Milbrandt had proposed an ATG 84 nucleotides downstream from this site [14].

Cardiomyocytes were isolated from the heart of adult Wistar-Kyoto rats (200-250 g) by the collagenase method [16]. 10^5 cells in medium BM 86 were attached (60 min, 37 °C) to a 10 cm^2 Petri dish precoated with laminin (1 mg/cm^2). Contamination by non-myocytes was less than 0.5 %. 1.5 mM unmodified oligodeoxynucleotide (synthesized on a Pharmacia Gene Assembler and purified over a NAP 10 column) were added. Cells were kept at 37 °C in a CO$_2$-incubator for 18 hrs. Insulin (10^{-8}M) or buffer (control) were added 5 min after ^{3}H-phenylalanine (Phe, 1mCi) and incubation continued for 3hrs. Cells were then precipitated and washed 3x with 4 % perchloric acid, the pellet resuspended in 1n NaOH and counted. Preincubation with T$_3$ (3',3',5-triiodo-L-thyronine; 0.8 nM) was for 24 hours to allow for the slower induction of protein synthesis by T$_3$. ^{3}H-Phe was added for 3 hours and acid precipitation performed as above. ^{3}H-Phe transport into the cells was assessed in the presence of 3×10^{-5}M cycloheximide.

For analysis of the function of the sarcolemmal calcium-transporting ATPase (SL-ATPase), a similar approach was taken except that cells had to be isolated and cultured under sterile conditions and kept on laminin coated (1 mg/cm^2) coverslides in M199 for 48 hrs. This procedure was necessary because an effect of the antisense sequence complementary to the mRNA of this enzyme was only seen after 24 hrs and was maximal after 48 hrs. This was presumably due to the fact that in contrast to the short-lived Egr-1 gene product [15], the SL-ATPase is a structural protein with a longer half-life. The antisense oligonucleotide used was complementary to the first 6 codons of the rat sequence of isoform 1 of the enzyme [17].

The contraction/relaxation pattern of the cells was assessed using a system that has previously been described by Rose et al. [18]. In short, cells were stimulated under an inverted microscope. At preset time points (every 5 ms from 10 to 175 ms) after electrical stimulation of the cells a stroboscope flash was triggered by a computer system and the number of picture elements (pixels) occupied by the cell assessed. This value was then subtracted from the number of pixels in diastole. The results were transferred to a data bank (Lotus 1,2,3) which allowed averaging and statistical treatment of the data. Stimulation rate was 120/min in all experiments investigating the calcium-ATPase.

Results

Fig. 1 shows that the antisense sequence completely inhibited insulin-induced protein synthesis. Basal synthesis and cell morphology were unaffected indicating that the antisense oligonucleotides were not toxic. Introduction of a single mismatch at position 8 of the 15mer abolished the inhibitory effect of the antisense sequence; the same was true for an oligonucleotide containing two mismatches at positions 4 and 10 (Fig. 1). Controls using the sense sequence were no different from buffer alone indicating that there was no unspecific effect of the oligonucleotides (not shown).

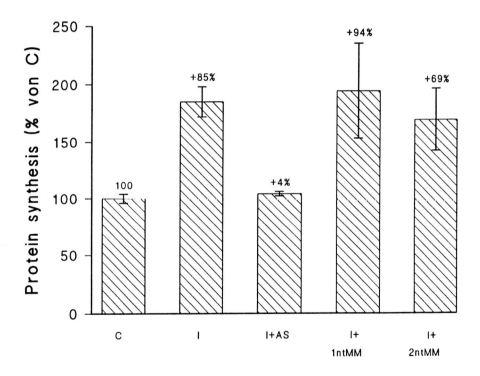

Fig. 1: Effect of Egr-1 antisense oligonucleotides on protein synthesis. Insulin (I, 10^{-8}M) stimulated ^{3}H-phenylalanin incorporation almost 2-fold (C=control without insulin). An antisense oligodeoxynucleotide complementary to the first 15 bases of the Egr-1 mRNA coding region completely abolished this stimulation (AS). A single or double mismatch in the antisense sequence (1 and 2nt MM) resulted in an ineffective oligonucleotide. C (=Control, no hormone). n=7 independent experiments (in duplicate). Mean ± SEM, p<0.01 for differences between control and insulin incubation.

The well-known induction of myocardial protein synthesis by T_3 [19] was not affected by the antisense oligonucleotide (not shown). This demonstrated that Egr-1 has no direct role in the T_3 signal transduction pathway and excludes unspecific toxicity of the antisense sequence. To exclude that endothelin and T_3 inhibited ^{3}H-phenylalanine (^{3}H-Phe) transport into the cell thus altering the specific activity of the intracellular isotope, ^{3}H-Phe transport was studied in the presence of cyclohexamide. No influence of the oligonucleotides was observed. A minimum of 6 hours preincubation was required for uptake of the antisense oligonucleotides into the cells, but more consistent results were obtained after 12-18 hours preincubation (data not shown). This time course is in agreement with other work using antisense oligodeoxynucleotides [7].

These data indicated that Egr-1 is a transcription factor which is essential for the induction of growth processes in the adult myocardium. Furthermore, they suggested that isolated adult myocardial cells were exquisitely sensitive to unmodified antisense oligonucleotides.

Therefore, we wondered whether the expression of long-lived structural gene proteins - as opposed to short-lived transcription factors - could also be inhibited by antisense DNA in this system. Many attempts to target structural genes by antisense technology have failed up to now for reasons that are not entirely clear [7]. The gene we chose was the sarcolemmal calcium-pumping ATPase, mainly because its role in intracellular calcium homeostasis and its physiological properties as well as its changes in cardiac hypertrophy remain unclear [1]. Fig. 2 shows that inhibition of the expression of this enzyme had a dramatic effect on the contractile behaviour of the cells as measured by the percentage of shortening (i.e. diastolic length was set 100 %, 97 % refers to a shortening of the cell by 3 %). The contraction maximum increased from 97 ± 0.3 % to 93 ± 0.8 %. This represented a 133 % increase in fractional shortening ($p < 0.01$). In antisense-treated cells, relaxation was complete only after 125 ± 10 ms, whereas controll cells were completely relaxed after 90 ± 6ms ($p < 0.01$). At higher calcium concentrations, these effects were even more pronounced and relaxation was incomplete at calcium concentrations above 4mM, resulting in cell death at this stimulation rate (120/min).

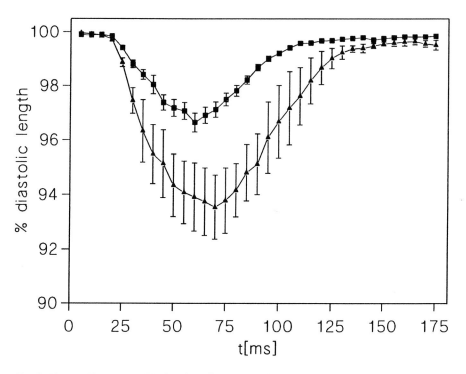

Fig. 2: Contractile pattern of isolated cardiomyocytes in the presence and absence of an antisense oligonucleotide complementary to the first 6 codons (downstream of the translation start site) of isoform 1 of the sarcolemmal calcium ATPase. Cells were preincubated with the antisense sequence for 48 hrs and the contraction/relaxation pattern analysed in the presence of 2mM Ca^{2+}. n=15 cells from 3 independent experiments. p<0.01 for the difference in contraction between controls and antisense-incubated cells.

Discussion

The most surprising finding of this study is the extreme susceptibility of adult cardiac myocytes in culture to unmodified DNA antisense oligonucleotides. This technique permitted, for the first time, to target single genes in these cells which have proven to be largely refractory to classical transfection techniques employing calcium phosphate, electroporation, and other methods (own results and K. Chien, personal communication). In feline adult cardiomyocytes, transfection has been achieved by the calcium phosphate method [20], but transfection efficiency was very low with only about 2-3 % of all cells taking up the transgene. Therefore, this approach can be used only for studying the effect of overexpression of transcription factors on strong promoters driving reporter genes such as the luciferase or the chloramphenicol acetyl transferase gene. In contrast, the antisense approach is potentially able to target genes in the vast majority of cells as demonstrated by the fact that the effect of insulin on protein synthesis was completely abolished. In the case of the SL calcium ATPase, analysis of about 200 cells revealed that only a subset of 10-15 % of all cells did not show abnormal contractile behaviour when incubated with the antisense oligonucleotide. These cells have been included in Fig. 2; therefore, the effect of the antisense sequence on the ATPase may have been even 10-15 % stronger in cells that had taken up the oligonucleotide.

The two other results of this study are concerned with the two aspects of cardiac growth and hypertrophy our laboratory is currently interested in. Firstly, the intracellular signal transduction pathway of endo/-paracrine substances that are relevant in -at least some forms of- hypertension on cardiac growth and secondly abnormalities in the contractile pattern of the hypertrophied heart. As to the first aspect, hyperinsulinism has been shown to occur in essential hypertensives, even if the effect of overweight is eliminated by matching lean hypertensives with lean control subjects [21]. We therefore investigated the effect of this hormone on the myocardium. Our results suggest that insulin may contribute to cardiac hypertrophy to the extent that the short-term measurement of protein synthesis we used can be extrapolated to the hormone's long-term effects. Clearly, more studies are needed on this issue, but the prominent role of insulin in muscle development and growth [19] invites to the speculation that the hyperinsulinemia may play a decisive role in the development of cardiac hypertrophy. The intracellular pathway of insulin action is only partially known [22] but our results establish that the gene product of the early growth response gene-1 is a necessary -albeit not necessarily sufficient - intermediate step in insulin-mediated signal transduction.

The second interest of our laboratory is concerned with the function of the sarcolemmal calcium ATPase in the hypertrophied myocardium. While it is clear that this enzyme is one of the two systems (together with the Na^+/Ca^{2+}-exchanger) capable of extruding calcium from excitable cells [1], its function remains elusive. Although the hypothesis that the gene is required for fine tuning of the intracellular calcium level based on its high affinity for calcium, but relatively low capacity for transport [1], others have challenged this hypothesis on the grounds that these kinetic parameters were assessed in reconstituted systems using the isolated pump and therefore not reflecting the in vivo situation. The results demonstrated here favour the original hypothesis [1] since the decline in the expression of the pump in vivo increased the maximum contraction and relaxation time markedly. This suggests that, under these conditions, calcium is being pumped out of the cell more slowly, resulting in a higher maximum of contraction and slower relaxation.

Future prospects of the antisense approach in this system include studying the function of other growth - or contraction - related gene(s). Although many hurdles have yet to be taken, it is conceivable that therapeutic strategies will evolve from this approach. First steps in this direction are currently being undertaken by us and others [12].

Summary

In this report we describe the use of antisense oligodeoxyribonucleotides to selectively inhibit gene expression in the myocardium. Isolated adult cardiomyocytes were used to study the role of the early growth response gene-1 (Egr-1) in the induction of protein synthesis by insulin. Inhibiting expression of Egr-1 by an antisense sequence resulted in an almost complete inhibition of insulin-mediated protein synthesis. This demonstrated that induction of Egr-1 is a necessary (although not necessarily sufficient) event in the stimulation of protein synthesis in the myocardium by insulin.

In a second experimental series, we attempted to target the sarcolemmal calmodulin-dependent Ca^{2+}-ATPase (calcium pump), a long-lived structural protein by this approach. Reducing expression of this enzyme resulted in a marked increase in contraction and a considerable delay in relaxation. These results established an important in vivo function for this calcium transport system. Because the contraction abnormalities induced by this approach closely resemble the abnormalities observed in cardiac hypertrophy, future studies will try to elucidate the modification of the calcium pump that might occur in this disease. Thus antisense oligonucleotides provide a means for selective inhibition of single genes in adult cardiomyocytes.

References

1. CARAFOLI, E., M. CHIESI, & P. GAZZOTTI (1990): The membrane carriers related to intracellular calcium regulation. In: LARAGH, J.H. & B.M. BRENNER (eds): Hypertension Pathophysiology. Diagnosis and Management Raven Press, New York.
2. O'BRIEN, T.X., J.J. HUNTER, E. DYSON & K.R. CHIEN (1991): Heart to heart. Circulation 83, 2133-2136.
3. AUSUBEL, F.M., R. BRENT, R.E. KINGSTON, D.D. MOORE, J.G. SEIDMAN, J.A. SMITH & K. STRUHL (1989): Current protocols in molecular biology. Vol. 1-2, Wiley Greene, New York.
4. SAMBROOK, J., E.F. FRITSCH & T. MANIATIS (1989): Molecular cloning, 2nd ed. Cold Spring Harbor Laboratory Press, New York.
5. CAPECCHI, M.R. (1989): Altering the genome by homologous recombination. Science 244, 1288-1292.
6. DOLNICK, B.J. (1990): Antisense agents in pharmacology. Biochem. Pharm. 40, 671-675.
7. WICKSTROM, E. (ed) (1991): Prospects for antisense nucleic acid therapy of cancer and AIDS. Wiley Greene, New York.
8. ZAMECNIK, P.C. & M.L. STEPHENSON (1978): Inhibition of rous sarcoma virus replication and cell transformation by a specific olgodeoxynucleotide. Proc. Natl. Acad. Sci. USA 75, 280-284.
9. LOKE, S.L., C.A. STEIN, X.H. ZHANG, K. MORI, M. NAKANISHI, C. SUBASINGHE, J.S. COHEN & L.M. NECKERS (1989): Characterization of oligonucleotide transport into living cells. Proc. Natl. Acad. Sci. USA 86, 3474-3478.
10. IRIBARREN, A.M., B.S. SPROAT, P. NEUNER, I. SULSTON, U. RYDER & A.I. LAMOND (1990): 2'-o-alkyl oligoribonucleotides as antisense probes. Proc. Natl. Acad. Sci. USA 87, 7747-7751.
11. STEIN, C.A. & J.S. COHEN (1988): Oligodeoxynucleotides as inhibitors of gene expression: a review. Cancer Res. 48, 2659-2668.
12. SIMONS, M., E.R. EDELMAN, J.L. DeKEYSER, R. LANGER & R.D. ROSENBERG (1992): Antisense c-myb oligonucleotides inhibit arterial smooth muscle cell accumulation in vivo. Nature 359, 67-70.
13. BASTIE DE LA, D., D. LEVITSKY, L. RAPPAPORT, J.J. MERCADIER, F. MAROTTE, C. WISNEWSKY, V. BROVKOVICH, K. SCHWARTZ & A.M. LOMPRE (1990): Function of the sarcoplasmic reticulum and expression of its Ca^{2+}-ATPase gene in the pressure overload-induced cardiac hypertrophy in the rat. Circ. Res. 66, 554-564.
14. MILBRANDT, J. (1987): A nerve growth factor-induced gene encodes a possible transcriptional regulatory factor. Science 238, 797-799.
15. SUKHATME, V.P., X. CAO, L.C. CHANG, C.H. TSAI-MORRIS, D. STAMENKOVICH, P.C. FERREIRA, D.R. COHEN, S.A. EDWARDS, T.B. SHOWS, T. CURRAN, M.M. LE BEAU & E.D. ADAMSON (1988): A zinc finger-encoding gene coregulated with c-fos during growth and differentiation, and after cellular depolarization. Cell 53, 37-43.
16. PIPER, H.M., A. VOLZ & P. SCHWARZ (1990): Adult ventricular rat muscle cells. In: (PIPER, H.M., ed.) Cell culture techniques in heart and vessel research. Springer, Berlin, New York, London.
17. SHULL, G.E. & J. GREEB (1988): Molecular cloning of two isoforms of the plasma membrane Ca^{2+}-transporting ATPase from rat brain. J. Biol. Chem. 263, 8646-8657.

18. ROSE, H. & H. KAMMERMEIER (1989): Contraction and metabolic activity of electrically stimulated cardiac myocytes from adult rats. Plügers Arch. 407, 116-118.
19. MORGAN, H.E., E.E. GORDON, Y. KIRA, B.H.L. CHUA, L.A. RUSSO, C.J. PETERSON, P.J. MCDERMOTT & P.A. WATSON (1987): Biochemical mechanisms of cardiac hypertrophy. Annual Rev. Physiol. 49, 533-545.
20. LA PRES, J., N. SHIMIZU, R. DECKER, R. ZAK & W. CLARK (1991): Beta-adrenergic regulation of myosin heavy chain promoter activity in the adult feline cardiomyocyte. UCSD Asilomar Conference.
21. FERRANINNI, E., S.M. HAFFNER & M.P. STERN (1990): Insulin sensitivity and hypertension. J. Hypertens 8, 169-173.
22. MOLLER, D.E. & J.E. FLIER (1991): Insulin resistance - mechanisms, syndromes, and implications. New Engl. J. Med. 13, 938-948.

Effects of diltiazem on cellular redox-state and capillary perfusion in the hypoperfused myocardium of the anesthetized rat

F. Vetterlein, P.N. Tran and G. Schmidt

Zentrum Pharmakologie und Toxikologie der Universität Göttingen

Introduction

A restriction of coronary flow induces metabolic alterations in the myocardium characterized by decreases in tissue concentrations of ATP and increases in lactate and NADH. It is well known that pathological rhythms may be generated in such substrate-depleted specialized as well as ordinary muscle cells. For this reason the observation has gained much interest that in the heart anoxic areas develop not only during complete occlusion of a coronary artery but also during partially reduced perfusion [4]. During the latter condition, inhomogeneously distributed groups of myocytes have been found to become anoxic.

Cellular anoxia may be detected by the phenomenon of NADH-fluorescence [1]. The deficiency of oxygen leads to the accumulation of reduced substrates in the respiratory chain, one of which is NADH. The reduced nucleotid can be detected by its bright blue fluorescence in UV light; this phenomenon does not exist when the substrate is oxydized to NAD.

The anoxic areas observed in isolated hearts with this technique have been considered to be the result of localized ischemic zones [4].

Aim of the present study was to answer the question whether such inhomogeneities may be detected under in vivo conditions with respect to NADH-fluorescence as well as the state of capillary perfusion and whether such irregularities in tissue supply may be influenced pharmacologically.

Methods

The principle approach was similar to that described earlier [6]. Rats of 210 g b.w. were anesthetized and thoracotomized. An anastomosis was inserted which connected the left carotid artery via the right carotid artery to the left coronary artery. An electromagnetic flowprobe, a side-branch for pressure measurement and an occlusor were inserted into this system and allowed the controlled reduction of coronary flow and perfusion pressure.

After insertion of the system the perfusion pressure was reduced to 80 mmHg for 5 min first; a value of 50 mmHg was then adjusted and maintained for 10 min. In part of the experiments diltiazem was i.v. infused in a dose of 0.2 mg/kg during the second half of the occlusion period. For demonstration of the pattern of capillary blood flow, two albumin conjugated fluorochromes were applied at the end of the period of reduced perfusion pressure. FITC-albumin, injected i.v., was allowed to circulate for 60 s, lissamine rhodamine B200 (RB200) albumin was infused into the left atrium during 20 s. Subsequently a biopsy was cut from the myocardium and rapidly frozen.

Frozen sections were prepared, freeze-substituted and analysed in the fluorescence microscope for the intravascular dyes FITC and RB200 as well as intracellular NADH. Values are given as $x \pm SD$.

Results and discussion

With respect to the general circulatory parameters the following observations were made. In the non-diltiazem-treated group (n=6) the adjustment of the coronary perfusion pressure to 50 mmHg led to a decrease in coronary flow from 2.6 ± 0.3 to 1.2 ± 0.3 ml • min^{-1}. This measure led to a slight decrease in blood pressure (122 ± 21 to 106 ± 26 mmHg). The atrial pressure increased from 8.3 ± 2.8 to 13.8 ± 8.3 mmHg; the heart rate did not change significantly (353 ± 24 and 342 ± 34 min^{-1}, respectively). When diltiazem was applied (n=6), the reduction in coronary flow was much less pronounced; a value of 1.7 ± 0.4 ml/min was attained at the end of the occlusion period. At the same time the blood pressure was 97 ± 20 mmHg, the atrial pressure 5.8 ± 3.0 mmHg and the heart 296 ± 22 min^{-1}.

Evaluation of the histological preparations showed the following results. In the non-diltiazem-treated group blue fluorescent areas were found to be irregularly distributed throughout the myocardial tissue. When the tissue was scanned for the intensity of NADH-fluorescence in myocardial cells (10 µm measuring diaphragm, 100 points per tissue section and exp.) it be-

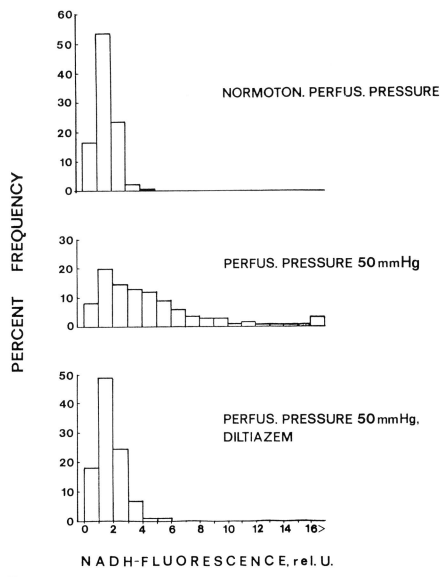

Fig. 1: Percent frequency of NADH-fluorescence intensity in the myocardium of the rat during normotonic perfusion, reduced coronary perfusion pressure with and without diltiazem treatment. Each of the 3 experimental groups n=6; the values of about 100 measuring points per experiment were summarized for each group.

came evident that the percent frequency was shifted towards significantly higher intensities as compared to the preparations of a non-occluded group (n=6) (Fig. 1). As a reference value the intensity of NADH-fluorescence in subendocardial cells which are oxygenated from the ventricular blood directly was used.

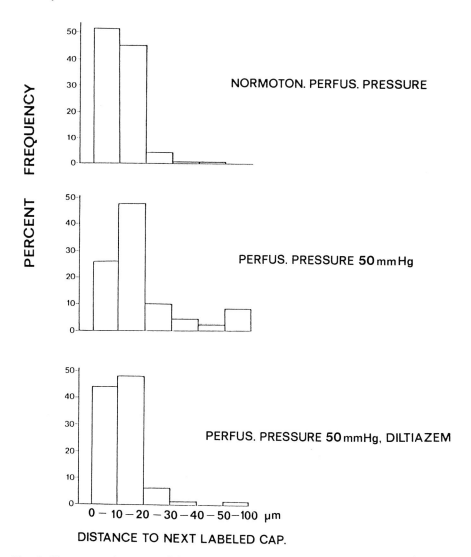

Fig. 2: The same points as used for measurement of NADH fluorescence (Fig. 1) were evaluated with respect to the distance to the next dye (RB200) labeled capillary and summarized in an analogous way.

The distribution of dye-labeled capillaries also pointed to the development of irregularities in capillary flow. Localized areas were found which had not taken up the intravascular dyes. When applying the concentric-circles method for quantification of the distribution [3], we found significant increases in the distances of the measuring points (used for NADH-fluorescence measurement) to the next labeled capillary (Fig. 2).

When comparing the distributions of the two labels with each other, it became evident that the pattern of ischemic areas was rather stable. If the zones of lacking capillary labeling had changed with time, FITC which had circulated for 60 s, would have gained access to much more capillaries than the short-time label RB200. However, since the distributions were nearly identical, a rather stable alteration in the pattern of capillary flow may be assumed.

When the distribution of capillary flow and cellular NADH-fluorescence were compared, it was found that both changes - the signs of ischemia and anoxia - did not occur in a congruent pattern. Large areas were observed having taken up the intravascular label but nevertheless showed increases in NADH-fluorescence. Evidently in such areas the capillary flow was insufficient with respect to oxygen supply. In areas of lacking capillary labeling most myocytes showed an increased NADH-signal.

Diltiazem significantly influenced the described effects of reducing coronary perfusion. As shown in Fig. 1 and 2, increases in tissue NADH as well as the signs of lacking capillary flow were found greatly diminished. The appearance nearly resembled that of the non-occluded control hearts.

Several factors are supposed to have contributed to this effect. Reduction in heart rate and systemic blood pressure both reduce the myocardial oxygen demand and facilitate coronary perfusion due to increased diastolic perfusion time and reduced tissue pressure [e.g. 5]. In addition, vasodilation of coronary resistance vessels is expected to have been involved in the observed changes in capillary perfusion and cellular redox state. It has been found that poststenotic vascular segments do not develop maximal relaxation since sympathetic reflexes and other mechanisms counteract vasodilation in such vessels despite inadequacy of flow [e.g. 2]. Therefore it appears conceivable that a diltiazem-induced reduction in coronary tone had contributed to the improvement in tissue supply which was observed during severely restricted coronary blood flow.

Acknowledgement

Supported by the "Deutsche Forschungsgemeinschaft",
SFB 330 Organprotektion

References

1. CHANCE, B., J.R. WILLIAMSEN, D. JAMIESON, & B. SCHOENER (1965): Properties and kinetics ofreduced pyridine nucleotide fluorescence of the isolated and in vivo rat heart. Biochem. Z. 341, 357-377.
2. CHILIAN, W.M. & S.M. LAYNE (1990): Coronary microvascular responses to reductions in perfusion pressure. Evidence for persistent arteriolar vasomotor tone during coronary hypoperfusion. Circ. Res. 66, 1227-1238.
3. KAYAR, S., P.G. ARCHER, A.J. LECHNER, & N. BANCHERO (1982): Evaluation of the concentric-circles method for estimating capillary-tissue diffusion distances. Microvasc. Res. 24, 342-353.
4. STEENBERGEN, C., G. DELEEUW, C.H. BARLOW, B. CHANCE & J.R. WILLIAMSEN (1977): Heterogeneity of the hypoxic state in perfused rat heart. Circ. Res. 41, 606-615.
5. VANHOUTTE, P.M. (1988): Ca^{2+} antagonists and vascular disease. In: P.M. VANHOUTTE, R. PAOLETTI & S. GOVONI (eds.) Calcium Antagonists. Pharmacology and clinical research. Ann. N.Y. Acad. Sci. 522, 380-389.
6. VETTERLEIN, F. & G. SCHMIDT (1985): Dilatatory capacity of the coronary system of the anesthetized rat. Basic Res. Cardiol. 80, 661-669.

Hyperpolarization, relaxation, and ionic concentrations in hypoxic human coronary arteries

G. Siegel, F. Schnalke and R. Hetzer*

Department of Physiology, The Free University of Berlin, and German Heart Institute Berlin*

Introduction

The number of cardiac infarctions has not yet essentially subsided in our country. While in the Anglo-Saxon and Nordic countries the number of non-lethal and lethal heart attacks is substantially declining, it is still drastically increasing in the East European countries. This is also true for East Germany which belongs to the top flight of the highest risks. The strategies globally assigned for fighting against this disease set on to the removal of the risk constellation. The risks for coronary heart diseases can be ranked according to their importance as follows: hyperlipidemias, low HDL-cholesterol, smoking, high blood pressure etc. The coronary sclerosis implies a marked loss of the ability to produce the eicosanoid prostacyclin (PGI_2) and endothelium-derived hyperpolarizing factor (EDHF). Thus, evidence is provided for endothelial cells being the early target sites in the pathogenesis of atherosclerosis. In an arteriosclerotic vascular bed a diminished blood flow is often coupled to a limited oxygen distribution, therefore, we were particularly interested in the response of normal vs. arteriosclerotic vessels to a variable O_2 supply.

Materials and methods

Experimental Preparations and Solutions

Intracellular potential recordings and measurements of isometric tension were performed on the vascular smooth muscle of human coronary artery

[15-17,21]. Coronary arteries were taken from heart transplant patients who had been suffering from a dilative cardiomyopathy or extensive atherosclerosis. There was a clear differentiation between normal and atherosclerotic vessels where the preparations had been subjected to light and electron microscopic examination. All arterial segments were equilibrated in a Krebs solution of the following composition: Na^+ 151.16, K^+ 4.69, Ca^{2+} 2.52, Mg^{2+} 1.1, Cl^- 145.4, HCO_3^- 16.31, $H_2PO_4^-$ 1.38, glucose 7.77 mmol/l (temp. 37 °C, pH 7.35). The solution was usually aerated with a 95 % O_2 - 5 % CO_2 gas mixture (carbogen). Blood substitute solutions were equilibrated with $O_2/CO_2/N_2$ mixtures containing different oxygen fractions, but a constant fraction of carbon dioxide (5 ml/dl) to vary the oxygen tension. Microelectrodes consisting of platinum cathodes were used for continuous oxygen tension measurements in the Krebs solution close to the blood vessel strip [4]. Indomethacin (Vonum, Econerica, Germany) was applied in a concentration of 10^{-5} mol/l. Each solution was freshly prepared. Endothelium-denuded preparations were obtained by gently scraping off the endothelial layer. Whether the procedure was successful was verified using light and electron microscopy.

Mechanical and Electrical Recording

Cylinders from the coronary arteries, 4-5 mm long, were cut lengthwise. Because muscle cells of the arteries are arranged circularly, the folded-out vessel ring, 5-10 mm long, was attached at the cut ends to an isometric tension measuring device (KWS 522.C, K 52 C; Hottinger-Baldwin, Darmstadt, Germany) [15,17,21]. The specimens were superfused with a carbogen Krebs solution at 50-60 ml/min for 15 min at an initial tension of 2 g. This high flow rate was used in order to bring about quick changes in PO_2 and reach low pressures. After this time, the tension was steady and amounted to 0.995 ± 0.156 g (n=10). Then, solutions with first decreasing and then increasing oxygen partial pressures (reversibility) were applied for 15 min each. After these periods, the mechanical tension had reached a steady-state value at each concentration step [18]. All values are the means ± SEM of the indicated number of preparations. Statistical significance (error probability P) was calculated according to the one-tailed t-test for dependent or independent samples.

Intracellular recordings of membrane potential were made with glass capillary microelectrodes, filled with 3 mol/l KCl, simultaneously with the mechanical tension registration. The electrode resistances ranged from 60-

100 MΩ and the tip potentials from -40 to -80 mV [18,21]. Electrode resistances and tip potentials were measured before and after impalement. Only when these values were unchanged was the recorded membrane potential included in the evaluation. The electrodes were shielded to just below the tips; otherwise, conventional recording techniques were used [14]. The microelectrode was inserted into the arterial muscle cell from the intimal surface. Arteries in a normal Krebs solution with membrane potentials between -50 and -80 mV were selected for the final averaging. Membrane potentials more positive than -50 mV (20 % of all impalements) had to be discarded because, according to our own measurements and those of other authors [12,21], they stem from endothelial cells.

At each oxygen tension step, the membrane potential had attained a steady-state value after 3 min and the tension after 7 min at the most. In principle, intracellular recordings were carried out after the fifth minute. In all preparations, at least ten impalements per oxygen level were averaged. The mean values of the membrane potential of all the human coronary arteries at each oxygen tension were averaged and are represented in the figures.

Determination of Ion Concentrations

Isolated coronary segments were incubated in Krebs solution for one hour. The total ion concentrations were determined using an atomic absorption spectrometer. After determination of wet and dry weight, the preparation was placed in an ice-cold quartz Erlenmeyer flask containing pure oxygen and Pt catalyst and burnt ash-free. The gaseous products were dissolved in a defined volume of 1.3 % HNO_3 [14,18]. Atomic absorption measurements were made directly from this fluid for Na, K and Mg, and for Ca after addition of a 2 % lanthanum nitrate solution. The total method error is $< \pm 3$ %.

Results

Figs. 1a, 2a illustrate the effect of hypoxia on membrane potential and tension of normal and arteriosclerotic human coronary arteries. There was a continuous hyperpolarization and relaxation with a reduction of PO_2 from 535 to 30 mmHg, and a depolarization and contraction between 30 and 0 mmHg. It is striking that, in the case of atherosclerosis, vascular smooth muscle cells were more depolarized and had more tone. This was true for all O_2 tensions. In normal carbogen Krebs solution, the membrane potential amounted to -60.4 ± 0.3 mV (n=5) and the initial force to 0.985 ± 0.096 g (n=5). Arteriosclerotic coronary arteries were depolarized to -59.8 ± 1.0 mV

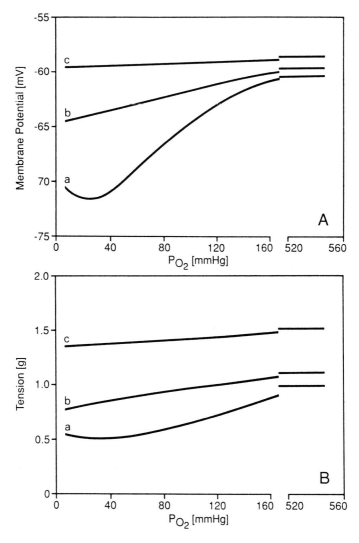

Fig. 1: Membrane potential (A) and tension (B) in isolated vascular strips of human coronary arteries in dependency on the oxygen partial pressure of the Krebs solution. Mean values from 15 experiments. *a:* Normal Krebs solution; *b:* Krebs solution with indomethacin (10^{-5} mol/l); *c:* Normal Krebs solution, endothelial layer of the coronary segments removed.

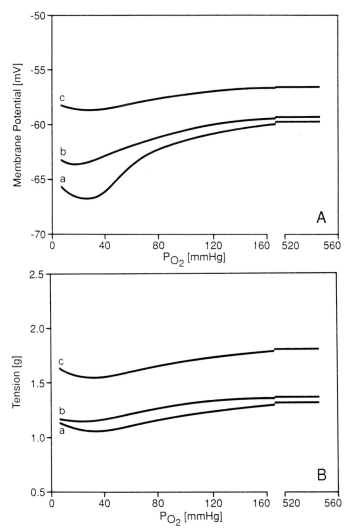

Fig. 2: Membrane potential (A) and tension (B) in isolated vascular strips of arteriosclerotic human coronary arteries in response to the oxygen partial pressure of the Krebs solution. Mean values from 15 experiments. *a:* Normal Krebs solution; *b:* Krebs solution with indomethacin (10^{-5} mol/l); *c:* Normal Krebs solution, endothelial layer of the coronary segments removed.

(n=5) and contracted to 1.316 ± 0.061 g (n=5; $P < 0.02$). During oxygen deficiency, control preparations showed a maximal hyperpolarization of 10.9 mV and a maximal relaxation of 0.466 g. Arteriosclerotic arteries, however, became hyperpolarized by merely 7.1 mV and relaxed by 0.258 g.

Two series of experiments, one with an application of indomethacin (Figs. 1b, 2b) and another one with deendothelialized blood vessels (Figs. 1c, 2c), confirmed the hypothesis that the endothelium of arteriosclerotic coronary arteries may produce less prostacyclin (PGI_2) and endothelium-derived hyperpolarizing factor (EDHF). For clarity, the points measured and their deviations were omitted. In normal coronary arteries, indomethacin reduced the hypoxic hyperpolarization and dilatation at 30 mmHg PO_2 by about 51 % (Fig. 1). The hyperpolarizing and dilatory contribution by PGI_2 was only about 32 % for a carbogen Krebs solution (resting, control conditions). Without mentioning that arteriosclerotic coronary arteries were more depolarized and contracted, they became less hyperpolarized and relaxed by a fall in oxygen partial pressure (Fig. 2). With indomethacin, the hypoxic hyperpolarization and vasorelaxation was attenuated by only 27 % (Tab. 1). The share of prostacyclin in dilatory vascular reactivity was restricted to 12 % in normal Krebs solution. These results can be qualitatively realized by the closed up curves *a* and *b* for arteriosclerotic blood vessels (Fig. 2) compared with the normal ones (Fig. 1). Thus, it may be concluded that in arteriosclerotic blood vessels, PGI_2 synthesis and release are predominantly diminished or its effectivity is impaired [16].

Table 1: Proportional distribution of the hyperpolarizing and relaxing effects of PGI_2 and EDHF in normal and arteriosclerotic coronary arteries.

PO_2	536	30		mmHg
Human coronary artery			19 (VSM)	
PGI_2	32	51		%
EDHF	68	49	32 (EC)	%
Arteriosclerotic human coronary artery			10 (VSM)	
PGI_2	12	27		%
EDHF	88	73	17 (EC)	%

VSM vascular smooth muscle
EC endothelial cell

Table 2: Structural compartmentation, transmembrane Na^+/K^+ distribution and Na^+/K^+ equilibrium potential in normal and arteriosclerotic human coronary arteries

	Human coronary artery	Arteriosclerotic human coronary artery	
Water content	75,9 ± 0.8 (8) (P<0.05)	70.0 ± 2.3 (8)	[%]
$[Na^+]_o$	151.2	151.2	[mmol/l]
$[Na^+]_t$	97.8 ± 1.0 (6) (P<0.005)	113.7 ± 3.8 (7)	[mmol/kg wet wt.]
$[Na^+]_i$	16.6	60.9	[mmol/l]
E_{Na} [1)	+64.2 (P<0.005)	+29.5	[mV]
$[K^+]_o$	4.7	4.7	[mmol/l]
$[K^+]_t$	36.8 ± 2.3 (5) (P<0.0001)	19.0 ± 1.4 (7)	[mmol/kg wet wt.]
$[K^+]_i$	134.6	95.0	[mmol/l]
E_K	-89.7	-80.4	[mV]
V	-64.9 ± 0.3 (5) (P<0.02)	-61.4 ± 1.0 (5)	[mV]

[1] Calculated with the freely ionized Na^+ fraction [cf.19]

Besides the imbalance between vasodilating and vasoconstricting factors another impairment could be jointly responsible for the depolarized state of arteriosclerotic vessels, namely a transmembrane redistribution of monovalent cations. From Tab. 2 follows that arteriosclerotic coronary vessels contained not only a lower water content but also a significantly increased internal Na^+ concentration together with an internal K^+ concentration diminished by 30 %. Thus, a K^+ equilibrium potential more positive by 9.3 mV correlated to the membrane depolarization by 3.5 mV. E_{Na} was reduced to about half. The membrane potential of arteriosclerotic blood vessels should adjust itself to a more depolarized value even with unchanged Na^+/K^+ permeabilities.

Discussion

The response of vascular smooth musculature to a decline in oxygen tension presents itself as a balanced interplay between hyperpolarizing-vasodilatory (PGI_2, EDHF) and depolarizing-vasoconstrictory factors (noradrenaline, 20-HETE, endothelin). The same holds true for the adjustment of muscle tone under stationary resting conditions because all of these compounds have a basal release [14,17,21]. This balance between relaxing and constricting factors seems to be disturbed and shifted to the constriction side in arteriosclerosis. Since atheromatous plaques contain high concentrations of lipid peroxides, which are known to inhibit prostacyclin synthetase [5,10], it was suggested that the PGI_2 production might be severely impaired in this disease [8]. Human arteriosclerotic iliac and femoral arteries form less 6-keto-prostaglandin $F_{1\alpha}$ than arteries obtained from healthy controls [22]. Endothelium-dependent relaxations to acetylcholine were reduced or absent in isolated atherosclerotic human coronary arteries [3]. These findings are fully confirmed by our observations. Arteriosclerotic human coronary arteries were more depolarized (by 0.6 mV) and more contracted (by 0.331 g) compared to normal ones in a carbogen Krebs solution [16,17] (Figs. 1,2). This difference was even greater with a physiological PO_2 of 95 mmHg (ΔV = 3.5 mV; ΔT = 0.552 g; $P < 0.02$) or a PO_2 of 30 mmHg (ΔV = 4.5 mV; ΔT = 0.539 g; $P < 0.05$). The endothelial function is possibly limited in this tissue. Apparently, less PGI_2 and/or EDHF are produced by arteriosclerotic vessels. The distribution of both substances was changed as well. Under resting conditions, the contribution of PGI_2 toward the basal release of hyperpolarizing and relaxing factors was 32 % in normal coronary arteries, but only 12 % in arteriosclerotic coronary arteries [15]. The remainder can be attributed to the basal release of the endothelial dilator EDHF (Tab. 1). In principle, a decline in O_2 tension shifts this ratio to the side of PGI_2. At 30 mmHg PO_2, PGI_2 contributed by 51 % to the hypoxic hyperpolarization and relaxation in normal coronary arteries, but only by 27 % in arteriosclerotic coronary arteries. Therefore, in arteriosclerotic blood vessels, PGI_2 synthesis and release may be restricted. An alternative explanation could be that impairment of PGI_2-dependent hyperpolarization and relaxation in the circulation of arteriosclerotic coronaries is not due to diminished PGI_2 formation but, in spite of an unchanged or even enhanced synthesis and release, due to a reduced action (increased inactivation, reduced sensitivity of the vasculature) of liberated PGI_2 [16]. Finally, the proportional distribution of the hyperpolarizing and relaxing factors in a normal blood vessel at an oxygen partial pressure of 30 mmHg was analyzed to be 18.7 % smooth muscle PGI_2, 31.6 % endothelial PGI_2, and 49.7 % EDHF. Corresponding values in an arteriosclerotic blood vessel were 10.3 % smooth muscle PGI_2, 17.3 % endothelial PGI_2, and 72.4 % EDHF.

Within the context of an explanation for hypoxic membrane hyperpolarization, we would like to discuss about K^+ channel opening. The cause of hypoxic hyperpolarization is probably an increase in K^+ conductance with both compounds, PGI_2 and EDHF [14,16,17,20,21]. The central starting point of the physiological mode of action of K^+ channel openers is the hyperpolarization of smooth muscle cells, which leads to relaxation by closing T- and/or L-type Ca^{2+} channels without, in the classical sense, the participation of cAMP or cGMP [20]. In the case of PGI_2, cAMP plays a part in the increase in the Ca^{2+}-activated K^+ outward current [20,21,23]. As suggested by Sadoshima et al. [13], the cAMP-dependent protein kinase seems to increase the Ca^{2+} sensitivity of the Ca^{2+}-activated K^+ channel. Obviously, one or two types of K^+ channels are stimulated by phosphorylation with cA-PK. Therefore, the hyperpolarizing and relaxing effect of PGI_2 may be explained by interventions of cA-PK at the Ca^{2+}-activated K^+ channel (stimulation), the sarcolemmal Ca^{2+} pump (stimulation), and the $I_{Ca(s)}$ (inhibition) [23]. In principle, the effect of EDHF seems to be the same, but its effector chain proceeds via cyclic GMP-dependent protein kinase. We presume that, with respect to the effect of prostacyclin, the Ca^{2+}-activated and perhaps the ATP-sensitive K^+ channel are responsible for the K^+ channel opening resulting in the hypoxic hyperpolarization [17,20,21]. The effect of the vasodilator EDHF, however, might be mediated by an ATP-sensitive K^+ channel [11].

From Figs. 1,2 and Tab. 1 it can be seen that the depolarized membrane potential observed in arteriosclerotic coronary arteries and the muscle tone consequently increased can be traced back to a reduced synthesis and release of PGI_2 or its diminished efficacy at the receptor site. Thus, the balance between vasodilating and vasoconstricting factors is disturbed with arteriosclerosis. Tab. 2 shows that an impaired transmembrane cation distribution additionally contributes to this depolarization. Arteriosclerotic vessel alterations are often preceded by hypertension having lasted for years. The process of hypertension is frequently paralleled by a restricted Na^+/K^+-ATPase activity, i.e. the electrogenic pump efficiency is lowered [1,6,7]. The increase of the intracellular Na^+ concentration and the decrease of the intracellular K^+ concentration found in arteriosclerotic blood vessels can be considered as being a late consequence of these active transport processes partly blocked (Tab. 2). The rise in $[Na^+]_i$ leads inevitably to a rise in $[Ca^{2+}]_i$ and thus to an increase in muscle tension [1]. Since the electrogenic ion pump normally supplies a hyperpolarizing contribution to the membrane potential, a membrane depolarization will arise with its impairment under arteriosclerosis. The passive potential genesis is disturbed as well. The K^+ redistribution leads to a K^+ equilibrium potential E_K more positive by 9.3 mV. Even with cation permeabilities remaining the same, the E_K depolarization is followed by a depolarization of the membrane resting potential. In summary, it shall be emphasized that the electrogenic ion pump efficiency impaired under arteriosclerosis results in a redistribution of transmembrane ion concentrations, which itself contributes to membrane depolarization and increased tension in arteriosclerotic vessels.

Summary

Human coronary arteries were taken from heart transplant patients. Arteriosclerotic arteries were more depolarized and constricted over the whole PO_2 range between 535 and 0 mmHg. During oxygen deficiency, control preparations showed a maximal hyperpolarization of $\Delta V = 10.9$ mV and a maximal relaxation of $\Delta T = 0.466$ g. Arteriosclerotic arteries, however, became hyperpolarized by merely $\Delta V = 7.1$ mV and relaxed by $\Delta T = 0.258$ g. In normal coronary arteries, indomethacin reduced the hypoxic hyperpolarization and dilatation at 30 mmHg PO_2 by about 51 %. The reduction was 27 % in arteriosclerotic vessels. The complete removal of the endothelium caused a 49 % (73 % in arteriosclerotic coronaries) restriction of dilatory vascular reactivity. The relationship was quite similar for a carbogen Krebs solution. The hyperpolarizing and dilatory contribution by prostacyclin was 32 % in normal and 12 % in arteriosclerotic coronary arteries. The remainder could be attributed to the basal release of endothelium-derived hyperpolarizing factor (EDHF). Thus, it may be concluded that in arteriosclerotic blood vessels, prostacyclin (PGI_2) synthesis and release are predominantly diminished. Finally, we found that the ratio PGI_2/EDHF in the voltage and tension changes strongly shifted to the PGI_2 side with a declining oxygen tension. This is true for normal and arteriosclerotic vessels. Supplementarily, a disturbed transmembrane cation distribution in the arteriosclerotic coronary vessels comes into question as an additional explanation for the depolarized membrane potential and increased muscle tone. $[Na^+]_i$ of normal arteries amounted to 16.6, of arteriosclerotic arteries to 60.9 mmol/l; $[K^+]_i$ values were 134.6 in normal and 95.0 mmol/l in arteriosclerotic coronaries, respectively. Therefore, the K^+ equilibrium potential of arteriosclerotic vessels was more positive by 9.3 mV. Besides this influence on the passive potential genesis in positive direction, the reduced electrogenic ion pump efficiency (inhibition of the Na^+/K^+-ATPase activity) contributes to the membrane depolarization as well. In accordance with the activation curve for vascular smooth muscle, the hyperpolarization leads to relaxation via a closure, the depolarization to constriction via an opening of Ca^{2+} channels. Hyperpolarization or depolarization of 2.5 mV reduces or augments the tension developed by one-half.

Acknowledgements

The authors thank Mrs. I. Krukenberg for her excellent technical assistance and Mr. H. Ewald from the mechanical workshop for his constant help. We are grateful to Mrs. M. Krawczynski for her outstanding work in preparing the illustrations and Mr. P. Holzner for the photographs. We are indebted to Mrs. A. Scheuermann and Mrs. E. Hofmann for the translation and editorial elaboration of the manuscript.

References

1. BLAUSTEIN, M.P. (1977): Sodium ions, calcium ions, blood pressure regulation, and hypertension: a reassessment and a hypothesis. Am. J. Physiol., 232, C165-C173.
2. COLLINS, R., R. PETRO, S. MACMAHON, P. HERBERT, N.H. FIEBACH, K.A. EBERLEIN, J. GODWIN, N. QIZILBASH, J.O. TAYLOR & C.H. HENNEKENS (1990): Blood pressure, stroke, and coronary heart disease. Part 2, Short-term reductions in blood pressure: overview of randomised drug trials in their epidemiological context. Lancet, 335, 827-838.
3. GINSBURG, R. & P.H. ZERA (1984): Endothelial relaxant factor in the human epicardial coronary artery. Circulation, 70 (Suppl. II), 122.
4. GROTE, J., G. SIEGEL, K. ZIMMER & A. ADLER (1988): The influence of oxygen tension on membrane potential and tone of canine carotid artery smooth muscle. Adv. Exp. Med. Biol., 222, 481-487.
5. GRYGLEWSKI, R.J., S. BUNTING, S. MONCADA, R.J. FLOWER & J.R. VANE (1976): Arterial walls are protected against deposition of platelet thrombi by a substance (prosta-

glandin X) which they make from prostaglandin endoperoxides. Prostaglandins, 12, 685-713.
6. HAMLYN, J.M., M.P. BLAUSTEIN, S. BOVA, D.W. DUCHARME, D.W. HARRIS, F. MANDEL, W.R. MATHEWS & J.H. LUDENS (1991): Identification and characterization of a ouabain-like compound from human plasma. Proc. Natl. Acad. Sci. USA, 88, 6259-6263.
7. HERMSMEYER, K. (1985): Membrane ATPase mechanism of K^+-return relaxation in arterial muscles of stroke-prone SHR and WKY. Am. J. Physiol., 250, C557-C562.
8. LÜSCHER, T.F. (1988): Endothelial vasoactive substances and cardiovascular disease. S. Karger, Basel, München, Paris, London, New York, New Delhi, Singapore, Tokyo, Sydney.
9. MACMAHON, S. (1990): Antihypertensive drug treatment: the potential, expected and observed effects on vascular disease. J. Hypertension, 8 (Suppl. 7), S239-S244.
10. MONCADA, S., R.J. GRYGLEWSKI, S. BUNTING & J.R. VANE (1976): A lipid peroxide inhibits the enzyme in blood vessel microsomes that generates from prostaglandin endoperoxides the substance (prostaglandin X) which prevents platelet aggregation. Prostaglandins, 12, 715-737.
11. NELSON, M.T., J.B. PATLAK, J.F. WORLEY & N.B. STANDEN (1990): Calcium channels, potassium channels, and voltage dependence of arterial smooth muscle tone. Am. J. Physiol., 259, C3-C18.
12. NORTHOVER, B.J. (1980): The membrane potential of vascular endothelial cells. Adv. Microcirc., 9, 135-160.
13. SADOSHIMA, J.-I., N. AKAIKE, H. KANAIDE & M. NAKAMURA (1988): Cyclic AMP modulates Ca-activated K channel in cultured smooth muscle cells of rat aortas. Am. J. Physiol., 255, H754-H759.
14. SIEGEL, G., J. GROTE, F. SCHNALKE & K. ZIMMER (1989): The significance of the endothelium for hypoxic vasodilatation. Z. Kardiol., 78 (Suppl. 6), 124-131.
15. SIEGEL, G., K. RÜCKBORN, F. SCHNALKE & J. GROTE (1992): Membrane physiological reactions of human arteriosclerotic coronary arteries to hypoxia. J. Cardiovasc. Pharmacol., 20 (Suppl. 12), S217-S220.
16. SIEGEL, G., F. SCHNALKE, K. RÜCKBORN, J. MÜLLER & R. HETZER (1992): Role of prostacyclin in normal and arteriosclerotic human coronary arteries during hypoxia. Agents Actions Suppl., 37, 320-332.
17. SIEGEL, G., F. SCHNALKE, J. SCHAARSCHMIDT, J. MÜLLER & R. HETZER (1991): Hypoxia and vascular muscle tone in normal and arteriosclerotic human coronary arteries. J. Vasc. Med. Biol., 3, 140-149.
18. SIEGEL, G., A. WALTER, M. BOSTANJOGLO, A.W.H. JANS, R. KINNE, L. PICULELL & B. LINDMAN (1989): Ion transport and cation-polyanion interactions in vascular biomembranes. J. Membrane Sci., 41, 353-375.
19. SIEGEL, G., A. WALTER, K. RÜCKBORN, F. SCHNALKE, E. BUDDECKE, A. SCHMIDT & B. LINDMAN (1993): Maintenance of the Na^+ distribution in the arterial wall. In: KAKIHANA, H., H.R. HOSHI JR., T. HOSHI & K. TOYOKURA: Seventh symposium on salt, Vol. II, pp. 395-407. Elsevier Science Publ. Amsterdam, London, New York, Tokyo.
20. SIEGEL, G., A. WALTER, F. SCHNALKE, A. SCHMIDT, E. BUDDECKE, G. LOIRAND & G. STOCK (1991): Potassium channel activation, hyperpolarization, and vascular relaxation. Z. Kardiol., 80 (Suppl. 7), 9-24.

21. SIEGEL, G., K. WENZEL, F. SCHNALKE, J. MIRONNEAU, G. SCHULTZ, G. SCHRÖDER, E. SCHILLINGER, O. GRAUHAN & R. HETZER (1990): Prostacyclin analogues as K^+ channel openers. Clin. Pharmacol., 7, 72-96.
22. SINZINGER, H., W. FEIGL & K. SILBERBAUER (1979): Prostacyclin generation in atherosclerotic arteries. Lancet, II, 469.
23. SPERELAKIS, N. & Y. OHYA (1990): Cyclic nucleotide regulation of Ca^{2+} slow channels and neurotransmitter release in vascular muscle. Prog. Clin. Biol. Res., 327, 277-298.

Six histamine H_1, H_2 or H_3 receptor-mediated effects in the cardiovascular system of pithed rats

E. Schlicker and B. Malinowska

Institut für Pharmakologie und Toxikologie, Universität Bonn

Introduction

Histamine H_3 receptors were first characterized in 1983 in the rat cortex by Arrang et al. [1] as autoreceptors, i. e. receptors located on the histaminergic neurones themselves. In the meantime, the occurrence of H_3 heteroreceptors has also been shown, both in the central [15] and autonomic nervous system [2,4]. With respect to the cardiovascular system, inhibitory presynaptic H_3 receptors have been demonstrated in vitro on the postganglionic sympathetic nerve fibres innervating the blood vessels [7,13] and the heart [6,9]. Evidence for the existence of postsynaptic H_3 receptors has also been presented [5,14]. It was the first aim of our study to examine whether H_3 receptors play any role under in situ conditions in the cardiovascular system of pithed rats.

Since the occurrence of H_3 receptors could indeed be shown in the pithed rat we tried to determine whether H_1 and H_2 receptor-mediated effects are also detectable in this model. Hypotensive and, less frequently, biphasic blood pressure effects of histamine have been shown in the pithed rat [3]. We further analyzed the effect of histamine on diastolic blood pressure using selective agonists for each of the three histamine receptor subtypes. Since both an H_1 and an H_2 receptor-mediated hypotensive effect could be shown, additional experiments were carried out to determine the mechanism(s) involved in both effects. The present article represents a short review of our recent work related to this topic [10-12].

Methods

Male Wistar rats weighing 180-380 g were anaesthetized with methohexitone 300 µmol/kg i.p., injected with atropine 2 µmol/kg, pithed and vagotomized. Arterial blood pressure was measured from the right carotid artery; the pressure wave triggered a ratemeter. The left femoral vein was cannulated for i.v. injections of drugs. Electrical stimulation was generated between the pithing rod and an indifferent electrode placed ventrally. (+)-Tubocurarine 1.3 µmol/kg was injected i.v. 5-10 min before administration of the histamine agonist or the first electrical stimulation. For further details of the method, see legend to Fig. 1 or Tab. 1 and Tab. 2.

Results

The electrically induced increase in basal diastolic blood pressure (BDBP) and heart rate (HR) was decreased by the H_3 receptor agonist R-(-)-α-methylhistamine (RαMeHA) but not changed by the H_1 receptor agonist 2-(2-thiazolyl)ethylamine (2TEA) and the H_2 receptor agonist dimaprit; the effect of RαMeHA was attenuated by the H_3 receptor antagonist thioperamide (Fig. 1a, b). RαMeHA did not affect the increase in BDBP and HR induced by exogenously added noradrenaline and isoprenaline, respectively (not shown).

BDBP was not affected by RαMeHA through the activation of H_3 receptors (not shown). 2TEA (studied in the presence of propranolol in order to block the increase in HR induced by high doses of this substance) and dimaprit decreased BDBP; these hypotensive responses were abolished by the H_1 receptor antagonist dimethindene and the H_2 receptor antagonist ranitidine, respectively (Tab. 1). The effects of 2TEA and dimaprit were also studied after the administration of N^ω nitro-L-arginine methyl ester (NAME; an inhibitor of the biosynthesis of nitric oxide by endothelial cells) and indomethacin (an inhibitor of the biosynthesis of prostaglandins). Since NAME increased BDBP by about 50 mmHg (not shown), controls and animals treated with indomethacin or its vehicle received vasopressin to adjust diastolic blood pressure to the level obtained in NAME-treated rats. NAME reduced the magnitude of the hypotensive response to 2TEA by 45 % and its duration by 36 % without attenuating the vasodepressor response to dimaprit. Indomethacin did not affect the hypotensive response to 2TEA and dimaprit (Tab. 1).

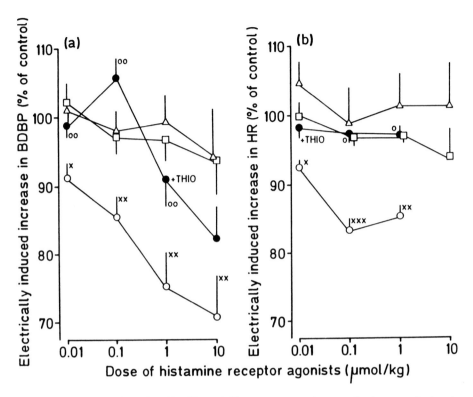

Fig. 1: Effects of histamine H_1, H_2 and H_3 receptor agonists on the increase in basal diastolic blood pressure (BDBP) and heart rate (HR) induced by electrical stimulation of preganglionic sympathetic nerves. Four or five (S_1-S_4 or S_1-S_5) 15-s periods of electrical stimulation (0.5 Hz, 1 ms, 50 V) were administered to pithed and vagotomized rats at intervals of 7 min. 2-(2-Thiazolyl)ethylamine (□), dimaprit (Δ) or R-(-)-α-methylhistamine (circles) was injected in increasing doses 5 min before S_2, S_3, S_4 and S_5. Thioperamide (THIO) 1 μmol/kg was injected alone (part a) or together with rauwolscine 1 μmol/kg (part b) 5 min before S_1. S_1 was 36.8 ± 2.1 mmHg (part a) and 83.1 ± 3.2 beats/min (part b) and was not changed by thioperamide. The ratios of the increase in BDBP or HR evoked by S_2, S_3, S_4 and S_5 over that evoked by S_1 are expressed as percentages of the respective S_n/S_1 values in controls (saline injected 5 min before S_2, S_3, S_4 and S_5). Means ± S.E.M. of 4-9 rats. $^x p<0.05$, $^{xx} p<0.01$, $^{xxx} p<0.001$ compared to the corresponding controls. $^o p<0.05$, $^{oo} p<0.01$ compared to the group without thioperamide.

The unselective histamine receptor agonist $N^α$-methylhistamine ($N^α$MeHA; studied after administration of propranolol in order to block the increase in HR induced by this substance) had a biphasic effect on BDBP. The initial vasodepressor phase was blocked by combined administration of dimethindene and ranitidine (not shown). The subsequent vasopressor phase reached its maximum at 1 μmol/kg (Tab. 2). Ranitidine enhanced the

Table 1: Effects of dimethindene, ranitidine, N$^\omega$-nitro-L-arginine methyl ester (NAME) and indomethacin on the decrease in basal diastolic blood pressure (BDBP) induced by 2-(2-thiazolyl)ethylamine (2TEA) and dimaprit in pithed rats.

	BDBP before first dose of agonist (mmHg)	Decrease in BDBP after administration of			
		2TEA 1 μmol/kg		Dimaprit 1 μmol/kg	
		Magnitude (mmHg)	Duration (s)	Magnitude (mmHg)	Duration (s)
I.					
P	57.4 ± 2.4	12.6 ± 2.3	24.0 ± 4.2	n.e.	n.e.
Dimethindene	54.5 ± 4.6	0**	0**	n.e.	n.e.
0.9 % NaCl	52.4 ± 4.6	n.e.	n.e.	13.5 ± 1.5	63.0 ± 4.6
Ranitidine	50.5 ± 2.4	n.e.	n.e.	3.4 ± 0.9***	24.5 ± 5.4**
II.					
VP+P	106.4 ± 3.8	36.3 ± 4.5	21.5 ± 2.5	35.0 ± 4.6	112.0 ± 20.6
NAME+P	104.1 ± 5.4	19.8 ± 3.3*	13.8 ± 1.8*	32.2 ± 3.6	159.7 ± 14.6
VP+Tris+P	97.8 ± 2.3	36.6 ± 5.5	25.2 ± 2.5	30.2 ± 3.2	109.0 ± 18.3
VP+INDO+P	97.5 ± 3.1	38.7 ± 7.6	27.4 ± 4.3	36.8 ± 4.3	156.8 ± 32.3

In the first group of experiments (I), 2TEA and dimaprit, administered i.v. in 4 increasing doses (0.1-10 μmol/kg), caused a dose-dependent decrease in BDBP; (only the data for 1 μmol/kg are shown). Dimethindene (1 μmol/kg) plus propranolol (P; 3 μmol/kg) or ranitidine (10 μmol/kg) were/was administered 5 min before the first dose of agonist. In the second group of experiments (II), NAME (370 μmol/kg) was injected first or the infusion of vasopressin (VP; 0.04-0.4 I.U./kg/h) was initiated. The remaining drugs (μmol/kg) were injected according to the following protocol: indomethacin 14 or its vehicle (Tris buffer): 5 min later; propranolol 3. 10 min later; 2-TEA or dimaprit 1: 15 min later. Means ± S.E.M. or 5-6 rats. *p<0.05, **p<0.01, ***p<0.001. n.e. - not examined. Note that NAME produced a marked and sustained increase in BDBP (suggesting that endogenously released nitric oxide accounts for the low level of BDBP) and that the hypotensive effects of 2TEA and dimaprit were strongly enhanced at high levels of BDBP (e.g., after administration of NAME or during infusion of VP). The hypotensive response to dimaprit was markedly longer than that to 2TEA, both at low (I) and high (II) levels of BDBP.

vasopressor response to N$^\alpha$MeHA 10 μmol/kg. Dimethindene and combined administration of dimethindene and ranitidine abolished the vasopressor phase (Tab. 2). In adrenalectomized animals, N$^\alpha$MeHA showed a vasodepressor response only (not shown), whereas the subsequent vasopressor phase was abolished (Tab. 2).

Basal HR was not changed by the activation of H_2 and H_3 receptors (not shown) but was increased by N^{a}MeHA; this response was totally or subtotally blocked by adrenalectomy, propranolol or dimethindene (Tab. 2).

Table 2: Increase in basal diastolic blood pressure (BDBP) and heart (HR) induced by N^a-methylhistamine (N^aMeHA) in pithed rats.

	Values before first dose of N^αMeHA	Increase in BDBP or HR after administration of N^αMeHA at a dose of		
		0.1	1	10 μmol/kg
		BDBP (mmHg)		
N^αMeHA+P	44.1 ± 4.6	8.3 ± 2.4	27.4 ± 5.3	10.9 ± 1.4
N^αMeHA+P+D	42.7 ± 2.3	0**	0**	0***
N^αMeHA+P+R	42.9 ± 1.2	2.5 ± 1.8	24.5 ± 5.9	27.9 ± 5.1**
N^αMeHA+P+D+R	39.8 ± 3.7	0.6 ± 0.6**	4.1 ± 1.2**	2.3 ± 0.8**
N^αMeHA+A	44.8 ± 1.8	0**	1.4 ± 0.8**	0.5 ± 0.3**
		HR (beats/min)		
N^αMeHA	326.8 ± 9.6	13.8 ± 6.1	32.4 ± 9.2	51.9 ± 10.1
N^αMeHA+D	333.0 ± 9.1	1.0 ± 1.0*	6.0 ± 3.8*	10.8 ± 4.3**
N^αMeHA+P	313.0 ± 2.3	0**	0**	0***
N^αMeHA+A	348.0 ± 9.1	0**	0**	0***

Each rat received four increasing doses of N^αMeHA (0.01, 0.1, 1 and 10 μmol/kg i.v.). N^αMeHA 0.01 μmol/kg did not increase BDBP and HR. Propranolol (P; 3 μmol/kg), dimethindene (D; 1 μmol/kg) or ranitidine (R; 10 μmol/kg) were administered 5 min before the first dose of N^αMeHA. Some experiments were performed in adrenalectomized rats (A). Means ± S.E.M. of 4-9 rats. *p<0.05, **p<0.01, ***p<0.001 compared to "N^αMeHA+P" (upper part of the table) and "N^αMeHA" (lower part). Note that N^αMeHA had a biphasic effect on BDBP (hypotensive effect, followed by vasopressor response) and that only the second phase is shown here. The low vasopressor response to N^αMeHA 10 μmol/kg (1st line) is probably due to the preceding hypotensive effect; consequently, attenuation of the H_2 receptor-mediated hypotensive effect by ranitidine markedly increased the vasopressor effect of N^αMeHA 10 μmol/kg.

Discussion

The first and the second histamine receptor-mediated effects presented in our study are the attenuation of the electrically induced increase in BDBP and HR by RαMeHA. Both effects of RαMeHA (which were not mimicked by 2TEA and dimaprit) were diminished by thioperamide, demonstrating that H_3 receptors are involved. The lack of influence of RαMeHA on the pressor response and tachycardia induced by exogenously added noradrenaline and isoprenaline, respectively, suggests that the H_3

receptors are not located postsynaptically on the vascular smooth muscle and the heart; they may be located presynaptically on the postganglionic sympathetic nerve fibres. The present results demonstrate that inhibitory presynaptic H_3 receptors on the sympathetic nerve fibres, which have been previously shown in blood vessels as well as in the heart in vitro [6,7,9,13], are operative also under in situ conditions.

The third and the fourth histamine receptor-mediated effects are the decrease in BDBP induced by the activation of both H_1 and H_2 receptors. NAME (an inhibitor of the synthesis of nitric oxide) markedly reduced the fall in blood pressure produced by 2TEA without affecting the response to dimaprit; indomethacin (an inhibitor of cyclooxygenase) did not change the hypotensive response to 2TEA and dimaprit. These results, which are in harmony with previous findings obtained in vitro [for review see ref. 8], suggest that the H_1 receptors are located in the endothelial cells and mediate relaxation of the resistance vessels by inducing release of nitric oxide, whereas the H_2 receptors produce vasorelaxation by a direct effect on vascular smooth muscle.

The fifth and the sixth histamine receptor-mediated effects are represented by the increase in BDBP and HR produced by NαMeHA. Since both effects were blocked by dimethindene or adrenalectomy, we suggest that these effects are connected with the release of catecholamines from the adrenal medulla through the activation of H_1 receptors [16].

No evidence could be obtained in our study for the occurrence of presynaptic H_1 and H_2 and postsynaptic H_3 receptors in the resistance vessels and the heart in pithed rats.

Conclusions

In the cardiovascular system of the pithed rat, a total of 6 histamine receptor-mediated effects could be detected: inhibition of (1) the neurogenic vasopressor response and (2) the neurogenic tachycardia via **H_3** receptors, probably located on the postganglionic sympathetic nerve fibres innervating the resistance vessels and the heart, respectively; (3) a vasodepressor response via **H_2** receptors, located on the vascular smooth muscle cells of the resistance vessels and (4) a vasodepressor response via NO-releasing endothelial **H_1** receptors; (5) vasopressor response and (6) tachycardia via catecholamine-releasing H_1 receptors in the adrenal medulla.

References

1. ARRANG, J.-M., M. GARBARG & J.-C. SCHWARTZ (1993): Auto-inhibition of brain histamine release mediated by a novel class (H_3) of histamine receptor. Nature, 302, 832-837.
2. BARNES, P.J. & M. ICHINOSE (1989): H_3 receptors in airways. Trends Pharmacol. Sci., 10, 264.
3. BELESLIN, D.B. (1962): The action of histamine on the blood pressure of the rat. Arch. int. Pharmacodyn., 138, 19-31.
4. BERTACCINI, G., G. CORUZZI & E. POLI (1991): The histamine H_3-receptor - a novel prejunctional receptor regulating gastrointestinal function. Aliment. Pharmacol. Therap., 5, 585-591.
5. EA-KIM, L. & N. OUDART (1988): A highly potent and selective H_3-agonist relaxes rabbit middle cerebral artery, in vitro. Eur. J. Pharmacol., 150, 393-396.
6. FUDER, H., M. EGENOLF & M. TORZEWSKI (1990): Inhibitory prejunctional histamine H_3-receptors on noradrenergic nerves of guinea-pig atria. Naunyn-Schmiedeberg's Arch. Pharmacol., 341 (Suppl.), R87.
7. ISHIKAWA, S.& N. SPERELAKIS (1987): A novel class (H_3) of histamine receptors on perivascular nerve terminals. Nature, 327, 158-160.
8. LEVI, R., L.E. RUBIN & S.S. GROSS (1991): Histamine in cardiovascular function and dysfunction: recent developments. In: UVNÄS, B. (ed.), Histamine and histamine antagonists. pp. 347-383, Springer, Berlin, Heidelberg, New York.
9. LUO, X.-X., Y.-H. TAN & B.-H. SHENG (1991): Histamine H_3-receptors inhibit sympathetic neurotransmission in guinea pig myocardium. Eur. J. Pharmacol., 204, 311-314.
10. MALINOWSKA, B. & E. SCHLICKER (1991): H_3 receptor-mediated inhibition of the neurogenic vasopressor response in pithed rats. Eur. J. Pharmacol., 205, 307-310.
11. MALINOWSKA, B. & E. SCHLICKER (1993): Identification of endothelial H_1, vascular H_2 and cardiac presynaptic H_3 receptors in the pithed rat. Naunyn-Schmiedeberg's Arch. Pharmacol., 347, 55-60.
12. MALINOWSKA, B. & E. SCHLICKER (1993): Effects of H_1, H_2 and H_3 agonists on the neurogenic vasopressor response in the pithed rat. Agents Actions, 38, C254-C256.
13. MOLDERINGS, G.J., G. WEISSENBORN, E. SCHLICKER, J. LIKUNGU & M. GÖTHERT (1992): Inhibition of noradrenaline release from the sympathetic nerves of the human saphenous vein by presynaptic histamine H_3 receptors. Naunyn-Schmiedeberg's Arch. Pharmacol., 346, 46-50.
14. ROSIC, M., C.S. COLLIS, I.Z. ANJELKOVIC, M.B. SEGAL, D. DJURIC & B.V. ZLOKOVIC (1991): The effects of (R)α-methylhistamine on the isolated guinea pig aorta. In: TIMMERMAN, H. & H. VAN DER GOOT (eds.), New perspectives in histamine research. Agents and actions supplements, pp. 283-287, Birkhäuser, Basel.
15. SCHLICKER, E., R. BETZ & M. GÖTHERT (1988): Histamine H_3 receptor-mediated inhibition of serotonin release in the rat brain cortex. Naunyn-Schmiedeberg's Arch. Pharmacol., 337, 588-590.
16. VON EULER, U.S. (1966): Relationship between histamine and the autonomous nervous system. In: ROCHA E SILVA, M. (ed.), Histamine and antihistaminics, pp. 318-333, Springer, Berlin, Heidelberg, New York.

On the mechanism of the coronary dilator response to ACE inhibitors

M. Hecker, A.T. Bara, F. Nestler, I. Pörsti and R. Busse

Institut für angewandte Physiologie der Universität Freiburg

Introduction

Angiotensin-converting enzyme (ACE) inhibitors are widely used in the treatment of essential hypertension and congestive heart failure due their unique mechanism of action and favorable safety profile. Their acute blood pressure-lowering effect in patients with an activated renin-angiotensin system, but not in those with normal or low levels of renin, can be explained by an inhibition of systemic and local angiotensin II formation. Since ACE or kininase II (EC 3.4.15.1) also catalyzes the degradation of the potent vasodilator bradykinin [1], it has long been suspected, but not yet proven, that an increase in the concentration of endogenous kinins within the vascular wall [2] also plays an important role in the antihypertensive effect of this class of compounds [3]. Indeed, vascular endothelial and smooth muscle cells contain considerable amounts of high-molecular weight ininogen which upon activation of kallikrein-like serine proteases can be cleaved to yield bradykinin [4,5].

The potent dilator action of bradykinin is mainly brought about by the subsequent release of nitric oxide (NO) and prostacyclin (PGI_2) from the endothelium through activation of B_2-receptors (6). Both ACE and the B_2-receptor are located in the luminal plasma membrane of endothelial cells [7]. It is conceivable, therefore, that the proteolytic activity of this enzyme influences the concentration of bradykinin in the vicinity of the receptor and hence the amounts of NO and PGI_2 being formed in response to receptor occupancy.

By promoting the accumulation of endogenous kinins, presumably bradykinin, ACE inhibitors can enhance the basal release of both PGI_2 and NO from cultured endothelial cells, an effect which is mediated by a B_2-receptor-dependent increase in the intracellular concentration of free Ca^{2+} in these cells [8,9]. To evaluate the functional consequences of this kinin accumulation in native endothelial cells, we have studied the effects of different ACE inhibitors on the tone and cyclic GMP content of isolated bovine coronary arteries and on the vasodilator response to exogenously administered bradykinin in the isolated saline-perfused rabbit heart.

Methods

Materials. Hoe 140 (D-Arg[Hyp^3,Thi^5,D-Tic^7,Oic^8]-bradykinin) and ramiprilat were kindly provided by Hoechst AG (Frankfurt/Main, Germany), moexiprilat by Schwarz Pharma AG (Monheim, Germany), and the cyclic GMP antibody by Dr. B. Brüne (University of Konstanz, Germany).

Bioassay - Bovine coronary arteries were cleaned of adipose and connective tissue and cut into ring segments of ~5 mm width which were mounted between a force transducer and a rigid support for measurement of isometric force. Two segments were simultaneously superfused (20 ml/h) with warmed (37 °C), oxygenated (95 % O_2/5 % CO_2) Tyrode's solution (pH 7.4; composition in mM: Na^+ 144.3; K^+ 4.0; Cl^- 138.6; Ca^{2+} 1.7; Mg^{2+} 1.0; HPO_4^{2-} 0.4; HCO_3^- 11.9; glucose 10.0) and basal (passive) tension was adjusted over a 30 min equilibration period to 1 g. Thereafter, the segments were preconstricted to 2-3 g of tension by superfusions of 1-5 μM prostaglandin $F_{2\alpha}$ ($PGF_{2\alpha}$). In a separate series of experiments, the segments were incubated in 10 ml of warmed (37 °C), oxygenated (95 % O_2/5 % CO_2) Krebs-Henseleit solution (pH 7.4; composition in mM: Na^+ 142.0; K^+ 5.2; Cl^- 127.0; Ca^{2+} 2.5; Mg^{2+} 1.0; KPO_4^{2-} 1.2; HCO^{3-} 24.0; D-glucose 5.0; pyruvate 2.0) and passive tension was adjusted over a 30 min equilibration period to 5 g. Thereafter, the segments were preconstricted to 10 g of tension with U46619 (9,11-dideoxy-11α,9α-epoxymethano-prostaglandin $F_{2\alpha}$, 10-30 nM).

Cyclic GMP determination - The concentration of cyclic GMP in these segments was determined by using a specific radioimmunoassay [10].

Isolated rabbit heart (Langendorff preparation) - Hearts from anesthetized mongrel rabbits (1.0-1.5 kg body weight) of either sex were excised and perfused with warmed (37 °C), oxygenated (95 % O_2/5 % CO_2)

Krebs-Henseleit solution, pH 7.4 as described previously [11]. Coronary perfusion pressure (CPP) and isovolumetric left ventricular pressure (LVP) were measured by means of pressure transducers connected to a sidearm of the aortic perfusion cannula and to a fluid-filled latex balloon inserted into the left ventricle, respectively. Heart rate was derived from the LVP signal by a cardiotachometer, and the flow rate (20-30 ml/min) was adjusted to obtain a coronary perfusion pressure of approximately 60 mmHg.

The concentration of 6-keto-PGF$_{1\alpha}$, the stable hydrolysis product of PGI$_2$, in the coronary effluent (collected for 20 s before and during the infusion of each substance at various intervals) was measured by using a specific radioimmunoassay [11]. The release of NO was estimated by monitoring the increase in the intracellular concentration of cGMP in washed human platelets after passage through the coronary vascular bed as described in detail elsewhere [11].

Statistical analysis - Unless indicated otherwise, all data in the figures are expressed as mean ± SEM. Statistical evaluation was performed by using the unpaired two-tailed Student's *t*-test with a P-value <0.05 considered statistically significant.

Results and discussion

ACE inhibitors and vascular tone

In the presence of a cyclooxygenase inhibitor (diclofenac 1 µM) PGF$_{2\alpha}$-preconstricted bovine coronary artery segments substantially relaxed (~63 %) when they were superfused with bradykinin at a concentration of 3 nM (n>10). Moexiprilat alone (0.1 µM) and without previous exposure of these segments to bradykinin also caused a distinct relaxation (~23 %, Figure 1a). Almost complete dilatation was obtained in the presence of both bradykinin and the ACE inhibitor. Another ACE inhibitor, ramiprilat, elicited a relaxant response, the degree of which (~18 %, n=6) was similar to that caused by moexiprilat. Removal of the endothelium totally blunted the relaxant response to bradykinin or the ACE inhibitors [12].

Neither moexiprilat nor ramiprilat in concentrations up to 3 µM had any effect on coronary artery tone when the segments were incubated in organ chambers [12]. Other ACE inhibitors have also been reported to be unable to elicit an endothelium-dependent relaxation in bovine [13] or canine [14] coronary arteries under no-flow conditions, whereas perindoprilat induced the release of an endothelium-derived relaxing factor from luminally perfused canine carotid arteries [15]. Flow or mass transport may thus sensitize isolated arterial segments to the dilator activity of ACE inhibitors.

The relaxant response to moexiprilat in superfused segments, like that caused by bradykinin (~93 % inhibition, n>10), was strongly attenuated in the presence of the specific B_2-receptor antagonist Hoe 140 (0.1 µM, Fig. 1a). The NO synthase inhibitor, N^G-nitro-L-arginine (30 µM), also inhibited the moexiprilat-induced relaxation to the same extent as Hoe 140 (Fig. 1a), suggesting that this response was mediated by an activation of B_2-receptors on the coronary endothelium and the subsequent enhanced release of NO from these cells. Interestingly, N^G-nitro-L-arginine only partially inhibited the relaxant response to bradykinin (~45 % inhibition) which was, however, completeley suppressed when both N^G-nitro-L-arginine and a high (depolarizing) concentration of potassium chloride ($\geq$20 mM) were added to the superfusate (n$\geq$4). Thus, in addition to stimulating the release of NO from the coronary endothelium, bradykinin caused an endothelium-dependent hyperpolarization of the coronary smooth muscle. Similar findings have also been reported for indomethacin-treated canine [14] and porcine [16] coronary arteries. It is, however, not clear as to whether this hyperpolarization is mediated by an endothelium-derived humoral factor or based on an electrotonic coupling between endothelium and vascular smooth muscle [14,16,17].

ACE inhibitors and endothelial NO release

To substantiate the notion that the relaxant response to the ACE inhibitor(s) was mediated by an enhanced release of NO from the endothelium, we determined the cGMP content of endothelium-intact and -denuded bovine coronary artery segments. Moexiprilat (0.3 µM) elicited a significant increase in the cGMP content of endothelium-intact segments (Figure 1b). Removal of the endothelium as well as inhibition of NO biosynthesis strongly attenuated the cGMP content of unstimulated (~86 % decrease) and moexiprilat-treated segments (Fig. 1b). Hoe 140 (0.1 µM) also blunted the stimulatory effect of moexiprilat (Fig. 1b).

These results suggest that, as with cultured endothelial cells *in vitro* [8,9], ACE inhibitors unmask an endogenous production of vasoactive kinins also in native endothelial cells *in situ*. As a consequence of the accumulation of these kinins in or at the vascular wall, the release of relaxing factors from

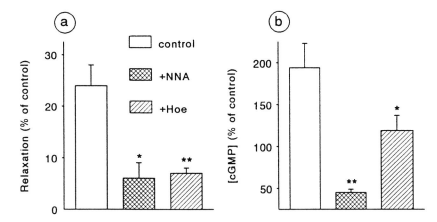

Fig. 1: (a) Relaxations of superfused endothelium-intact ring segments of bovine coronary artery induced by moexiprilat (Mxp, 0.1 µM) before (control) and after treatment with N^G-nitro-L-arginine (+NNA, 30 µM) or Hoe 140 (+Hoe, 0.1 µM). (b) Effects of moexiprilat (0.3 µM) on the cGMP content of endothelium-intact bovine coronary artery segments incubated in the absence (control) or presence of N^G-nitro-L-arginine or Hoe 140 for 10 min at 37 °C in Tyrode's solution. The asterisks denote significant differences (*P<0.05, **P<0.01) from the corresponding control values (n≥5).

the endothelium, namely that of NO, is enhanced. Due to the cyclooxygenase blockade, PGI_2 release from the coronary artery segments was not determined, but usually parallels that of NO.

One finding that argued against the hypothesis that the ACE inhibitor-induced dilatation was solely mediated by an accumulation of endothelium-derived vasoactive kinins, however, was that the time course of the relaxant response to bradykinin and the ACE inhibitors was virtually identical. Moreover, besides causing a slow prolonged increase in intracellular calcium ($[Ca^{2+}]_i$) in cultured endothelial cells, ACE inhibitors can also elicit an immediate transient rise in $[Ca^{2+}]_i$ in these cells in the absence of exogenous bradykinin, which is blocked by Hoe 140 [18]. ACE inhibitors can also evoke profound relaxant responses in bovine [12,13], porcine [12] and human [13] coronary arteries under no-flow conditions when administered ~10 min after the exposure of these vascular preparations to a threshold concentration of bradykinin (≥0.3 nM). Since the ACE activity present in these freshly isolated coronary arteries is considered to be too low to exert a major influence on the dilator response to bradykinin [13], it seems that apart from protecting endothelium-derived vasoactive kinins from proteolytic degradation, ACE inhibitors can also modulate the action

ACE inhibitors and the intact coronary microcirculation

In the isolated rabbit heart perfused at constant flow, administration of ramiprilat or moexiprilat in concentrations up to 3 μM had no significant effect on coronary perfusion pressure (CPP, n≥3). Ramiprilat and Hoe 140 also did not affect the basal release of NO from the heart (Fig. 2). In a different series of experiments, moexiprilat also failed to augment the basal release of PGI_2 from the isolated perfused heart of the rat [19]. Moreover, increasing the flow rate, hence elevating the level of shear stress the coronary endothelium is exposed to, also did not reveal a release of vasoactive kinins from the perfused rat [19] or rabbit heart [20]. Thus, in contrast to isolated bovine and porcine coronary [12] and canine carotid arteries [15], there is no evidence to suggest that endothelium-derived kinins are involved in the control of resting vascular tone or endothelial autacoid release in the coronary microcirculation of the rabbit and the rat.

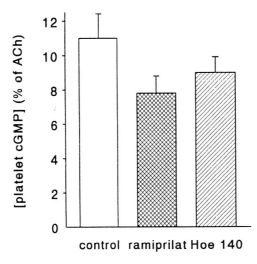

Fig. 2: Basal release of NO from the intact coronary vascular bed of the rabbit in the absence (control) and presence of either ramiprilat (0.1 μM) or Hoe 140 (0.1 μM) NO release was determined by monitoring the increase in intracellular cyclic GMP (cGMP) in washed human platelets (expressed as percent of the platelet cGMP level during an infusion of 1 μM acetylcholine) passing through the coronary bed of the saline-perfused rabbit heart (n=6).

However, administration of ramiprilat [19] or moexiprilat (0.3 μM) significantly augmented the dilator response to exogenously administered bradykinin in the perfused rabbit heart (Fig. 3). This potentiating effect was much more pronounced when sub-threshold (0.3 nM) or threshold (1 nM) concentrations of bradykinin were used. Administration of Hoe 140 (0.1

μM) before bradykinin and/or moexiprilat completely prevented the decrease in CPP induced by both compounds. Moexiprilat also significantly enhanced the bradykinin-induced release of 6-keto-PGF$_{1\alpha}$ from the isolated perfused rat heart, and this effect as well as that of bradykinin was completely abolished by pretreatment of the hearts with Hoe 140 [19]. Neither ramiprilat nor Hoe 140 affected the fall in CPP in the perfused rabbit heart caused by another endothelium-dependent vasodilator, acetylcholine [11,19]. This finding argues against the possibility that ACE inhibitors interfere with the receptor-dependent formation of vasoactive autacoids from the coronary endothelium in a non-specific manner.

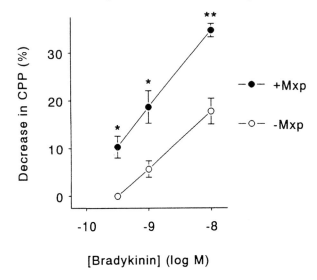

Fig. 3: Potentiation by moexiprilat (0.3 μM) of the decrease in coronary perfusion pressure (CPP) elicited by sub-threshold and threshold concentrations of bradykinin (5 min infusion) in the isolated perfused rabbit heart. The asterisks denote significant differences (*$P<0.05$, **$P<0.01$) between the changes in CPP in the absence (-Mxp) and presence (+Mxp) of the ACE inhibitor (n≥3).

Continuous infusion of bradykinin at a dose of 10 nM (half-maximal effective concentration, see Fig. 3) elicited a rapid but transient dilator response with coronary perfusion pressure (CPP) returning to baseline values at ~30 min. Subsequent co-infusion of moexiprilat (0.3 μM), after a lag phase of ~1 min, elicited another fall in CPP, the magnitude and time course of which was very similar to the response elicited by bradykinin before (Fig. 4). Bradykinin alone and the subsequent co-infusion of moexiprilat also caused a substantial increase in the release of PGI_2 from the rabbit heart, which was ~2-fold higher in the presence of the ACE inhibitor (Fig. 4). Both of these effects of bradykinin and moexiprilat were completely abrogated in the presence of Hoe 140 (0.1 µM, n=3). Interestingly, moexiprilat failed to elicit a fall in CPP or increase in PGI_2 release when administered 10 min after stopping the infusion of bradykinin, but did so when the perfusate contained 1 µM bradykinin instead of 10 nM (n=3). It seems, therefore, that a critical kinin concentration in or at the vascular wall is necessary to unmask the vasodilator action of the ACE inhibitor.

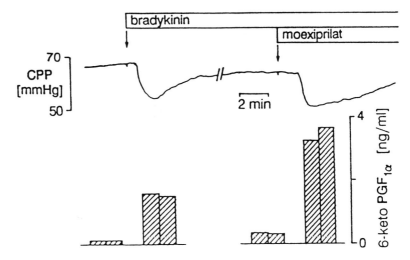

Fig. 4: Changes in coronary perfusion pressure (CPP, *top*) and basal PGI_2 release (determined as ng 6-keto-$PGF_{1\alpha}$/ml effluate, double determination, *bottom*) during the continuous infusion of bradykinin (10 nM) into the isolated rabbit heart and effect of the subsequent co-infusion of moexiprilat (0.3 µM). The figure shows a representative experiment typical for at least three experiments with different hearts.

ACE inhibitors are bradykinin-potentiating factors

As with the freshly isolated coronary preparations, the time course of the dilator response to moexiprilat during the continued presence of bradykinin was very rapid, again poiting to a mode of action of the ACE inhibitor different from just promoting the accumulation of bradykinin in or at the vascular wall. Indeed, recent findings from our laboratory suggest that ACE inhibitors can act as bradykinin-potentiating factors in the coronary circulation. In the 1960s, *Ferreira* and colleagues found that the venom of pit vipers contains factors that intensify the vascular responses to bradykinin [21]. These were subsequently identified as a familiy of peptides of 5 to 13 amino acid residues and shown to block the conversion of angiotensin I to angiotensin II [1]. Drug design based on the structure of these bradykinin-potentiating peptides provided the first generation of ACE inhibitors for clinical use in the treatment of hypertension. An action of these compounds at the bradykinin receptor level has been proposed as far back as 1975 [22], but was not established. In contrast, an increase in the concentration of endogenous kinins within the vascular wall has usually been assumed to play a role in the antihypertensive effect of this class of compound which could not be attributed to the inhibition of local or systemic angiotensin II formation [2]. However, most of the clinical evidence provided thus far can also be interpreted as indicating that ACE inhibitors potentiate the action of endogenously formed or exogenously administered kinins. It can be inferred from the present study, that the contribution of this kinin-potentiating effect to the dilator action of ACE inhibitors *in vivo* will vary between different vascular beds, since it is likely to be governed by the relative degree of kinin synthesis in these blood vessels.

In summary, our findings suggest that ACE inhibitors can amplify the dilator response to endogenously produced or exogenously administered kinins in the coronary circulation, and that this effect is at least in part mediated by an interaction of these agents with the endothelial B_2-receptor or its signal transduction cascade. In addition to blocking vascular angiotensin II formation and protecting endogenously produced kinins from inactivation by ACE, this direct action of ACE inhibitors may play an important role in their blood pressure-lowering and cytoprotective activity.

Acknowledgements

This work was supported by the *Deutsche Forschungsgemeinschaft* (He 1587/2-1) and the *Alexander-von-Humboldt Stiftung* (I.P.). We are indebted to Dr. Thomas Dambacher for his help with the isolated rabbit heart preparation and to Christine Kircher and Isabel Winter for expert technical assistance.

References

1. REGOLI, D. & J. BARABE (1980): Pharmacology of bradykinin and related kinins. Pharmacol. Rev. 32, 1-46.
2. KIOWSKI, W., L. LINDER, C. KLEINBLOESEM, P. VAN BRUMMELEN & F.R. BÜHLER (1992): Blood pressure control by the renin-angiotensin system in normotensive subjects - assessment by angiotensin converting enzyme and renin inhibition. Circulation 85, 1-8.
3. IIMURA, O. & K. SHIMAMOTO (1989): Role of kallikrein-kinin system in the hypotensive mechanisms of converting-enzyme inhibitors in essential hypertension. J. Cardiovasc. Pharmacol. 13 (Suppl. 3), S63-S66.
4. SCHMAIER, A.H., A. KUO, D. LUNDBERG, S. MURRAY & D.B. CINES (1988): The expression of high molecular weight kininogen on human umbilical vein endothelial cells. J. Biol. Chem. 263, 16327-16333.
5. BHOOLA, K.D., C.D. FIGUEROA & K. WORTHY (1992): Bioregulation of kinins: kallikrein, kininogens, and kininases. Pharmacol. Rev. 44, 1-80.
6. SCHINI, V.B., C. BOULANGER, D. REGOLI & P.M. VANHOUTTE (1990): Bradykinin stimulates the production of cyclic GMP via activation of B_2-kinin receptors in cultured porcine aortic endothelial cells. J. Pharmacol. Exp. Ther. 252, 581-585.
7. ERDÖS, E.G. (1990): Some old and some new ideas on kinin metabolism. J. Cardiovasc. Pharmacol. 15 (Suppl. 6), S20-S24.
8. WIEMER, G., B.A. SCHÖLKENS, R.M.A. BECKER & R. BUSSE (1991): Ramiprilat enhances endothelial autacoid formation by inhibiting breakdown of endothelium-derived bradykinin. Hypertension 18, 558-563.
9. BUSSE, R. & D. LAMONTAGNE (1991): Endothelium-derived bradykinin is responsible for the increase in calcium produced by angiotensin-converting enzyme inhibitors in human endothelial cells. Naunyn-Schmiedeberg's Arch. Pharmacol. 344, 126-129.
10. JACKSON, W.F. & R. BUSSE (1991): Elevated guanosine 3':5'-cyclic monophosphate mediates the depression of nitrovasodilator reactivity in endothelium-intact blood vessels. Naunyn-Schmiedeberg's Arch. Pharmacol. 345, 345-350.
11. LAMONTAGNE, D., A. KÖNIG., E. BASSENGE & R.. BUSSE. (1992): Prostacyclin and nitric oxide contribute to the vasodilator action of acetylcholine and bradykinin in the intact rabbit coronary bed. J. Cardiovasc. Pharmacol. 20, 652-657.
12. HECKER, M., A.T. BARA. & R. BUSSE (1993): Relaxation of isolated coronary arteries by angiotensin-converting enzyme inhibitors: role of endothelium-derived kinins. J. Vasc. Res. 30, 257-262.
13. AUCH-SCHWELK, W., C. BOSSALLER, M. CLAUS, K. GRAF, M. GRÄFE & E. Fleck (1993): ACE inhibitors are endothelium dependent vasodilators of coronary arteries during submaximal stimulation with bradykinin. Cardiovasc. Res. 27, 312-317.
14. MOMBOULI, J.V., S. ILLIANO, T. NAGAO, T. SCOTT-BURDEN & P.M. VANHOUTTE, P.M. (1992): Potentiation of endothelium-dependent relaxations to bradykinin by angiotensin I converting enzyme inhibitors in canine coronary artery involves both endothelium-derived relaxing and hyperpolarizing factors. Circ. Res. 71, 137-144.
15. MOMBOULI, J.V. & P.M. VANHOUTTE (1991): Kinins and endothelium-dependent relaxation to converting enzyme inhibitors in perfused canine arteries. J. Cardiovasc. Pharmacol. 18, 926-927.

16. MYERS, P.R., R. GUERRA & D.G. HARRISON (1992): Release of multiple endothelium-derived relaxing factors from porcine coronary arteries. J. Cardiovasc. Pharmacol. 20, 392-400.
17. COWAN, C.L. & R.A. COHEN (1991): Two mechanisms mediate relaxation by bradykinin of pig coronary artery - NO-dependent and NO-independent responses. Am. J. Physiol. 261, H830-H835.
18. BUSSE, R., I. FLEMING & M: HECKER (1993): Endothelium-derived bradykinin: implications for ACE inhibitor therapy. J. Cardiovasc. Pharmacol. 22 (Suppl. 5), 531-536.
19. HECKER, M., T. DAMBACHER & R. BUSSE (1992): Role of endothelium-derived bradykinin in the control of vascular tone. J. Cardiovasc. Pharmacol. 20 (Suppl. 9), S55-S61.
20. BUSSE, R., A. MÜLSCH, I. FLEMING & M. HECKER (1993): Mechanisms of nitric oxide release from the vascular endothelium. Circulation 87 (Suppl. V), V18-V25.
21. FERREIRA, S.H. (1965): A bradykinin potentiating factor (BPF) present in the venom of *Bothrops jararaca*. Br. J. Pharmacol. 24, 163-169.
22. TOMINAGA, M., J.M. STEWART, T.B. PAIVA & A.C.M. PAIVA (1975): Synthesis and properties of new bradykinin potentiating peptides. J. Med. Chem. 18, 130-133.

Endothelium-dependent regulation of arteriolar tone in skeletal muscle *in vivo*

A.R. Pries and P. Gaehtgens

Institut für Physiologie, Freie Universität Berlin

Introduction

Following the publication by Furchgott and Zawadzki [1] on the obligatory role of endothelium in the relaxation of vascular smooth muscle caused by acetylcholine, the knowledge about the contribution of endothelium to the regulation of smooth muscle tone has greatly expanded. Most of the information obtained relates to vasoactive substances released by the endothelium, the chemical and mechanical factors stimulating this release, and the mechanisms of their action on vascular smooth muscle cells. It is of great importance for the understanding of the physiology and pathophysiology of tissue perfusion to understand how these pathways of smooth muscle control are integrated, *in vivo*, with myogenic, metabolic, and neuronal mechanisms influencing vascular smooth muscle tone. The relevance of the quantitative balance between these mechanisms is for instance obvious for the interaction between flow-dependent vasodilation which is mediated by EDRF and myogenic autoregulation: It has been postulated that the flow-dependent secretion of EDRF counteracts myogenic regulation and suppresses it completely in a number of tissues [2,3].

Current understanding of the interplay between different mechanisms influencing vascular smooth muscle tone *in vivo* is limited and available data are partially inconsistent. As an example, it has been described by some investigators that flow-dependent vasodilation depends on the release of EDRF [4,5] or prostanoids [6] from the endothelium, while others [7] report that this reaction is still seen after removal of the endothelium. Such discrepancies on one hand reflect the variability of vessels taken from different tissues and different species. On the other hand, however, the preparation of the tissue and the experimental conditions chosen could have an equally important influence.

The present study attempts to identify the quantitative contribution of the two most relevant endothelium-dependent vasodilatory mechanisms, i.e. the secretion of EDRF and prostanoids (PGI_2) to the control of the basal tone in arteriolar resistance vessels in resting skeletal muscle of the rat. In addition, the influence of blood flow and oxygen partial pressure on these mechanisms is investigated.

Materials and methods

The spinotrapezius muscle of Sprague-Dawley rats (body weight ranging from 85 to 95 g) was prepared for intravital microscopy as described by Klotz and coworkers [8]. After induction of anaesthesia by i.m. injection of pentobarbital (20 mg/kg b.w.) and ketamine (100 mg/kg b.w.), trachea, carotid artery and jugular vein were cannulated using PE tubing. Systemic arteriolar blood pressure was continuously measured and recorded. Through the venular catheter a continuous infusion of pentobarbital (9 mg/kg b.w./h) in physiological saline (25 ml/kg b.w./h) was given to maintain a constant level of anaesthesia and hydration.

After removing a square window of skin on the back of the animal, the fascia was removed under stereomicroscopic control from the spinotrapezius muscle in an area of about 10 to 8 mm by careful microsurgery. For a length of about 5 mm, the spinotrapezius muscle was separated atraumatically from the deeper muscles starting at its lateral rim. A small strip of cover glass fixed to a micromanipulator was inserted under the muscle lifting the spinotrapezius by about 40° from the thorax wall. After transferring the animal stage to an intravital microscope [9], the small prism of a C-shaped illumination unit was advanced into the space below the cover glass supporting the muscle (Fig. 1). Observations of the microcirculation were made with a 25'/0.6 salt water immersion objective and transmitted via a CCD video camera (type MX, HCS) to a video tape recorder.

The diameter of selected arterioles was measured off-line from the video recordings using an interactive image shearing module of a computerized video image analysis system, and blood flow velocity was determined with a spatial correlation module [10,11]. To allow reliable measurements of high flow velocities from video recordings, an asynchronous double strobe illumination was employed [12].

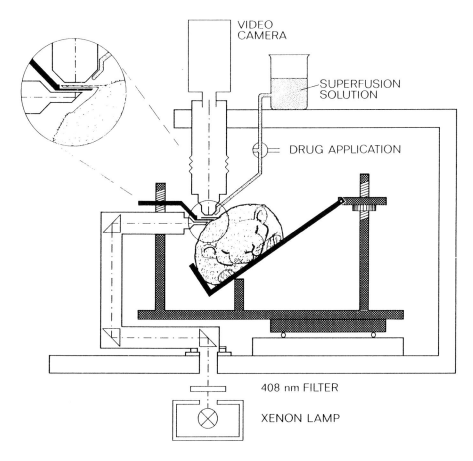

Fig. 1: Schematic drawing of the experimental setup. The rat is positioned on a special animal stage which, in addition, holds the micromanipulator operated glass slip supporting the spinotrapezius muscle (see insert). The 'C'-shaped illuminating unit allows Köhler type of illumination in the muscle area supported by the glass slip (approx. 5'5 mm).

Immediately following surgical exposure, the muscle was continuously superfused with temperature controlled (38 °C) bicarbonate buffered tyrode solution. In order to maintain a low PO_2, the superfusate was continuously equilibrated with 5 % CO_2 in N_2. At the level of the tissue, the oxygen partial pressure under these conditions was 15 mmHg, as measured with an oxygen electrode (model 57, YSI, USA). By equilibration with gas mixtures containing 20 % oxygen, the PO_2 of the superfusing solution could be raised to 150 mmHg within 1 min.

The blood flow velocity in the arteriolar segment under observation was manipulated using a microglass pipette with a spherical tip which was bent at right angles relative to the shaft. With a micromanipulator, the spherical tip of this pipette was lowered onto the vessel at a site just outside of but close to the field of observation. Thereby, blood flow through the vessel could be suddenly reduced to almost zero. However, blood flow was not completely stopped in order to avoid unduly high pressure with the micropipette on the tissue and to minimize damage to vessel walls. The flow reduction was maintained for about 2.5 min and repeated up to 3 times during any given experimental condition, with interposed control phases of 3 min each.

To block the production of cyclooxygenase-dependent prostanoids, indomethacin (10^{-5} M) was added to the superfusate starting 20 min before the respective measurement. In order to block the release of EDRF, N-Nitro-L-arginine (L-NNA, 35 mg/kg b.w.) was injected intravenously. The effectiveness of this block was tested by recording the response of vessel diameter to the topical application of acetylcholine (10^{-5} M). In all experiments reported here, the reaction to this compound was significantly reduced (by about 60 %) after L-NNA administration.

Results

a. Effect of flow interruption

The experiments in which blood flow in the investigated arterioles was manipulated, these vessels showed initial basal diameters of 19 ± 8 μm (n=14, mean ± SD). The mean blood flow velocity averaged 1180 ± 520 μm/s and was reduced during micropipette occlusion to 180 ± 150 μm/s (i.e. to 15 ± 12 % of the control value). Fig. 2 shows the results of the occlusion experiments. Interruption of flow led to vasoconstriction by 34 ± 4 % and 23 ± 7 % (n=7 for each group) of the basal diameter in the two groups of experiments shown. Upon release of the occlusion, the vessel diameter returned to 105 ± 5 % and 101 ± 6 % of the original value.

After i.v. injection of L-NNA and the addition of indomethacin to the superfusing solution, respectively, control arteriolar diameter was reduced by 23 ± 6 % (L-NNA) and 26 ± 5 % (indomethacin) compared to the original value. After injection of L-NNA, microocclusion of the vessel led to an additional constriction by only 11 ± 3 % of the control value. By contrast, reduction of blood flow after addition of indomethacin led to additional constriction of the vessel by 23 ± 6 % of the control diameter.

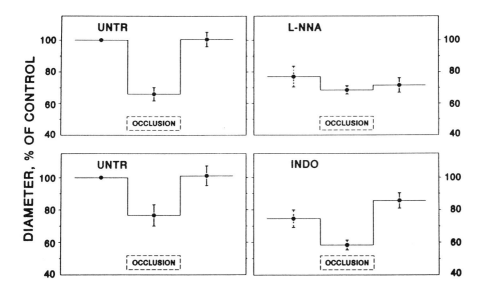

Fig. 2: Diameter changes following partial occlusion before (UNTR, upper left panel, n=7) and after injection of L-NNA (upper right panel) as well as before (UNTR, lower left panel, n=7) and during addition of indomethacin (INDO, lower right panel). All values are normalized with respect to the basal diameter in the untreated state during spontaneous flow. Shown are mean values with standard errors. The dashed error bars indicate the variation with respect to the basal diameter (100 %), while the continuous ones give the variation regarding the control diameter (first data point) of the respective panel which differs from 100 % for L-NNA and INDO.

b. Effect of increased PO_2

In the experiments in which the oxygen partial pressure was elevated the basal diameter of the vessels studied averaged 35 ± 12 μm (n=19). Increasing the PO_2 to 150 mmHg led to arteriolar constrictions by 25 ± 3 %. Both the injection of L-NNA (n=8) as well as the addition of indomethacin to the superfusate (n=5) led to comparable reductions of the control diameter by 26 ± 7 % and 23 ± 10 %, respectively. After L-NNA the response to oxygen was nearly abolished (3 ± 2 % of the control diameter), while it

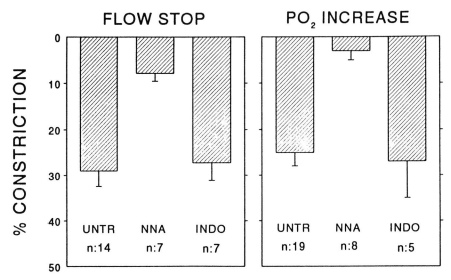

Fig. 3: Constrictor responses of untreated arterioles (UNTR) after injection of L-NNA (NNA) and during application of indomethacin (INDO) to a drastic reduction of blood flow velocity (left panels) and an increase of local PO_2 from 15 mmHg to about 150 mmHg (right panels). For both procedures, the resulting constriction is about 25-29 % in the UNTR groups. An additional constriction of the same magnitude is seen during application of indomethacin (which itself leads to a constriction of about 25 %). By contrast, the injection of L-NNA nearly abolishes an additional vasoconstriction by either stimulus.

remained nearly unchanged (27 ± 8 % of the control diameter) during application of indomethacin.

Figure 3 combines the results of both experimental series. Both the flow stop induced by arteriolar occlusion as well as by an increase of PO_2 in the superfusate led to reductions of arteriolar diameter by 25 to 29 % in the untreated state. After injection of L-NNA, the constrictor response to both stimuli was drastically reduced, while constrictions under indomethacin were equally strong compared to those observed in the untreated vessels.

Discussion

The present results demonstrate that resistance arterioles in the rat skeletal muscle at rest are exposed to a substantial dilatory influence by endothelium-dependent autacoids. If both of these stimuli are abolished by blocking the production of EDRF and cyclooxygenase-dependent prostanoids (probably PGI_2), the average vessel diameter decreases by up to

50 %. EDRF and the prostanoid system are therefore responsible for equal parts of the vasodilatory tone seen in control conditions. Both the combined and the individual vasoconstrictor effects seen after blocking the production of EDRF and prostanoids averaged about 25 % and thus are somewhat higher in the present study than those seen by de Wit and Pohl [13] in similar sized arterioles of the hamster cremaster. These authors report constrictions by 12 % and 21 % following application of N^G-Nitro-L-Arginine and indomethacin, respectively, while the combined treatment led to diameter reductions of 22 to 27 %. In the present study, no significant effect of basal vessel diameter on the vasodilatory effect of EDRF and prostanoids was found. With regard to EDRF, this finding is in contrast to results reported by Faraci [14], who found vasoconstriction of 10.4 % after application of N^G-Monomethyl-L-Arginine in "large" cerebral arteries (275 µm diameter) decreasing to 3.7 % in arterioles (diameter 65 µm).

There is some discrepancy in the literature as to the pathways and mechanisms of both flow- and PO_2-dependent changes of arteriolar tone. The effects of blood flow have been attributed to the production of EDRF on the basis of studies using isolated perfused segments of large canine arteries [4], coronary resistance arterioles (diameter about 110 µm) [5], and *in situ* perfused small arteries in the rabbit mesentery (diameters about 221 µm) [3]. On the other hand, Koller and Kaley [6] found complete suppression of flow-dependent diameter changes of arterioles (diameter about 20 µm) in the cremaster muscle of the rat under indomethacin, while N^G-Monomethyl-L-Arginine did not affect the response to flow changes. Finally, Bevan and coworkers [7] described that removal of the endothelium in a resistance artery (diameter 150 µm) was followed by only a partial (about 50 %) reduction of flow-dependent vasodilation.

A similar discrepancy exists with regard to the published results describing the effect of local PO_2 on vascular smooth muscle tone. Jackson [15] reported that arteriolar oxygen reactivity is not mediated by prostaglandins in the hamster cheek pouch and in the hamster and rat cremaster muscle [15] and is not mediated by EDRF in the hamster cheek pouch [16]. According to Messina and coworkers (17), however, the oxygen reactivity of isolated rat cremaster arteries (diameter 50-90 µm) is effected by prostaglandins. These results are in line with earlier observations of Busse et al. [18] on vascular resistance in the rat tail. For isolated rabbit femoral arteries and aortas, Pohl and Busse [19] demonstrated a vasodilation with hypoxia which they concluded to depend on the release of EDRF.

In the present study, the effects of blood flow and local PO_2 are both transmitted to the vascular smooth muscle via the production and release of EDRF. The mechanisms inducing an increased endothelial EDRF production are still hypothetical. It might, however, be significant that under the conditions prevailing in the present experiments, both a certain level of blood flow velocity *and* low levels of local PO_2 were needed to support the production of vasoactive quantities of EDRF. This observation would suggest that both mechanisms are not independently capable to increase EDRF production, possibly due to interactions at the receptor level or within the endothelial cell. By contrast, the production and release of prostanoids led to a dilatation of microvessels independent of and additive to that mediated by EDRF.

The discrepancies between the present results and some of the findings reported in the literature is striking. In principle, this could be explained by biological differences of the vessels and tissues investigated or by differences in experimental conditions. It is e.g. conceivable that no response to a given stimulus is observed, if the mechanism involved is investigated far away from its maximal response. If, in addition, the activation of more than one stimulus is necessary to provoke a response, as concluded here for the production of EDRF in response to low PO_2 and high blood flow velocity, it is even more likely that different experimental approaches will lead to different observations.

Summary

The influence of endothelial production of EDRF and cyclooxygenase-dependent prostanoids on the control of basal smooth muscle tone in arterioles with resting diameters ranging from 10 to 60 µm was quantified in the spinotrapezius muscle of the rat *in situ*. In addition, the response to changes of blood flow in the investigated vessel and the oxygen partial pressure in the superfusing solution was analyzed. The following procedures were used: blockade of EDRF synthesis by i.v. infusion of N-Nitro-L-arginine (L-NNA, 35 mg/kg b.w.); blockade of cyclooxygenase-dependent synthesis of prostanoids (PGI_2) by adding indomethacin (10 mM) to the superfusing solution; reduction of blood flow through the investigated arteriole to about 15 % of the resting level by micropipette occlusion; elevation of PO_2 in the superfusate from 15 to 150 mmHg. If used individually, all of these procedures led to vasoconstrictions of about 25 % of the resting diameter. After previous blockade of the cyclooxygenase pathway, the reactions upon a reduction of blood flow or an increase of PO_2 were well maintained. By contrast, the constrictor effects of blood flow reduction and elevation of oxygen partial pressure were nearly abolished (8 % and 3 % constriction) after blockade of EDRF synthesis. From these results the following conclusions are derived:

- Production of EDRF and cyclooxygenase-dependent prostanoids significantly modify the basal tone of small arterioles in the resting spinotrapezius muscle of the rat.
- The relaxations of arteriolar smooth muscle caused by both mediators are independent and additive. They are each responsible for about 25 % of the basal vessel diameter.
- The release of EDRF is controlled by the local oxygen partial pressure and by the blood flow in the individual vessel.
- In the animal model used the dilatory effect of EDRF can be abolished by a drastic reduction of blood flow *or* a significant increase in local PO_2.

References

1. FURCHGOTT, R.F. & J.V. ZAWADZKI (1980): The obligatory role of endothelial cells in the relaxation of arterial smooth muscle by acetylcholine. Nature, 288, 373-376.
2. GRIFFITH, T.M. & D.H. EDWARDS (1990): Myogenic autoregulation of flow may be inversely related to endothelium-derived relaxing factor activity. Am. J. Physiol., 258, H1171-H1180.
3. POHL, U., K. HERLAN, A. HUANG & E. BASSENGE (1991): EDRF-mediated shear-induced dilation opposes myogenic vasoconstriction in small rabbit arteries. Am. J. Physiol., 261, H2016-H2023.
4. RUBANYI, G.M., J.C. ROMERO & P.M. VANHOUTTE (1986): Flow-induced release of endothelium-derived relaxing factor. Am. J. Physiol., 250, H1145-H1149.
5. KUO, L., W.M. CHILIAN & M.J. DAVIS (1991): Interaction of pressure- and flow-induced responses in porcine coronary resistance vessels. Am. J. Physiol., 261, H1706-H1715.
6. KOLLER, A. & G. KALEY (1990): Prostaglandins mediate arteriolar dilation to increased blood flow velocity in skeletal muscle microcirculation. Circ. Res., 67, 529-534.
7. BEVAN, J.A., E.H. JOYCE & G.C. WELLMAN (1988): Flow-dependent dilation in a resistance artery still occurs after endothelium removal. Circ. Res., 63, 980-985.
8. KLOTZ, K.-F., A.R. PRIES, H. JEPSEN, R. GOSSRAU & P. GAEHTGENS (1991): A new approach to intravital videomicroscopy of rat spinotrapezius muscle. Int. J. Microcirc.: Clin. Exp., 10, 205-218.
9. LEY K., A.R. PRIES & P. GAEHTGENS (1987): A versatile intravital microscope design. Int. J. Microcirc.: Clin. Exp., 6, 161-167.

10. PRIES & P. GAEHTGENS (1987): Digital video image shearing device for continuous microvessel diameter measurement. Microvasc. Res., 34, 260-267.
11. PRIES (1988): A versatile video image analysis system for microcirculatory research. Int. J. Microcirc.: Clin. Exp.,7, 327-345.
12. PRIES, A.R., S.E. ERIKSSON & H. JEPSEN (1990): Real-time oriented image analysis in microcirculatory research. SPIE, 1357, 257-263.
13. DE WIT, C. & U. POHL (1992): Effects of prostaglandins and EDRF in the microvascular response to acetylcholine in the hamster cremaster. Pflügers Arch. Europ. J. Physiol., 420 (Suppl. 1), R118.
14. FARACI, F.M. (1991): Role of endothelium-derived relaxing factor in cerebral circulation: large arteries vs. microcirculation. Am. J. Physiol., 261, H1038-H1042.
15. JACKSON, W.F. (1986): Prostaglandins do not mediate arteriolar oxygen reactivity. Am. J. Physiol., 250, H1102-H1108.
16. JACKSON, W.F. (1991): Nitric oxide does not mediate arteriolar oxygen reactivity. Microcirc. Endothelium Lymphatics, 7, 199-215.
17. MESSINA, E.J., D. SUN, A. KOLLER, M.S. WOLIN & G. KALEY (1991): Role of the endothelium in skeletal muscle arteriolar reactivity to hypoxia. Proceedings of 5th World Congress for Microcirculation, Louisville/KY, USA, p 75, 1991.
18. BUSSE, R., U. FÖRSTERMANN, H. MATSUDA & U. POHL (1984): The role of prostaglandins in the endothelium-mediated vasodilatory response to hypoxia. Pflügers Arch., 401, 77-83.
19. POHL, U. & R. BUSSE (1989): Hypoxia stimulates release of endothelium-derived relaxant factor. Am. J. Physiol., 256, H1595-H1600.

Nitric oxide (NO) acting as an endothelial and parenchymal vasodilating factor in cerebral arteries

M. Wahl, L. Schilling and **A. Parsons***

Department of Physiology, University of Munich, and Smith Kline Beecham Pharma, Harlow*

Introduction

Evidence has accumulated that vascular endothelium modulates the vasomotor response of smooth muscle cells [1]. The concept that the endothelium is important for the mediation of vasomotor response elicited by several agents was created by Furchgott and Zawadzki [2]. Employing the sandwich technique the release of the endothelium derived relaxing factor (EDRF) was detected. Later, EDRF was identified as nitric oxide [3,4] or a NO containing moiety like nitrosothiol [5] which is derived from the terminal guanido group of L-arginine by the NO-synthase [6]. The relaxing effect of NO is due to activation of the soluble guanylate cyclase and formation of cGMP in the smooth muscle cell [7] where it may act by a reduction of either the cytosolic Ca^{2+} concentration or the Ca^{2+} sensitivity of contractile proteins [8,9]. Meanwhile several constrictor and dilating compounds have been found to be released from the endothelium. Constrictor factors are endothelin and TxA_2 besides the still hypothetical endothelium derived constrictor factor [10]. TxA_2 can probably be released by noradrenaline [11]. Endothelin which is a potent and long acting constrictor of cerebral arteries in situ [12,13] and in vitro [14,15] is released during subarachnoid hemorrhage where it obviously participates in the development of long lasting vasospasm [16]. EDRF can be released by shear stress [17], by neurotransmitters such as acetylcholine (Ach), [18] or autacoids like bradykinin (BK), [19] or serotonin (5-HT), [20]. However, ACh has been reported to release not only EDRF but also endothelium derived hyperpolarizing factor (EDHF), [21-23] and prostacyclin [24].

Recent findings demonstrate that NO is not only released from the endothelium but can also be formed in the smooth muscle cell under distinct conditions [25,26]. Since NO is also released from astrocytes and neurons [27-33] and from perivascular nerves [34,35] it may also act like a local chemical factor and a neurotransmitter, respectively.

Therefore, it was one aim of the present study to analyze by which mechanisms ACh induces relaxation of the rabbit isolated basilar artery. In the second part of the paper in situ data will be presented dealing with the role of NO in the regulation of pial artery resting tone and in the mediation of functional hyperemia.

Methods

In vitro experiments were performed using ring segments of rabbit basilar artery. After anesthesia with pentobarbitone (30 mg/kg i.v.) male New Zealand white rabbits were exsanguinated, the brain was removed, and placed in ice-cold Krebs-Henseleit buffer. After cutting the vascular ring segments they were set up in 5 ml baths for isometric recording of tension. The Krebs-Henseleit solution [18] was warmed up to 37 °C and equilibrated with 90 % O_2 and 10 % CO_2 to keep constant pH of 7.27. The vessels were allowed a 60 to 90 min equilibration period with repeated washing and adjustment of resting force to 3.0 - 3.5 mN. After testing the reactivity of the vessels to histamine (10^{-6} - 10^{-4} M) and a further 60 min wash period concentration-effect (C-E) curves to ACh (10^{-7} to 10^{-4} M) were formed on (s. Tab. 1) contraction to 5-HT (10^{-7} M). In separate experiments C-E curves were formed after 25 to 30 min incubation with either N^G-nitro-L-arginine (Nolag, 10^{-5} M), or indomethacin (10^{-6} M) or both compounds. Indomethacin was dissolved in ethanol and diluted by Krebs-Henseleit solution.

In situ experiments were performed in anaesthetized and immobilized rats and cats with artificial ventilation [36]. Blood pressure, body temperature, and endtidal CO_2 content were recorded continuously. The acid base status of the arterial blood was controlled intermittently. Craniotomy using a cooled dental drill and opening of the dura under a layer of warmed (37 °C) paraffin oil enabled access to pial arteries in the left parietal region. The vasomotor response of individual pial arteries was measured employing an image splitting device [37]. Artificial cerebrospinal fluid (CSF, for composition see [36] containing test compounds was infused into the perivascular space employing a microperfusion device [38] at a rate of 5ml/40s (rat, 0.5ml/40s). Normally, the duration of application was 40 s but in the experiments with cortical spreading depression (CSD) it lasted 2 to 2.5 min after eliciting CSD by intracortical injection of 5 µm 150 mM KCl. The appearance of the CSD wave was recorded in the immediate vicinity of the artery under investigation at a depth of approximately 500 µm as published previously [36].

Results are expressed as mean ± SD with relaxant responses given as percent of precontraction (in vitro) or of resting diameter (in situ). Differences between groups were assessed by paired t-test or by one way analysis of variance and Duncan's test for multiple comparisons. A value p < 0.05 was taken as significant.

Results and discussion

In order to test whether the relaxing effect of ACh in rabbit isolated basilar artery is mediated by an endothelial release of NO and relaxing prostanoids the inhibitors of NO-synthase, Nolag, and cyclooxygenase, indomethacin, were employed. As shown in Tab. 1 ACh (10^{-7} - 10^{-4} M) induced relaxation of the arteries precontracted by 10^{-7} M 5-HT. This relaxation was only partially blocked by either 10^{-5} or 10^{-4} M Nolag or 10^{-6} M indomethacin. However, the relaxation was completely suppressed in the presence of both inhibitors indicating that NO and a relaxing prostanoid, probably prostacyclin, mediate the relaxing effect of ACh in rabbit basilar artery. Species and vessel differences appear to be important since the dilating effect of ACh in rat isolated basilar and rabbit isolated middle cerebral artery is exclusively mediated by NO [18,39]. EDHF which may act upon ATP-sensitive K^+ channels or Na-K-ATPase in the smooth muscle cell membrane thus inducing hyperpolarization and closure of voltage dependent Ca^{2+} channels [40] also appears to be involved in the mediation of the ACh induced dilatation of rabbit or cat isolated middle cerebral artery [21,22]. However, the functional meaning of this mechanism has been questioned by others [18,41]. Furthermore, recently [23] an uncoupling between hyperpolarization and dilatation due to ACh has been found in rabbit basilar artery, thus also questioning the causal role of EDHF.

Inhibitiors of NO synthase like Nolag (10^{-5} M) contract rat isolated basilar artery (0.5 ± 0.4 mN) and rabbit isolated middle cerebral (0.5 ± 0.3 mN) and basilar artery (0.3 ± 0.2 mN). Similarly, constriction of large cerebral arteries has also been found in situ [42-44] thus indicating that the resting tone of these arteries is mediated partially by a continuous release of NO. However, perivascular microapplication of Nolag (10^{-5} - 10^{-3} M) did not significantly change the diameter of rat pial arteries (20-55 m). This finding is in agreement with observations obtained in other species [43-46] and may indicate that either NO-synthase is not present in the small cerebral resistance arteries or not involved in the regulation of resting diameter.

Table 1: Effect of NOLAG and indomethacin on acetylcholine-induced relaxation of isolated rabbit basilar artery. Mean ± SD, n = number of observations, negative values indicate contraction.

Relaxation (% precontraction)	Acetylcholine			
	10^{-7} M	10^{-6} M	10^{-5} M	10^{-4} M
Control (n=23)	12.6 ± 9.9	56.7 ± 22.6	82.2 ± 20.7	81.7 ± 20.8
In the presence of				
- NOLAG (10^{-5} M) (n=8)	11.1 ± 10.2	34.4 ± 12.3*	69.3 ± 15.2	61.8 ± 22.0
- NOLAG (10^{-4} M) (n=7)	-3.5 ± 12.2*	20.3 ± 21.8*	57.0 ± 34.5	35.1 ± 42.2*
- Indomethacin (10^{-6} M) (n=10)	0.3 ± 0.9	27.7 ± 17.8*	68.0 ± 25.6*	71.3 ± 24.4
- Indomethacin (10^{-6} M) + NOLAG (10^{-5} M) (n=5)	-5.4 ± 13.8	6.4 ± 17.2*	-7.0 ± 12.0*	-6.3 ± 17.2*

* $p < 0.05$ vs Control.

In order to test whether NO-synthase is present the endothelium dependent dilatation of 10^{-4} M ACh, 10^{-6} M BK and 10^{-8} M 5-HT was tested in the absence and presence of 10^{-5} or 10^{-4} M Nolag in rat pial arteries employing perivascular microapplication. The sequence of application was 1. agonist, 2. Nolag, and 3. agonist together with Nolag. The results summarized in Tab. 2 demonstrate that the dilating effect of ACh and 5-HT, but not of BK, are blocked by Nolag. This indicates that the NO-synthase is present in the wall of the small arteries and that the dilating effect of BK is mediated by another endothelial factor which appears to be H_2O_2 in rat pial arteries [47].

Since NO can also be released from brain parenchyma cells it may act like a local chemical factor. To test this and its possible involvement in the regulation of cerebral vascular resistance during functional hyperemia we used the model of cortical spreading depression (CSD). The initial phase of CSD is characterized by a neuronal excitation as indicated by a negative shift in the DC potential which is accompanied by arteriolar dilatation [36]. In order to test whether this transient dilatation is mediated partially by a release of NO we infused 10^{-4} M Nolag perivascularly to the artery under investigation. The period of application started with the remote initiation of a CSD wave by intracortical injection of KCl and lasted to the end of the vasodilatation. It is very likely that the adjacent brain parenchyma was equilibrated with the infusion fluid within this time. The CSD induced dilatation (44.0 ± 11.2 %) could be reduced significantly by Nolag (22.4 ± 10.6 %). In time matched controls the CSD induced dilatations (35.7 ± 21.9 and 32.5 ± 15.1) were not reduced by perivascular infusion of inert CSF. This indicates that NO obviously is one factor mediating functional hyperemia. The same was concluded from results obtained during cortical activation during sciatic nerve stimulation [48]. Thus, several local chemical factors, perivascular transmitters and autacoids appear to be involved in the regulation of cerebrovascular resistance during functional hyperemia [49].

Table 2: Effect of perivascular microapplication of acetylcholine, bradykinin and serotonin (5-HT) in the absence and presence of NOLAG (10^{-4} M with acetylcholine and bradykinin, 10^{-5} M with 5-HT) on rat pial arterioles diameter in situ. Mean ± SD, n = number of observations, * p < 0.05 vs Control.

	Control	+NOLAG
Acetylcholine (10^{-4} M)	+15.4 ± 9.1 (n=7)	+1.9 ± 5.5* (n=7)
Bradykinin (10^{-6} M)	+20.4 ± 13.2 (n=14)	+19.7 ± 6.2 (n=7)
5-HT (10^{-8} M)	+15.9 ± 10.9 (n=8)	+2.9 ± 7.5 (n=4)

References

1. VANHOUTTE, P.M., E.M. RUBANYI, V.M. MILLER & D.S. HOUSTON (1986): Modulation of vascular smooth muscle contraction by the endothelium. Annu.Rev.Physiol.48, 307-320.
2. FURCHGOTT, R.F. & J.V. ZAWADZKI (1980): The obligatory role of endothelial cells in the relaxation of arterial smooth muscle by acetylcholine. Nature 288, 373-376.

3. IGNARRO, L.J., G.M. BUGA, K.S. WOOD, R.E. BYRNS & G. CHAUDHURI (1987): Endothelium-derived relaxing factor produced and released from artery and vein is nitric oxide. Proc.Natl.Acad.Sci. 84, 9265-9269.
4. PALMER, R.M.J., A.G. FERRIGE & S. MONCADA (1987): Nitric oxide release accounts for the biological activity of endothelium-derived relaxing factor. Nature 327, 524-526.
5. MARSHALL, J. & H.A. KONTOS (1990): Endothelium-derived relaxing factors. A perspective from in vivo data. Hypertension 16, 371-386.
6. MONCADA, S., R.M.J. PALMER & E.A. HIGGS, (1989): Biosynthesis of nitric oxide from L-arginine. A pathway for the regulation of cell function and communication. Biochem.-Pharmacol. 38, 1709-1716.
7. FÖRSTERMANN, U., A. MÜLSCH & R. BUSSE (1986): Stimulation of soluble guanylate cyclase by an acetylcholine-induced endothelium-derived factor from rabbit and canine arteries. Circ.Res. 58, 531-538.
8. EGGERMONT, J.A., L. RAEYMAEKERS & R. CASTEELS (1989): Ca^{2+} transport by smooth muscle membrane and its regulation. Biomed.Biochim.Acta 48, S370-S381.
9. YANAGISAWA, T., M. KAWADA & N. TAIRA (1989): Nitroglycerin relaxes canine coronary arterial smooth muscle without reducing intracellular Ca^{2+} concentration measured with fura-2. Br.J.Pharmacol. 98, 469-482.
10. KATUSIC, Z.S., J.T. SHEPHERD & P.M. VANHOUTTE (1988): Endothelium-dependent contractions to calcium ionophore A23187, arachidonic acid, and acetylcholine in canine basilar arteries. Stroke 19, 476-479.
11. USUI, H., K. KURAHASHI, H. SHIRAHASE, K. FUKUI & M. FUJIWARA (1987): Endothelium-dependent vasoconstriction in response to noradrenaline in the canine cerebral artery. Japan J.Pharmacol. 44, 228-231.
12. FARACI, F.M.(1989): Effects of endothelin and vasopressin on cerebral blood vessels. Amer.J.Physiol. 257, H799-H803.
13. ROBINSON, M.J. & J. MCCULLOCH (1990): Contractile responses to endothelin in feline cortical vessels in situ. J.Cereb.Blood Flow Metab. 10, 285-289.
14. JANSEN, I., B. FALLGREN & L. EDVINSSON (1989): Mechanisms of action of endothelin on isolated feline cerebral arteries: in vitro pharmacology and electropyhsiology. J.Cereb.Blood Flow Metab. 9, 743-747.
15. KAUSER, K., G.M. RUBANYI & D.R. HARDER (1990): Endothelium-dependent modulation of endothelin-induced vasoconstriction and membrane depolarisation in cat cerebral arteries. J.Pharmacol.Exp.Ther. 252, 93-97.
16. SHIGENO, T., T. MIMA, M. YANAGISAWA, A. SAITO, A. FUJIMORI, R. SHIBA, K. GOTO, S. KIMURA, K. YAMASHITA, Y. YAMASAKI, T. MASAKI & K. TAKAKURA (1991): Possible role of endothelin in the pathogenesis of cerebral vasospasm. J.Cardiovasc.Pharmacol. 17, Suppl. 7, S480-S483.
17. LAMONTAGNE, D., U. POHL & R. BUSSE (1992): Mechanical deformation of vessel wall and shear stress determine the basal release of endothelium-derived relaxing factor in the intact rabbit coronary vascular bed. Circ.Res. 70, 123-130.
18. PARSONS, A.A., L. SCHILLING & M. WAHL (1991): Analysis of acetylcholine-induced relaxation of rabbit isolated middle cerebral artery: Effects of inhibitors of nitric oxide synthesis, NaK-ATPase, and ATP-sensitive K channels. J.Cereb.Blood Flow Metab. 11, 700-704.
19. MAYHAN, W.G. (1990): Impairment of endothelium-dependent dilatation of basilar artery during chronic hypertension. Amer.J.Physiol. 259, H1455-H1462.

20. PARSONS, A.A., Q. WANG, L. SCHILLING, N.A. LASSEN & M. WAHL (1991): Effects of N^G-nitro-L-arginine (NOLAG) on rat pial arterioles in situ. Pflügers Arch.Eur.J.Physiol. 419, Suppl.1, R112.
21. BRAYDEN, J.E. & G.C. WELLMAN (1989): Endothelium-dependentdilation of feline cerebral arteries: role of membrane potential and cyclic nucleotides. J.Cereb.Blood Flow Metab. 9, 256-263.
22. BRAYDEN, J.E. (1990): Membrane hyperpolarization is a mechanism of endothelium-dependent cerebral vasodilation. Amer.J.Physiol. 259, H668-H673.
23. RAND, V.E. & C.J. GARLAND (1992): Endothelium-dependent relaxation to acetylcholine in the rabbit basilar artery: importance of membrane hyperpolarization. Br.J.Pharmacol. 106, 143-150.
24. JAISWAL, N., R.K. JAISWAL & K.U. MALIK (1991): Muscarinic receptor-meditated prostacyclin and cGMP synthesis in cultured vascular cells. Mol.Pharmacol. 40, 101-106.
25. BUSSE R. & A. MÜLSCH (1990): Induction of nitric oxide synthase by cytokines in vascular smooth muscle cells. FEBS Lett. 275, 87-90.
26. SCHINI, V.B. & P.M. VANHOUTTE (1991): L-arginine evokes both endothelium-dependent and endothelium-independent relaxations in L-arginine depleted aortas of the rat. Circ.Res. 68, 209-216.
27. BREDT, D.S. & S.H. SNYDER (1989): Nitric oxide mediates glutamate-linked enhancement of cGMP levels in the cerebellum. Proc.Natl.Acad.Sci.USA 86, 9030-9033.
28. BREDT, D.S., P.M. HWANG & S.H. SNYDER (1990): Localization of nitric oxide synthase indicating a neural role for nitric oxide. Nature 347, 768-769.
29. FÖRSTERMANN, U., H.H.H.W. SCHMIDT, J.S. POLLOCK, M. HELLER & F. MURAD (1991): Enzymes synthesizing guanylate cyclase-activating factors in endothelial cells, neuroblastoma cells, and rat brain. J.Cardiovasc.Pharmacol. 17, Suppl. 3, S57-S64.
30. GARTHWAITE, J. (1991): Glutamate, nitric oxide and cell-cell signalling in the nervous system. Trends Neurosci. 14, 60-67.
31. GARTHWAITE, J., G. GARTHWAITE, R.M.J. PALMER & S. MONCADA, (1989): NMDA receptor activation induces nitric oxide synthesis from arginine in rat brain slices. Eur.J.Pharmacol. 172, 413-416.
32. SCHMIDT, H.H.H.W., P. WILKE, B. EVERS & E. BÖHME (1989): Enzymatic formation of nitrogen oxides from L-arginine in bovine brain cytosol. Biochem. Biophys. Res. Commun. 165, 284-291.
33. MURPHY, S., R.L. MINOR JR., G. WELK & D.G. HARRISON (1990): Evidence for an astrocyte-derived vasorelaxing factor with properties similar to nitric oxide. J.Neurochem. 55, 349-351.
34. LEE, T.J.-F. & S.J. SARWINSKI (1991): Nitric oxidergic neurogenic vasodilation in the porcine basilar artery. Blood Vessels 28, 407-412.
35. TODA, N. & T. OKAMURA (1991): Role of nitric oxide in neurally induced cerebroarterial relaxation. J.Pharmacol.Exp.Ther. 258, 1027-1054.
36. WAHL, M., M. LAURITZEN & L. SCHILLING (1987): Change of cerebrovascular reactivity after cortical spreading depression in cats and rats. Brain Res. 411, 72-80.
37. WAHL, M., W. KUSCHINSKY, O. BOSSE & K.. THURAU (1973): Dependency of pial arterial and arteriolar diameter on perivascular osmolarity in the cat. A microapplication study. Circ.Res. 32, 162-169.
38. WAHL, M., A.R. YOUNG, L. EDVINSSON & F. WAGNER (1983): Effects of bradykinin on pial arteries and arterioles in vitro and in situ. J.Cereb.Blood Flow Metab. 3, 231-237.

39. MACKERT, J.R.L., A.A. PARSONS, E. KSOLL, L. SCHILLING & M. WAHL (1990): Methylene blue and N-w-nitro-L-arginine inhibition of acetylcholine induced relaxation of rat isolated basilar artery. Int.J.Microcirc.Clin.Exp. 9, 227.
40. TAYLOR, S.G. & A.H. WESTON (1988): Endothelium-derived hyperpolarizing factor: a new endogenous inhibitor from the vascular endothelium. Trends Pharmacol.Sci. 9, 272-273.
41. SCHILLING, L., A.A. PARSONS, J.R.L. MACKERT & M. WAHL (1991): Is K^+ channel activation, EDRF, or cyclooxygenase products involved in acetylcholine-induced relaxation of rabbit isolated basilar artery? J.Cereb.Blood Flow Metab. 11, Suppl.2, S-256.
42. FARACI, F.M. (1990): Role of nitric oxide in regulation of basilar artery tone in vivo. Amer.J.Phyisol. 259, H1216-H1221.
43. FARACI, F.M. (1991): Role of endothelium-derived relaxing factor in cerebral circulation: large arteries vs. microcirculation. Amer.J.Physiol. 261, H1038-H1042.
44. FARACI, F.M. & D.D. HEISTAD (1992): Endothelium-derived relaxing factor inhibits constrictor responses of large cerebral arteries to serotonin. J.Cereb.Blood Flow Metab. 12, 500-506.
45. HABERL, R.L., P.J. DECKER, A. PIEPGRAS & K. EINHÄUPL (1991): Is L-arginine the precursor of an endothelium-derived relaxing factor in the cerebral microcirculation? J.Cardiovasc.Pharmacol. 17, Suppl. 3, S15-S18.
46. BUSIJA, D.W., C.W. LEFFLER & L.C. WAGERLE (1990): Mono-L-arginine containing compounds dilate piglet pial arterioles via an endothelium derived relaxing factor like substance. Circ.Res. 67, 1374-1380.
47. YANG, S.-T., W.G. Mayhan, F.M. Faraci & D.D. Heistad (1991): Mechanism of impaired endothelium-dependent cerebral vasodilatation in response to bradykinin in hypertensive rats. Stroke 22, 1177-1182.
48. NORTHINGTON, F.J., G.P. MATHERNE & R.M. BERNE (1992): Competitive inhibition of nitric oxide synthase prevents the cortical hyperemia associated with peripheral nerve stimulation. Proc.Natl.Acad.Sci.USA 89, 6649-6652.
49. WAHL, M. (1992): Mechanisms of cerebral vasodilatation during neuronal activation by bicuculline: a review. In: Schmiedeck, P., K. Einhäupl, C.M. Kirsch (eds.): Stimulated cerebral blood flow, pp 50-54, Springer, Berlin.

Effects of endothelium-derived nitric oxide on cerebral cortical blood flow during normoxia and hypoxia in rats

M. Wehler and **J. Grote**

Physiologisches Institut der Universität Bonn

Introduction

In recent years, the importance of the endothelial lining of blood vessels in the metabolism and synthesis of vasoactive compounds has been demonstrated. Endothelium-dependent vascular smooth muscle relaxation, first reported by Furchgott and Zawadski [7], seems to be mainly mediated by endothelium-derived relaxing factors (EDRF), of which one has been identified as nitric oxide, or a closely related nitroso-thiol compound [20, 12, 19]. Nitric oxide is synthesized when the amino acid L-arginine is converted to L-citrulline and produces relaxation of vascular smooth muscle by the stimulation of soluble guanylate cyclase and accumulation of guanosine 3',5'-cyclic monophosphate (cGMP) [5, 16]. cGMP reduces contraction of vascular smooth muscle cells by decreasing the cytosolic free calcium concentration and by diminishing the sensitivity of contractile proteins [11].

The release of NO from endothelium appears to play an important role as an intrinsic modulator of vascular tone in various tissues [12]. Inhibition of NO synthesis, using analogues of L-arginine acting as false substrates, has shown that NO is a potent vascular smooth muscle relaxant as demonstrated in isolated vessel and organ preparations [26, 23, 28]. In the intact animal inhibitors of NO synthesis have a substantial pressor effect [27, 30]. Although several lines of evidence suggest that NO is not only released in response to a variety of physiological stimuli but also continuously under basal conditions, its role in regulating regional vascular responses to a pathophysiological stimulus such as hypoxia has not been elucidated. To date, no study has fully characterized the role of the L-arginine/NO/cGMP pathway to modulate cerebral vascular tone in the intact animal.

Therefore we investigated the effects of blocking NO synthesis, using the competitive inhibitor N^G-L-arginine (L-NNA), on tone of pial arteries and cortical cerebral blood flow during arterial normoxia and hypoxia.

Material and methods

Ten male Sprague-Dawley rats weighing 400-450 g were anesthetized with sodium thiopental (100 mg/kg) given intraperitoneally. A tracheotomy was performed and the animals were artificially ventilated (Animal-Respirator 4601, Rhema-Labortechnik, F.R.G.) with oxygen/nitrogen mixtures and paralysed with pancuronium bromide (0,4 mg/kg). Supplemental doses of thiopental and muscle relaxant were given as necessary to maintain anesthesia. Temperature was monitored intrarectally and maintained close at 38 °C with a heating pad. The right femoral vein was cannulated for intravenous fluid and drug administration, the right femoral artery was cannulated and connected to a pressure transducer (Gould Statham, P23Db, U.S.A.) for continuous recording of blood pressure and to collect blood samples for analysis of arterial PO_2, PCO_2 and pH (ABL 330, Radiometer Copenhagen). In each animal a constant infusion of 0.9 % sodium chloride (1.5 ml/h) was administered throughout the experiment to maintain hydration. For anticoagulation sodium heparin (100 I.U./100g) was given as an i.v. bolus. After these preparations the heads of the animals were fixed in a stereotaxic frame and a craniotomy was performed over the right parietal cortex. A plexiglas funnel was attached above the exposed brain area and filled with paraffin oil to maintain the intracranial pressure as previously decribed in detail [10]. The dura mater was stripped from the craniotomy site, and the pial vessels on the cerebral cortex were thus exposed.

Pial arteries ranging in diameter between 35 and 85 µm were visualized by a stereomicroscope (x40) (Wild Heerbrugg, C.H.) equipped with a television camera (Model WV-1550/G, Panasonic, Japan) coupled to a video monitor. Within the measuring field of each animal the diameter of ten arteries was studied. Images were recorded on videotape and vessel diameters were measured later using a microcomputer-based image analysis program.

Regional cerebral blood flow (rCBF) in the cortex of the right hemisphere was measured using laser-Doppler flowmetry (LDF) (BFM3D, Moor Instruments, G.B.). This method permits continuous recording of rCBF in vivo [3, 9] A needle probe attached to a micromanipulator was positioned under microscopic guidance approximately 0.5 mm above the cortical surface. Special care was taken not to place the probe close to large pial vessels and to avoid direct light to the preparation. The time constant of the probe was set at 1.0 s. Since LDF does not provide absolute flow values, the LDF recordings are expressed as percentage of baseline levels.

All experiments were performed after a 45 min stabilization period following surgery. Mean arterial blood pressure (MABP) was recorded continuously throughout the experiment, arterial blood gas tensions and pH were analysed before and after each measurement of pial artery diameter and rCBF. After the onset of hypoxic ventilation an equilibration period of 5 minutes was allowed. To assess the effect of NO on cerebral blood flow during normoxic and hypoxic conditions pial artery diameters and rCBF were measured four times: (1) under control conditions of normoxia, these CBF recordings served as baseline values, (2) during hypoxia, (3) 5 min after intravenous injection of 10 mg/kg L-NNA (Serva Feinbiochemica, Heidelberg, F.R.G.) during normoxia, (4) 25 min after injection of L-NNA during hypoxia.

Statistical analysis of the obtained data was performed with paired Student's t test. Significance was accepted at the 0.05 level of probability. All results are expressed as means ± SD.

Results

Systemic variables. The mean values for the respiratory gas tensions and pH of arterial blood and the mean arterial blood pressure as determined before and after application of L-NNA during arterial normoxia and hypoxia are summarized in table 1. In untreated rats lowering of arterial oxygen tension from 111 mmHg to a hypoxic level of 38 mmHg in the mean induced under normocapnic conditions a significant decrease in MABP from 108 to 80 mmHg. Following administration of L-NNA arterial blood pressure increased significantly during normoxia (157 mmHg, $p<0.001$). Stable values were reached within ten minutes. Additional initiation of arterial hypoxia resulted in a moderate fall in MABP from 157 to 144 mmHg.

Table 1: Systemic variables determined after L-NNA during normoxia and hypoxia in rats. Given are mean values ±SD, $n = 10$

	CONTROL		L-NNA	
	Normoxia	Hypoxia	Normoxia	Hypoxia
P_aO_2 (mmHg)	111 ± 14	38 ± 4	112 ± 9	42 ± 4
P_aCO_2 (mmHg)	38 ± 3	39 ± 3	39 ± 5	41 ± 4
pH_a	7.43 ± 0.02	7.37 ± 0.03	7.36 ± 0.03	7.35 ± 0.02
MABP (mmHg)	108 ± 11	80 ± 6	157 ± 15	144 ± 14

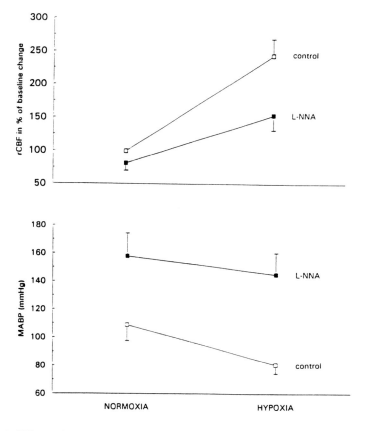

Fig. 1: Effects of L-NNA on pial artery diameter during arterial normoxia and hypoxia (open squares relate to controls, and closed squares to L-NNA treated animals). Given are mean values ± SD, $n = 103$.

Pial artery diameter and rCBF. As shown in Fig. 1 onset of hypoxia caused dilatation of the pial arteries with a 41 % increase in vessel diameter from 59 ± 14 μm to 83 ± 17 μm (p<0.05). During normoxia and blockade of NO synthesis all pial arteries measured were found to be constricted as compared to the control state. The mean artery diameter decreased to 50 ± 11 μm (p<0.05). Arterial hypoxia induced dilatation with a 32 % increase of the diameter to a mean value of 68 ± 15 μm (p<0.05).

The simultaneously performed rCBF measurements showed before inhibition of NO synthesis a blood flow increase of 242 ± 36 % of the baseline values recorded under normoxic conditions (Fig. 2). During normocapnic normoxia administration of L-NNA reduced rCBF to 82 ± 10 % of baseline, the following hypoxic state induced a blood flow increase to 153 ± 28 % above the control level.

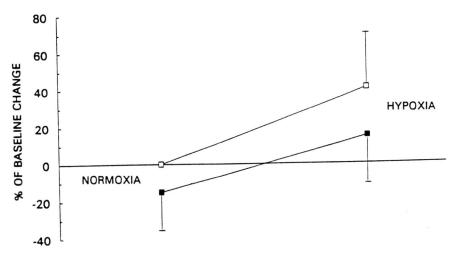

Fig. 2: Regional cerebral blood flow (rCBF) during arterial normoxia and hypoxia before (open squares) and after (closed squares) administration of 10 mg/kg L-NNA. Given are mean values ± SD,

Discussion

The present results demonstrate that the selective inhibitor of NO synthesis, L-NNA, significantly decreases pial arteriolar diameter and rCBF during normoxia. They also show that hypoxia-induced pial artery vasodilatation and increase in rCBF is markedly attenuated in the absence of NO synthesis. These findings indicate that pial artery diameter and cerebral blood flow in the brain cortex of rats during normoxic conditions and in response to arterial hypoxia are at least to some extent regulated by endothelium-derived nitric oxide.

The results of our in vivo studies are comparable to those of several other authors. Beckmann et al. [1] reported a 50 % decrease in cortical CBF of rats by nitroarginine hydrochloride infused i.v. at a rate of 30 mg/kg/hr. Macrae and coworkers [15] noted a significant blood flow decrease in the brain cortex of rats by 40 % induced by nitric oxide synthase inhibition with N^G-nitro meythyl ester hydrochloride (L-NAME). Recently, Prado and colleagues [25] showed that the intracarotid infusion of L-NAME at 3 mg/kg/min decreased rCBF in the brain cortex of rats by 20 %, whereas the intravenous administration of 15 mg/kg L-NAME reduced rCBF by 32 % of baseline values. Kozniewskia et al. [14] demonstrated in rats a decrease in CBF of 21 % by 100 mg/kg N^G-monomethyl-L-arginine (L-NMMA) intravenously. In addition, Moritz and Grote [18] observed a significant shift of the cortex tissue PO_2 of rats to lower values following L-NNA application. Thus, several in vivo studies have shown that NO contributes to the maintenance of cerebral blood flow and oxygen supply under normal conditions. Few data exist on wether NO participates in hypoxic cerebral vasodilatation and increase in CBF. The presented data suggest that NO moderates the hypoxic response of cerebral cortex circulation in rats. During blockade of NO synthesis rCBF increase in response to hypoxia reached lower maximal values but the relative increase of rCBF (+187 %) is comparable to that measured under control conditions. The results are consistent with those of Kozniewska and coworkers [14] who found that inhibition of NO synthesis by L-NMMA during hypoxia does not influence the magnitude in CBF increase but significantly reduces the maximum level if CBF compared to an untreated control group. In L-NNA treated rats a decrease in arterial oxygen pressure causes a significantly more pronounced tissue hypoxia in the brain cortex than in controls [18].

During normoxia the pial arteries studied showed a 18 % reduction in diameter following administration of L-NNA. Rosenblum and coworkers [29] demonstrated a dose-dependent constriction of mouse pial arteries with intact endothelium following topical application of L-NMMA. Effects of NO synthase inhibition does not only depend on intact endothelium but also on the initial diameter of the investigated arteries [4]. Faraci showed that topical application of L-NMMA in rats had a much greater effect on the basal tone of the basilar artery (diameter 275 μm) than on arterioles. Prado et al. [25] who studied large pial arteries (diameter 128 μm) in rats demonstrated a 60 % decrease of the vessel diameter by an intracarotid infusion of L-NAME.

Since the inhibition of NO synthesis induces a significant rise in systemic blood pressure without exceeding the limits of autoregulation one could argue that the observed constriction of pial arteries is in part an autoregulatory response. The simultaneous reduction in rCBF indicates, however, that the noted blood flow changes were directly caused by the restricted availability of vasodilating nitric oxide.

In the present study, pial artery diameter during hypoxia increased in the mean by 140 %, after administration of L-NNA changing from normoxic to hypoxic ventilation induced an increase by 135 %. As recently reviewed by Moncada [17] nitric oxide inhibitors are not very efficient in blocking vasodilation, suggesting that in vivo NO is just one among other relaxant factors. Findings by different groups lead to the conclusion that the effect of intraluminar oxygen tension on EDRF production is specific to certain vascular beds. In 1983 Busse and colleagues [2] demonstrated that endothelial cells are involved in the vasodilatory response to hypoxia. In vitro studies performed on canine and rabbit cerebral arteries showed that lowering of oxygen tensions induce hyperpolarization of vascular smooth muscle cells and a subsequent reduction in tone mediated by endothelium-derived factors [8, 21]. Pohl and Busse [24] noted that hypoxia stimulates the release of EDRF from the endothelium of native rabbit aortas and femoral arteries. In the pulmonary circulation of dogs EDRF seems to oppose pulmonary vasoconstrictor responses to hypoxia whereas in the renal vasculature inhibition of NO during hypoxia does not influence vascular reactions [22].

When comparing our results and observations of other groups to evaluate the extent by which NO regulates CBF under normoxic and hypoxic conditions several methodological differences, like the NO synthase inhibitor used, its concentration and route of administration, the time of observation, the species, the diameter of the vessels studied, differences in the spatial resolution of microcirculatory measurements (LDF, microspheres), have to be taken into account. To date, there seems to be no doubt that NO-mediated vasodilation contributes to the regulation of regional blood flow within the central nervous system of several species. Experimental data also suggest that NO has a modest effect on hypoxic vasodilation.

References

1. BECKMANN, J. S., K. A. CONGER, J. CHEN, M. J. TAN & J. H. HALSEY (1991): Nitric oxide helps regulate cerebral blood flow. J. Cereb. Blood Flow, 11 (Suppl 2), S629.
2. BUSSE, R., U. POHL, C, KELLNER & V. KLEMM (1983): Endothelial cells are involved in the vasodilatory response to hypoxia. Pflügers Arch., 397,78-80.
3. DIRNAGL, U., B. KAPLAN, M. JACEWICZ & W. PULSINELLI (1989): Continuous measurement of cerebral cortical blood flow by laser-Doppler flowmetry in a rat stroke model. J. Cereb. Blood Flow Metab., 9,589-596.
4. FARACI, F. M. (1991): Role of endothelium-derived relaxing factor in cerebral circulation: large arteries vs. microcirculation. Am. J. Physiol., 261,H1038-H1042.
5. FASEHUN, O. A., S. S. GROSS, L. E. RUBIN, E. A. JAFFE, O. W. GRIFFITH & R. LEVI (1990): L-arginine, but not N-benzoyl-L-arginine ethyl ester, is a precursor of endothelium-derived relaxing factor. J. Pharmacol. Exp. Ther., 255,1348-1353.
6. FLORENCE, G. & J. SEYLAZ (1992): Rapid autoregulation of cerebral blood flow: a laser-Doppler flowmetry study J. Cereb. Blood Flow Metab., 12,674-680.
7. FURCHGOTT, R. F. & J. V. ZAWADSKI (1980): The obligatory role of endothelial cells in the relaxation of arterial smooth muscle by acetylcholine. Nature, 288,373-376.
8. GROTE J., G. SIEGEL & K. ZIMMER (1988): The influence of oxygen tension on membrane potential and tone of canine carotid artery smooth muscle. Adv. Exp. Med., Biol. 222:481-487.
9. HABERL, R. L., M. L. HEIZER, A. MARMAROU & E. F. ELLIS (1989): Laser-Doppler assessment of brain microcirculation: effect of systemic alterations. Am. J. Physiol., 256, H1247-H1254.
10. HAGENDORFF, A., K. ZIMMER & J. GROTE (1990): A new model for long-term investigations in cerebral oxygen supply in rats. Adv. Exp. Med. Biol., 277,145-152.
11. IGNARRO,L. J. (1989):Biological actions and properties of endothelium-derived nitric oxide formed and released from artery and vein. Circ. Res., 65,1-21.
12. IGNARRO, L. J. & P. J. KADOWITZ (1985): The pharmacological and physiological role of cGMP in vascular smooth muscle relaxation. Annu. Rev. Pharmacol. Toxicol., 25,171-191.
13. IGNARRO, L. J. (1990):Biosynthesis and metabolism of endothelium-derived relaxing nitric oxide. Annu. Rev. Pharmacol. Toxicol., 30,535-560.
14. KOZNIEWSKA, E., M. OSEKA & T. STYS (1992). Effects of endothelium-derived nitric oxide on cerebral circulation during normoxia and hypoxia in the rat. J. Cereb. Blood Flow Metab., 12,311-317.
15. MACRAE, I. M., D. A. DAWSON, J. L. REID & J. MCCULLOCH (1991): Effects of nitric oxide synthetase inhibition on cerebral blood flow in the conscious rat. Soc. Neurosci., Abstr 17,475.
16. MONCADA, S. & E. A. HIGGS (1990): Nitric oxide from L-arginine: A Bioregulatory System. Amsterdam: Elsevier.
17. MONCADA, S. (1992): The 1991 Ulf von Euler lecture. The L-arginine:nitric oxide pathway. Acta Physiol. Scand., 145:201-227.
18. MORITZ, J. & J. GROTE (1991): Role of EDRF in regulation of cerebral oxygen supply during arterial normoxia and hypoxia. Pflügers Arch., 419 (Suppl 1):R112.

19. MYERS, P. R., R. L. MINOR, R. GUERRA, J. N. BATES & D. G. HARRISON (1990): Vasorelaxant properties of the endothelium-derived relaxing factor more closely resemble S-nitrosocysteine than nitric oxide. Nature, 345,161-163.
20. PALMER, R. M. J., D. S. ASHTON & S. MONCADA, S. (1988): Vascular endothelium cells synthesize nitric oxide from L-arginine. Nature, 333,664-666.
21. PEARCE, W. J., S. ASHWAL & J. CUEVAS (1989): Direct effects of graded hypoxia on intact and denuded rabbit cranial arteries. Am. J. Physiol., 257,H824-H833.
22. PERRELLA, M., E. S. EDELL, M. J. KROWKA, D. A. CORTESE & J. C. BURNETT, Jr. (1992): Endothelium-derived relaxing factor in pulmonary and renal circulation during hypoxia. Am. J..Physiol., 263, R45-50.
23. PERSSON, M. G., L. E. Gustafsson, N. P. Wiklund, P. Hedquist & S. MONCADA (1990): Endogenous nitric oxide as a modulator of rabbit skeletal muscle microcirculation in vivo. Br. J. Pharmacol., 100,463-466.
24. POHL, U.& R. BUSSE (1989): Hypoxia stimulates release of endothelium-derived relaxant factor. Am. J. Physiol., 256:H1595-H1600.
25. PRADO, R., B. D. WATSON, J. KULUZ, AND W. D. DIETRICH (1992): Endothelium-derived nitric oxide synthase inhibition: Effects on cerebral blood flow, pial artery diameter, and vascular morphology in rats. Stroke, 23,1118-1124.
26. REES, D. D., R. M. PALMER, H. F. HODSON & S. MONCADA (1989a): A specific inhibitor of nitric oxide formation from L-arginine attenuates endothelium-dependant relaxation. Br. J. Pharmacol., 96,418-424.
27. REES, D. D., R. M. J. PALMER & S. MONCADA (1989b): Role of endothelium-derived nitric oxide in regulation of blood pressure. Proc. Natl. Acad. Sci., USA 86,3375-3378.
28. ROBERTSON, B. E., J. B. WARREN & P. C. G. NYE (1990): Inhibition of nitric oxide synthesis potentiates hypoxic vasoconstriction in isolated rat lungs. Exper. Physiol., 75:255-257.
29. ROSENBLUM, W. I., H. NISHIMURA & G. H. NELSON (1990): Endothelium-dependent L-Arg and L-NMMA-sensitive mechanisms regulate tone of brain microvessels. Am. J. Physiol., 259, H1396-H1401.
30. WHITTLE, B. R., J. LOPEZ-BELMONTE & D. D. REES (1989): Modulation of the vasodepressor actions of acetylcholine, bradykinin, substance P and endothelin in the rat by a specific inhibitor of nitric oxide formation. Br. J. Pharmacol., 98,646-652.

Completness of brain capillary perfusion

U. Göbel, H. Theilen, and W. Kuschinsky

Department of Physiology, University of Bonn, and Department of Physiology, University of Heidelberg

Abstract

The density of the total and the perfused capillary network was determined in the brains of awake, normocapnic rats. Perfused capillaries were marked by i.v. fluoresceinisothiocyanate (FITC)-globulin or by Evans blue. Existing capillaries were made visible by antibodies directed against the fibronectin portion of the capillary walls. Comparison of perfused and existing capillaries in different brain sections by separate staining and in identical brain sections by double staining showed a high degree of congruence between perfused and existing brain capillaries. The results show a continuous perfusion of all capillaries in the brain of the awake normocapnic rat.

Introduction

The question whether or not all capillaries are perfused in the brain at any time point is discussed highly controversially. Several authors have reported inconsistent perfusion fractions varying from about 50 % to 100 %. The most extensive work has been presented by Weiss and his group [e.g. 1,8,9, for more references see 5]. They claim a perfusion of about half of the capillary bed in the brain at any time point. For their analysis they combine black and white photographs of alkaline phosphatase stained brain sections with the fluorescent pictures of the same air dried cryosections which were obtained after i.v. injection of the fluorescent marker (FITC dextran). Other techniques have yielded a higher percentage of perfused capillaries under normal conditions [2,6]. Indications for the perfusion of all or nearly all capillaries came from our previous study [5] which applied a technique of intravascular staining introduced for the heart by Vetterlein et al. [7]. When 2 intravascular fluorescent markers were injected i.v. at different time points before decapitation of the rat, identical patterns of capillary stains were obtained with circulation times ranging from 10 seconds to 30 minutes. Meanwhile, we have developed a method which allows us to stain, using the fluorescent microscope, the capillary morphology in addition to the intravascular perfusion marker.

Methods

The experiments were performed on male rats. Catheters were implanted during anesthetia into a femoral artery and vein. The animals recovered from anesthesia in a rat restrainer for 3 hours. Then the i.v. infusion of either FITC globulin or Evans blue was started. After 10, 30 or 60 seconds circulation time the animal was decapitated. The brain was rapidly removed and frozen in 2-methylbutane chilled to -40 °C with dry ice, embedded and stored in plastic bags at -70 °C. 6 m cryosections were obtained in a microtome. Details of the further processing of the tissue are given elsewhere [3]. An essential of the method is the fixation of the frozen brain tissue with cold acetone. The brain sections were photographed under the fluorescent microscope to detect perfused (FITC globulin or Evans blue) and existing (antibody or alkaline phosphatase method) capillaries. The color slides were then projected on a large glass screen and each perfused and / or existing capillary was documented and marked on transparent paper. From this, the numbers of perfused, existing, and -in double stain experiments- congruent capillaries were calculated for the area of 1 mm^2.

Results

Figure 1 corelates the local densities of perfused (FITC globulin) and total (fibronectin antibody) capillaries. Although different animals were taken for the detection of perfused and existing capillaries a high degree of identity was observed. This figure is a strong argument for the completeness of perfusion of all capillaries in the brain.

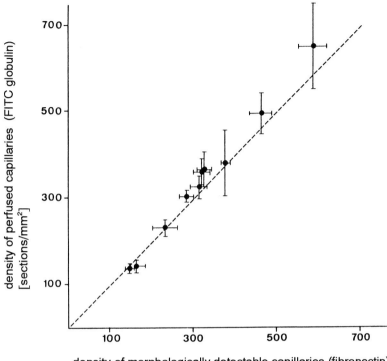

Fig. 1: Density of morphologically detectable capillaries (fibronectin antibody method) in relation to the number of perfused capillaries as measured after the i.v. injection of FITC globulin. It is evident that there exists a high degree of identity between the numbers of perfused and existing capillaries. Means ± SD.

Figure 2 compares the local densities of the capillaries measured by two different morphological methods. It is apparent that capillary densities as determined by the light microscopical alkaline phosphatase method were always lower than those determined by the fluorescent microscopical fibronectin antibody method.

This figure clearly demonstrates the high sensitivity of fluorescent microscopical methods in the detection of capillary morphology. It raised doubts against the light microscopical alkaline phosphatase method whenever it is used for the quantitative determination of capillary morphology or of perfusion fractions. This is pertinent for the studies of Weiss since they are based on the validity of the light microscopical alkaline phosphatase method.

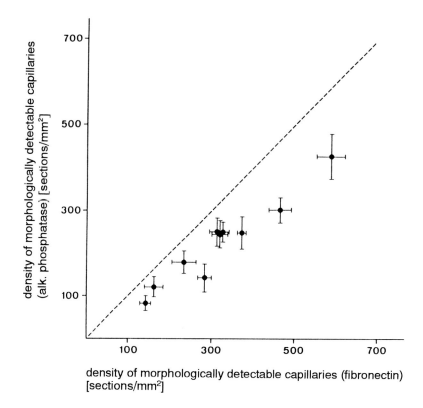

Fig. 2: Dependency of morphologically detectable capillaries in 10 different brain structures. Capillary counts obtained by the fibronectin antibody technique are related to the capillary densities measured by the alkaline phosphatase method. Significantly ($p < 0.01$) lower capillary counts were obtained in all 10 brain structures investigated when using the alkaline phosphatase method. Means ± SD.

Figure 3 shows typical photographs (converted to black and white) of the local capillary pattern within a brain section. In contrast to the data shown in fig. 1 and 2, in this figure the result of a fluorescent double staining of the same brain section is shown. The figure demonstrates the extensive congruence of the perfused and existing capillary network.

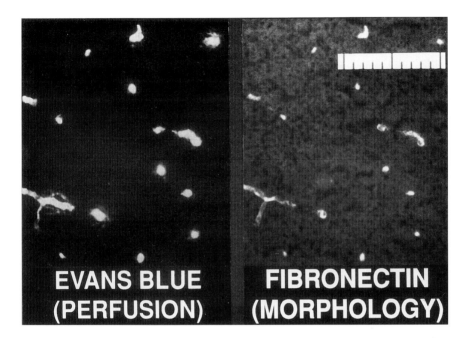

Fig. 3: Photomicrographs showing fluorescent double staining of perfused and morphologically existing capillaries. In both pictures the same location within a brain section of the visual cortex is shown. The identity of patterns in both pictures demonstrates the completeness of capillary perfusion in the brain.

Discussion

The present study demonstrates the completeness of capillary perfusion in the brains of awake rats when highly sensitive fluorescent microscopy is used to visualize both the perfused and the morphologically existing capillaries. This congruence could be demonstrated by comparing the counts of perfused and existing capillaries in the same brain structures of different animals, as demonstrated in fig 1. In addition, this congruence was verified directly by double staining of brain sections in which, as a first step, each single spot obtained from a perfused capillary (Evans blue) was documented by color photography. In a second step, existing capillaries were marked with FITC (fibronectin antibody) in the same sections which allowed a direct comparison between the local patterns of perfused and existing capillaries. Different filter combinations were used to separate the red fluorescence of Evans blue from the yellow-green fluorescence of FITC. The fact that a complete filling of all brain capillaries was obtained within 10 seconds after i.v. injection of the fluorescent marker shows that there is no perfusion reserve in the brain. Opening and closing of capillaries (capillary cycling) can also be excluded. The data lead to the conclusion that regulation of capillary flow is based on changes in the perfusion velocity of single capillaries.

Acknowledgment

Supported by the Deutsche Forschungsgemeinschaft

References

1. BUCHWEITZ, E. & H.R. WEISS (1986): Alterations in perfused capillary morphometry in awake vs anestetized brain. Brain Res. 377, 105-111.
2. COLLINS, R.C., I.L. WAGMANN, L. LYMER & J.M. MATTER (1987): Distribution and recruitment of capillaries in rat brain (abstract). J. Cereb. Blood Flow Metab. 7 (suppl1): S336.
3. GÖBEL, U., H. THEILEN & W. KUSCHINSKY (1990): Congruence of total and perfused capillary network in rat brains. Circ. Res. 66, 271-281.
4. KLEIN, B., W. KUSCHINSKY, H. SCHRÖCK & F. VETTERLEIN (1986): Interdependency of local capillary density, blood flow and metabolism in rat brains. Am. J. Physiol. 251, H1330-1340.
5. KUSCHINSKY, W. & O.B. PAULSON (1992): Capillary circulation in the brain. Cerebrovasc. Brain Metab. Rev. 4, 261-286.
6. PAWLIK, G., A. RACKL & R.J. BING (1981): Quantitative capillary topography and blood flow in the cerebral cortex of cats: an in vivo microscopic study. Brain Res. 208, 35-58.
7. VETTERLEIN, F., H. DAL RI & G. SCHMIDT (1982): Capillary density in rat myocardium during timed plasma staining. Am. J. Physiol. 242, H133-141.
8. WEISS, H.R. (1988): Measurement of cerebral capillary perfusion with a fluorescent label. Microvascular Res. 36, 172-180.
9. WEISS, H.R., E. BUCHWEITZ, T.J. MURTHA & M. AULETTA (1982): Quantitative regional determination of morphometric indices of the total and perfused capillary network in the rat brain. Circ. Res. 51, 494-503.

Regional cerebral and myocardial blood flow during ventricular pacing in rats

A. Hagendorff, C. Dettmers*, M. Manz, B. Lüderitz,
A. Hartmann* and J. Grote**

Departments of Cardiology, *Neurology and **Physiology, University of Bonn

Introduction

Ventricular tachyarrhythmias are commonly recognized as a possible cause of disorders of the circulation of the brain [1]. Loss of consciousness due to severe cerebral hypoperfusion is often observed in patients in the presence of tachycardias. Cerebral ischemia and sudden cardiac death might be caused by rapid ventricular tachycardia as well as ventricular flutter or fibrillation [2-4]. Systemic circulation is influenced by the hemodynamic effects of arrhythmias as well as of myocardial function. No marked hemodynamic effect is obvious during arrhythmias which do not cause symptoms, blood flow of brain and heart, however, might be altered. Directly after the onset of tachycardia arterial blood pressure markedly decreases followed by a variable period of hypotension depending on duration and rate of arrhythmia. The regional blood flow changes of brain and heart within this specific period are still targets of investigation. The purpose of the present study was to determine the hemodynamic effects of tachycardia induced by ventricular pacing on regional cerebral and myocardial blood flow as measured using the microsphere method.

Methods

The experiments were performed in 22 spontaneously breathing rats. Figure 1 shows the experimental set-up. After anaesthesia with thiobarbital

(Inactin-Byk 100mg/kg body weight) a polyethylene catheter was inserted into one femoral vein for administration of additional narcotics and for substitution of fluids. Both femoral arteries were catheterized, one for continuous blood pressure recording (Gould, Statham) and intermittent arterial blood sampling for blood gas analysis (BMS, Radiometer Copenhagen); the other for withdrawal of the reference flow during the microsphere injection. A heart catheter was introduced into the left ventricle through the right common carotid artery. The correct position of the catheter tip was documented by registration of the left ventricular pressure curve and by surgery at the end of the experiments. A lead for endocardial pacing was positioned through the lumen of the heart catheter.

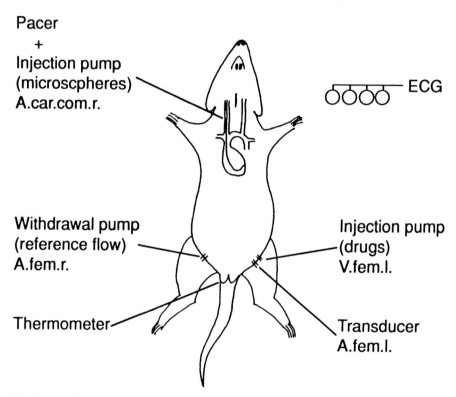

Fig. 1: Experimental set-up: Standard limb leads were placed for ECG recording. Catheters were inserted into the left femoral vein (Vfs) for drug and fluid administration, into the left femoral artery (Afs) for continuous blood pressure recording and intermittent blood sampling for blood gas analysis, into the right femoral artery (Afd) for withdrawal of reference flow and into the left ventricle for injection of microspheres via the right common carotid artery (Accd). An endocardial lead was placed through the heart catheter for pacing. Body temperature was rectally controlled.

Effective pacing was documented by ECG changes and by the decrease of arterial blood pressure. For regional tissue blood flow measurements the microsphere method was used [5-6]. During injection of the radioactive microspheres (Ruthenium-103) into the left ventricle no disturbances in systemic hemodynamics occured [7-8]. Regional cerebral and myocardial blood flow were determined during sinus rhythm (A) in eight experiments. In the following series measurements were performed between the first and second minute after onset of ventricular pacing at a rate of 11/s (B: n = 7) and 14/s (C: n = 7). Pacing energy was twice above the threshold. In order to prove homogeneous distribution of microspheres during injection, global renal blood flow measurements were additionally performed in some animals. At the end of the experiments the rats were sacrificed, brain and heart were removed, fixed in formaline and cut into samples. After weighing each sample its radioactivity was determined by a gamma-counter (Gamma Szint BF 5300, Berthold). Statistical comparison for differences of mean values was performed using the unpaired Students-t-test after analysis of variances and of normal distribution with the F-test. A P-value <0.05 was considered statistically significant. The tests were calculated with the SPSS.PC software package. Data are presented as mean value ± SD.

Results and discussion

The experiments were performed during arterial normoxia and normocapnia. Mean arterial oxygen tension ranged between 75 and 86 mmHg and mean carbon dioxide tension between 40 and 43 mmHg, respectively. Arterial pH was within normal limits during all measurements. In the control group A mean arterial blood pressure ranged from 95 to 115 mmHg. Whereas stimulation were continuously performed at the same rates mean arterial blood pressure was intraindividually reproducibly reduced but different reactions on blood pressure was observed between different rats. This might be partially due to the effect of different levels of anaesthesia [9]. In group B (11/s) arterial blood pressure ranged from 50 to 125 mmHg, in group C (14/s) from 20 to 65 mmHg. Table 1 displays the results of the tissue blood flow measurements. In group A the results of regional cerebral blood flow measurements ranged from 0.5 and 2.35 ml/g/min. The interhemispheric differences are possibly caused by the occlusion of the right common carotid artery during heart catheterization. The highest flow values were measured in the occipital regions, the cerebellum and the brainstem. Regional myocardial blood flow ranged from 0.5 to 8.75 ml/g/min. The interindividual variation was greater in myocardial than cerebral blood flow. Local perfusion of the right ventricle was lower than that of the septum and of the left ventricle. The marked differences in regional myocardial blood flow might in part be due to disturbances of microsphere influx into the coronary circulation during left ventricular injection caused by a partial obstruction of one coronary ostium by the catheter [10-11]. Since no differences in left and right renal blood flow could be found, one can assume a homogeneous distribution of microspheres in the systemic circulation.

Table 1: Regional cerebral and myocardial blood flow determined in rats during control conditions (A) and during left ventricular pacing at a heart rate of 11/s (B) and 14/s (C). Given are mean values ± SD.

Group:	A	B	C
	Regional tissue blood flow (ml/g·min)		
Brain:			
left rostral hemispherical region	1.01	0.78	0.44
	0.32	0.32	0.20
left medial hemispherical region	1.00	1.01	0.42
	0.39	0.44	0.20
left occipital hemispherical region	1.30	0.94	0.43
	0.55	0.32	0.30
right rostral hemispherical region	0.97	0.70	0.37
	0.30	0.30	0.14
right medial hemispherical region	0.88	0.60	0.28
	0.20	0.30	0.17
right occipital hemispherical region	0.97	0.76	0.34
	0.20	0.30	0.16
left cerebellum	1.40	1.35	0.53
	0.50	0.60	0.28
right cerebellum	1.46	1.35	0.52
	0.60	0.50	0.17
brainstem	1.13	0.83	0.43
	0.30	0.30	0.16
Heart:			
left ventricle lateral region	5.45	4.74	1.90
	1.70	3.00	1.00
left ventricle septal region	5.43	4.45	1.54
	1.50	2.60	0.71
right ventricle lateral region	4.90	4.34	2.02
	1.80	2.30	1.40
Mean arterial blood pressure	100	78	36
(mmHg)	9	18	12

Mean arterial blood pressure as well as mean regional cerebral and myocardial blood flow changed during high rate ventricular pacing (Tab. 1). The pattern of regional blood flow were comparable to that found in the control group. The regional blood flow values observed in the brain and heart were reduced by about 15 % in group B. In single experiments, in which mean arterial blood pressure was increased during ventricular pacing, regional myocardial blood flow was observed above control levels whereas regional cerebral blood flow remained unchanged. In case of reduction of mean arterial blood pressure, regional cerebral blood flow was distinctly decreased, whereas minor changes occured in regional myocardial blood flow. In group C blood flow of brain and heart was significantly reduced ($p < 0.01$) by about 65 % due to hypotension induced by ventricular pacing. Fig. 2 summarizes the effects of hypotension due to ventricular tachycardia on global cerebral blood flow.

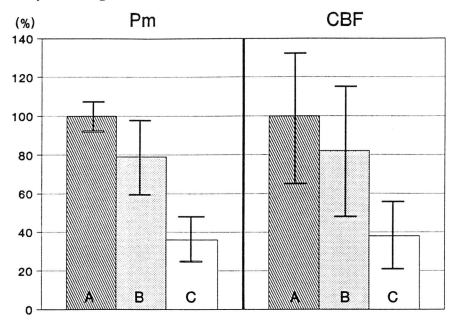

Fig. 2: Bar diagrams of mean arterial bood pressure and global cerebral blood flow (CBF) during control conditions (A) and ventricular pacing at a rate of 11/s (B) and 14/s (C).

Blood flow in the brain tissue is regulated by changes of arteriolar smooth muscle tone induced by myogenic reactions, by local release of vasoactive substances, by the activity of the autonomic nervous system and by humoral stimuli [4,12]. Furthermore, the flow resistance of the large arteries seem to play an important role in regional blood flow regulation, especially in the cerebral circulation [13]. Sudden hypotension causes a short term decrease in tissue blood flow [14-16]. If the blood pressure changes are within the range of autoregulation normalization of cerebral blood flow as well as myocardial blood flow usually occurs within one minute [14,17-18]. Experimental and clinical studies of the influence of ventricular dysrhythmias on systemic as well as on cerebral circulation showed an acute decrease of cardiac output of about 50 to 75 % as well as a significant reduction of blood flow velocity in the brain supplying arteries [19-22]. As our measurements were performed one minute after onset of high frequent ventricular pacing, one should expect normal tissue perfusion of the brain and heart muscle under conditions of normotension or mild hypotension. We observed, however, a decrease of regional cerebral blood flow during ventricular tachycardias in three experiments, even when mean arterial blood pressure was within the limits of autoregulation. In contrast to the behaviour of cerebral blood flow, myocardial blood flow showed an increase during normotensive pacing. These findings are explained as a consequence of increased myocardial oxygen consumption during elevated heart rate, which causes an improvement of coronary autoregulation [18]. Obviously, regional blood flow of the brain is more affected than regional blood flow of the heart under conditions of normotensive and borderline hypotensive pacing indicating a limitation of the capacity of brain blood flow regulation during tachyarrhythmias. Therefore a dissociation of cerebral and myocardial blood flow during tachycardias can be assumed. In addition, the results indicate that normalization of cerebral perfusion during mild hypotension requires more than two minutes.

When ventricular pacing induced pronounced hypotension regional blood flow of the brain tissue as well as of the myocardium were found to be decreased (Tab. 1).

Summary and conclusions

The present experimental set-up enables the quantification of hemodynamic effects induced by ventricular tachycardias. This model represents an acute normovolemic hypotension and differs from previous hypovolemic or drug induced hypotension models. During normotensive tachycardias regional myocardial blood flow increased while regional cerebral blood flow remained unchanged. If ventricular pacing caused blood pressure decrease cerebral blood flow as well as myocardial blood flow showed a sifgnificant reduction in comparison to control values. Since blood flow reactions in the cerebral circulation were more pronounced, neurological complaints may occur during tachyarrhythmias, even when arterial blood pressure is decreased within the normal range of autoregulation. The reduction of cardiac output due to arrhythmia seems to be an important determinant for the occurrence of neurological deficits.

Acknowledgement

Supported by Deutsche Forschungsgemeinschaft (Ha 1922/1-1 and De 425/2-1).

References

1. NORRIS, J.W. (1989): Cardiac arrhythmias in stroke In: TOOLE, J.F. (ed): Handbook of clinical neurology Vol. 11: Vascular diseases, Part III pp. 151-159, Elsevier Science Publishers B.V.
2. REFSUM, H., I.A. SULG & K.RASMUSSEN (eds.) (1989): Heart & Brain, Brain & Heart. Springer: Berlin, Heidelberg, New York.
3. LÜDERITZ, B. (ed.) (1990): Arrhythmiebehandlung und Hämodynamik. Springer: Berlin, Heidelberg, New York, London, Paris, Tokyo, Hong Kong.
4. KUSCHINSKY, W., & M. WAHL (1978): Local and chemical and neurogenic regulation of cerebral vascular resistance. Physiol.Rev. 58, 656-689.
5. HEYMANN, M.A., B.D. PAYNE, J.I.E. HOFFMANN & A.M. RUDOLPH (1977): Blood flow measurements with radionuclide-labeled particles. Prog.In Card. 20, 55-79.
6. TUMA, R.F., U.S. VASTHARE, G.L. IRION & M.P. WIEDEMAN (1986): Considerations in the use of microspheres for flow measurements in anaesthetized rat. Am.J.Physiol. 250, H137-H143.
7. MALIK, A.B., J.E. KAPLAN & T.M. SABA (1976): Reference sample method for cardiac output and regional blood flow determination in the rat. J.Appl.Physiol. 40, 472-475.
8. STANEK, K.A., T.L. SMITH, W.R. MURPHY & T.G. COLEMAN (1983): Hemodynamic disturbances in the rat as a function of the number of microspheres injected. Am.J.Physiol. 245, H920-H923.
9. MADSEN, J.B., & G.E. COLD (ed.) (1990): The effects of anesthetics upon cerebral circulation and metabolism - experimental and clinical studies. Springer: Wien, New York.
10. WICKER, P., & R.C. TARAZI (1982): Importance of injection site for coronary blood flow determinations by microspheres in rats. Am.J.Physiol. 242, H94-H97.

11. HOFFMANN, W.E., D.J. MILETICH, R.F. ALBRECHT & S. ANDERSON (1983): Regional cerebral blood flow measurements in rats with radioactive microspheres. Life Sci. 33, 1075-1080.
12. FEIGL, E.O. (1983): Coronary physiology. Physiol.Rev. 63: 1-205.
13. FARACI, F.M., & D.D. HEISTAD (1990): Regulation of large cerebral arteries and cerebral microvascular pressure. Circ.Res. 66, 8-17.
14. RAPELA, C.E., & H.D. GREEN (1964): Autoregulation of canine cerebral blood flow. Circ.Res. 15, Suppl.1, 205-211.
15. HARPER, A.M. (1964): Autoregulation of cerebral blood flow: influence of the arterial blood pressure on the blood flow through the cerebral cortex. J.Neurol.Psychiat. 29, 398-403.
16. KONTOS, H.A., E.P. WEI, R.M. NAVARI, J.E. LEVASSEUR, W.I. ROSENBLUM & J.L. PATTERSON (1978): Responses of cerebral arteries and arterioles to acute hypotension and hypertension. Am.J.Physiol. 234, H371-H383.
17. BETZ, E. (1972): Cerebral blood flow: Its measurement and regulation. Physiol.Rev. 52:, 595-630.
18. DOLE, W.P. (1987): Autoregulation of the coronary circulation. Prog.Cardiovasc.Dis. 29, 293-323.
19. CORDAY, E. & D.W. IRVING (1960): Effect of cardiac arrhythmias on the cerebral circulation. Am.J.Cardiol. 6, 803-809.
20. BENCHIMOL, A. & M.S. LIGGETT (1966): Cardiac hemodynamics during stimulation of the right atrium, right ventricle and left ventricle in normal and abnormal hearts. Circulation 33, 933-944.
21. MANZ, M., P. PFITZNER, J. NITSCH & B. LÜDERITZ (1988): Hämodynamische Messungen bei Patienten mit rezidivierenden persistierenden ventrikulären Tachykardien. Z.Kardiol. 77, Suppl. 1, 74.
22. COSIN, J., A. HERNANDIZ, J.M. SAEZ, J. SOLAZ, F. ANDRES, G. TORREGROSA, F.J. MIRANDA & E. ALBORCH (1990): Cerebral blood flow during tachyarrhythmias. New trends arrhyth. VI, 315-321.

Glial swelling and glial acidosis induced by arachidonic acid

A. Winkler*, F. Staub*, J. Peters*, O. Kempski** and A. Baethmann*

Institut für Chirurgische Forschung der Universität München* und Institut für Neurochirurgische Pathophysiologie der Universität Mainz**

Introduction

Arachidonic acid (AA) is a major constituent of membrane phospholipids in tissues including the brain. The concentration of the free fatty acid in the brain is increasing in pathophysiological conditions such as cerebral ischemia, from a normal level of about 0.005 mM/kg fresh weight (f.w.) to 0.5 mM/kg f.w. [16]. The release involves activation of phospholipases causing breakdown of membrane lipids. Arachidonic acid is considered to mediate a variety of pathophysiological processes in the brain, among others the formation of brain edema [2]. Arachidonic acid itself and/or its equally potent degradation products, such as the prostaglandins, leukotrienes or superoxide anions can be considered to have a pathophysiological function in this context [3]. As to the sequelae on cell metabolism, experiments of Hillered & Chan [6] have shown that arachidonic acid induces disturbances of the respiratory function of mitochondria thereby stimulating glycolysis. Other pathologically relevant reactions are induced by superoxide anions, which together with H^+-ions enhance formation of highly reactive oxygen-derived free radicals, as hydroyperoxy radicals ($^{\bullet}OOH$), a process which in turn initiates lipid peroxidation [15].

In order to analyze cytotoxic brain edema-inducing properties of arachidonic acid in greater detail, the present experiments were conducted for assessment of the volume response of C6 glioma cells to increasing concentrations of the fatty acid in vitro. Additional experiments were made to elucidate mechanisms involved in the swelling process elicited by the free fatty acid. The intracellular pH (pH_i) was investigated for that purpose during exposure of the glial cells to arachidonic acid. In order to assess the significance of metabolites generated from arachidonic adic, respective experiments were conducted in the presence of superoxide dismutase (SOD) or of an 21-aminosteroid (U-74389F).

Methods

An established cell line (C6 glioma) with glial-specific properties was utilized for the experiments [9]. The cells were grown in Petri dishes using Dulbeccos modified minimal essential medium (DMEM) buffered with bicarbonate (25 mM). The medium was supplemented with 10 % fetal calf serum (FCS), 100 IU/ml penicillin G, and 50 μg/ml streptomycin. The cells were cultivated in a humidified atmosphere in room air enriched with 5 % CO_2 at 37 °C. Cell cultures were used for the experiment upon reaching confluency. The C6 glioma cells were harvested from culture with 0.05 % trypsin/0.02 % EDTA in phosphate buffered saline. The cells were washed then three times and transferred to an incubation chamber [cf. 8].

Cell volume was determined by flow cytometry using an advanced Coulter system with hydrodynamic focusing. Alterations in cell size of only 1 % can be recognized with this method [7]. The cytosolic pH was also assessed by flow cytometry with employment of the pH-sensitive fluorochrome BCECF. Fluorescence of the indicator was excited with light of a Hg-lamp at < 500 nm wave length. Emission of the fluorescence indicator was measured at two wave lengths, 532 and 630 nm [13]. The ratio of the fluorescence intensities at 532 nm and 630 nm was utilized as measure of pH_i. For calibration, the intracellular pH was adjusted to that of the extracellular by addition of the ionophore nigericin (10 μM). In buffer medium with a K^+-concentration approximating that of the intracellular compartment, the intracellular pH follows the extracellular pH [14].

The experiments with arachidonic acid were preceded by a 45-min control period for determination of normal cell volume, intracellular pH, and medium osmolality. The glial cells were incubated during 30 min with BCECF (10 μM) prior to the control period for assessment of pH_i. Arachidonate (Na^+-arachidonate, Sigma) was added then in individual experiments in concentrations ranging from 0.01 mM to 1.0 mM (final concentration in medium). Cell volume and pH_i were frequently assessed then during an experimental observation period of 90 min. SOD and the 21-

aminosteroid were added in further experiments to the cell suspension 15 min prior to administration of arachidonic acid.

Results

During incubation of C6 glioma cells under control conditions, cell volume and pH_i remained constant. Addition of the fatty acid to the cell suspension led to a dose-dependent swelling of the C6 glioma cells. An arachidonic acid concentration of 0.01 mM sufficed already to induce a significant increase of the cell volume. 10 min after administration of AA cell volume attained 103.0 ± 1.0 % (mean ± SEM) of control (p <0.01) observed prior to addition of the fatty acid. Cell swelling of 112.2 ± 1.9 %, or of 121.1 ± 3.7 % resulted within 10 min when the cells were administered with AA at 0.1 mM, or 1.0 mM, respectively (p <0.001; Tab. 1). Cell volume remained increased at the level reached within 10-20 min after addition of AA during the entire experimental observation period.

Following addition of AA, the intracellular pH was found to immediately decrease. At 0.05 mM AA led to a fall of pH_i within 5 min from 7.3 ± 0.01 (obtained in the final three control measurements) to 7.12 ± 0.03 (p <0.05). At 0.1 mM arachidonic acid resulted in a pH_i of 7.06 ± 0.03 (p <0.01). In both groups, pH_i recovered subsequently to normal, reaching 7.31 ± 0.06, or 7.25 ± 0.01 after 90 min after injection of 0.05 or 0.1 mM of the fatty acid, respectively (Tab. 1).

Administration of SOD (300 U/ml) was found to reduce, but not completely prevent the arachidonic acid-induced glial swelling. The cell suspension was added with the enzyme 15 min prior to administration of arachidonic acid (0.1 mM). In the presence of SOD, the maximum of cell swelling attained at 20 min following administration of AA was 109.3 ± 1.3 % of control. Cell volume began thereafter to continuously decline, reaching 103.5 ± 0.8 % at termination of the experiment as compared to 106.9 ± 1.7 % in untreated controls (p <0.05; Tab. 1). The 21-aminosteroid (U-74389F) was found to afford complete inhibition of cell swelling by arachidonic acid (0.1 mM; p <0.01; Tab. 1), indicating a significant role of lipid peroxide formation from AA in the cell swelling process.

Table 1: Volume response of glial cells (% control; mean ± SEM) to administration of arachidonic acid (AA) at 0.1 mM (final concentration) to glial cell suspension. The cell volume response was studied at various time periods (min) following administration of the fatty acid alone, or in combination with either SOD or 21-aminosteroid (U-74389F).

Time	Control				Incubation with arachidonic acid						
	-15	-10	-5	1	5	10	20	40	60	90
Cell Volume	100.4	99.9	99.7	104.5	110.0	112.2	111.0	112.4	109.6	106.9
AA 0.1 mM	0.3	0.2	0.3	1.2	1.5	1.9	2.2	2.8	2.2	1.7
Cell Volume	99.8	100.3	99.9	104.6	108.3	109.4	109.3	104.9	103.2	103.1
AA 0.1 mM+SOD (300 U/ml)	0.1	0.4	0.4	2.0	2.0	1.2	1.3	0.8	1.0	0.8
Cell Volume	100.3	99.4	100.3	99.4*	100.2	98.9*	100.7	100.7	101.0	101.4
AA 0.1 mM+U74389F 0.1 mM	0.3	0.5	0.4	0.7	1.3	1.4	0.9	1.0	1.1	1.5

* $p < 0.05$ vs AA 0.1 mM
** $p < 0.01$ vs AA 0.1 mM

Discussion

The minimally effective concentration of arachidonic acid currently required to induce glial cell swelling was 0.01 mM. Concentrations of the free fatty acid at this magnitude are easily reached under pathophysiological conditions in the brain as in cerebral ischemia [16]. The swelling of glial cells by administration of arachidonic acid followed a dose-response-characteristic. It could be further shown that arachidonic acid causes a dose-dependent, yet transient decrease of the intracellular pH from 7.26 to 7.06 within 5 min after exposure of the glial cells to the fatty acid at a concentration of 0.1 mM. The pH_i was, however, subsequently found to spontaneously recover reaching 7.25 within 90 min. Concerning the mechanism underlying transient acidification of the glial cells from arachidonic acid, inhibition of the respiratory chain by the free fatty acid as observed in isolated mitochondria of brain tissue causing activation of glycolysis might have played a role [3, 6]. Consequently, accumulation of protons in the glial cells leading to a decrease of pH_i might have activated the Na^+/H^+-antiporter as a compensatory mechanism in an attempt to normalize the intracellular pH. This response is associated with accumulation of Na^+-ions in the cell in exchange against intracellular H^+-ions [5]. Thus, activation of the Na^+/H^+-antiporter was conceivably involved in the spontaneous recovery of pH_i after its initial decrease following administration of arachidonic acid.

A major question worth discussion is whether swelling of the glioma cells following administration of arachidonic acid is attributable to the fatty acid itself and/or to its degradation products, such as prostaglandins, leukotrienes, or oxygen radicals [4]. It should be noted in this context that formation of superoxide anions together with the increase of the H^+-ion concentration facilitates formation of hydroxyperoxy radicals ($^\bullet OOH$), a powerful reaction initiating lipid peroxidation. The latter has been reported to inflict damage to cell membranes, affecting ion channel function as a mechanism underlying the enhanced influx of Na^+-ions ultimately causing cell swelling [10]. The significance of oxygen radicals and of lipid peroxidation products from AA was presently studied by concurrent administration of either superoxiddismutase (SOD) or a 21-aminosteroid compound for inhibition of lipid peroxidation. As shown, the steroid compound was found to inhibit completely the arachidonic acid-induced swelling of glial cells, whereas administration of SOD was only partially effective. The limited efficacy of SOD may be associated with restrictions of entrance of the enzyme molecule into the intracellular compartment on account of its molecular size (MW: 31.000). Nevertheless, since intracellularly generated superoxide anions may be released into the extracelluar compartment probably involving specific anion channels, it is conceivable that inhibition of cell swelling by SOD was attributable to attenuation of respective effects of these agents at the membrane surface of the cells [11]. It is questionable, on the other hand, whether SOD had influenced formation or scavenging, respectively of free radicals which were generated in the cells. In contrast to SOD, the 21-aminosteroid compound as a lipophilic molecule can be considered to penetrate the lipid bilayer of the cell membrane. Consequently, lipid peroxides and other susceptible agents might be scavenged by the steroid agent inside the cell [1]. The complete inhibition of the arachidonic acid-induced cell swelling by the 21-aminosteroid indicates strongly that generation of lipid peroxides plays a major role in the swelling process induced by the fatty acid (Tab. 1).

Taken together, the present findings on arachidonic acid-induced swelling of glial cells demonstrate a dose-response characteristic of this process and provide experimental evidence concerning underlying mechanisms. Specific inhibition of the secondary processes following trauma or ischemia of the brain by direct antagonization of arachidonic acid and/or of its metabolites can be expected to have a beneficial function under clinical circumstances.

Acknowledgements

The excellent technical and secretarial assistance of Ulrike Goerke, Helga Kleylein, Ingrid Kölbl and Monika Stucky is gratefully acknowledged. We appreciate the generous gift of U-74389 by Dr. McCall, Upjohn Laboratories, Kalamazoo, MI, USA. Supported by Deutsche Forschungsgemeinschaft: Ba 452/6-7.

References

1. BRAUGHLER, J.M., R.L. CHASE, G.L. NEFF, P.A. YONKERS, J.S. DAY, E.D. HALL, V.H. SETHY & R.A. LAHTI (1988): A new 21-aminosteroid antioxidant lacking glucocorticoid activity stimulates adrenocorticotropin secretion and blocks arachidonic acid release from mouse pituitary tumor (AtT-20) cells. J. Pharmacol. Exp. Ther. 244, 423-427.

2. CHAN, P.H. & R.A. FISHMAN (1978): Brain edema: Induction in cortical slices by polyunsaturated fatty acids. Science 201, 358-360.
3. CHAN, P.H., S.F. CHEN & A.C.H. YU (1988): Induction of intracellular superoxide radical formation by arachidonic acid and by polyunsaturated fatty acids in primary astrocytic cultures. J. Neurochem. 50: 1185-1193.
4. ELSTNER., E.F. (1991): Oxygen radicals - Biochemical basis for their efficacy. Klin. Wochenschr. 69, 949-956.
5. GRINSTEIN, S. & A. ROTHSTEIN (1986): Mechanisms of regulation of the Na^+/H^+ exchanger. J. Membrane Biol. 90, 1-12.
6. HILLERED, L. & P.H. CHAN (1988): Role of arachidonic acid and other free fatty acids in mitochondrial dysfunction in brain ischemia. J. Neurosci. Res. 20, 451-456.
7. KACHEL, V., E. GLOSSNER, G. KORDWIG & G. RUHENSTROTH-BAUER (1977): Fluvo-Metricell, a combined cell volume and cell fluorescence analyser. J. Histochem. Cytochem. 25, 804-812.
8. KEMPSKI, O, L. CHAUSSY, U. GROSS, M. ZIMMER & A. BAETHMANN (1983): Volume regulation and metabolism of suspended C6 glioma cells: An in vitro model to study cytotoxic brain edema. Brain. Res. 279, 217-228.
9. KEMPSKI, O., F. STAUB, M. JANSEN, F. SCHÖDEL & A. BAETHMANN (1988): Glial swelling during extra cellular acidosis in vitro. Stroke 19, 385-392.
10. KOVACHICH, G.B. & O.P. MISHRA (1981): Partial inactivation of Na,K-ATPase in cortical brain slices incubated in normal Krebs-Ringer phosphate medium at 1 and at 10 Atm oxygen pressures. J. Neurochem. 36, 333-335.
11. LYNCH, R.E. & I. FRIDOVICH (1978): Permeation of the erythrocyte stroma by superoxide radical. J. Biol. Chem. 253, 4697-4699.
12. MACKNIGHT, A.D.C. (1984): Cellular volume under physiological conditions. In: STAUB, N.C. & A.E. TAYLOR (eds): Edema, pp 81-93, New York, Raven Press.
13. MUSGROVE HEDLEY, E., C. RUGG & D. (1986): Flow cytometric measurement of cytoplasmic pH: A critical evaluation of available fluorochroms. Cytometry 7, 347-355.
14. PRESSMANN, B.C. (1976): Biological application of ionophores. Annu. Rev. Biochem. 45, 501-530.
15. SIESJÖ, B.K., G. BENDEK, T. KOIDE, E. WESTERBERG & T. WIELOCH (1985): Influence of acidosis on lipid peroxidation in brain tissues in vitro. J. Cereb. Blood Flow Metab. 5, 253-258.
16. YOSHIDA, S., S. INOH, T. ASANO, K. SANO, M. KUBOTA, H. SHIMAZAKI & N. UETA (1980): Effect of transient ischemia on free fatty acids and phospholipids in the brain. J. Neurosurg. 53, 323-331.

The study of the microcirculation of islets of Langerhans: An *in vivo* microscopic approach

M.D. Menger, P. Vajkoczy, C. Beger and **K. Messmer**

Institute for Clinical and Experimental Surgery, University of Saarland, Homburg/Saar, and Institute for Surgical Research, University of Munich

In diabetes research the study of the microcirculation of islets of Langerhans gains more and more interest, inasmuch as vasomotor control has been suggested to be an essential component in regulation of insulin release [1,2]. However, little is known about regulatory mechanisms of microvascular perfusion of pancreatic islets. This may - in part - be due to the lack of adequate models, allowing the study of the microcirculation of the islets. Histomorphologic-, dye dilution-, and corrosion cast techniques [3-6] may be useful to investigate morphologic aspects of the islet's microangioarchitecture, however, are not appropriate to study dynamic parameters, such as the microcirculation. During the last decade a variety of experimental studies aimed to evaluate microvascular perfusion of pancreatic islets under physiologic and pathophysiologic conditions using non-radioactive microspheres [7-9]. However, the major draw back of this method remains the inability to visualize dynamic processes within the microvascular network.

In contrast, *in vivo* microscopy of pancreatic islets has the potential to analyze dynamic microcirculatory parameters, such as functional capillary density, red blood cell velocity, and individual vessel diameters [2,10,11]. The technique is limited by the quality of visualization of the microvasculature due to the thickness of the pancreas, and by the fact that repeated analyses during a prolonged period of time can hardly be performed on the pancreas in situ. In the following an implantation/transplantation model will be presented, which allows for quantitative analyses of the microcirculation of individual pancreatic islets over a prolonged period of time using *in vivo* fluorescence microscopy.

Model for in vivo analysis of the microcirculation of islets of Langerhans

Pancreatic islets are isolated from Syrian golden hamsters using a modified collagenase digestion technique [12]. Subsequently, the isolated islets are implanted into the dorsal skinfold chambers of syngeneic animals [13,14]. A hand-picking procedure guarantees exocrine-free islets for transplantation. The dorsal skinfold chamber of the Syrian golden hamster consists of subcutaneous and striated muscle tissue, the latter serves as host tissue for the islet implants [15].

Using *in vivo* fluorescence microscopy and epi-illumination techniques, the microvasculature of the transplanted islets is visualized after contrast enhancement with 5 % fluorescein isothiocyanate-labeled dextran (M_r 150.000, Sigma Chemical Co., St. Louis, MO) [14]. The high molecular weight of the fluorescent compound prevents extravasation from the microvessels, thus providing sharp images for quantitative analysis of microhemodynamic parameters. Microscopic images are recorded by a low-light-level CCD (charge coupled device) video camera (COHU FK6990; Prospective Measurements, San Diego, CA) and transferred to a video system for off-line analysis.

Quantitative analysis of the islet's microcirculation may include determination of functional capillary density (length of all red blood cell perfused capillaries per islet area), and red blood cell (RBC)-velocity, diameters and blood flow of individual microvessels (arterioles, capillaries, venules). In addition, microvascular permeability is assessed by the extravasation of high molecular weight compounds, and flow behaviour of white blood cells (WBC) and platelets may be analyzed after *in vivo* staining of those cells with acridine orange or rhodamin-6G (Sigma) [16].

Functional capillary density is determined by means of the Computer Assisted Microcirculation Analysis System (CAMAS; Zeintl, Heidelberg, FRG), including planimetric area measurement for the assessment of the size of individual islets. Red blood cell velocity is measured in the centerline of the microvessels using the dual slit technique, (Velocity Tracker Mod 102B; I.P.M. INC., San Diego, CA). Vessel diameters are analyzed by means of image shearing (Image Shearing Monitor Mod 907; I.P.M. INC., San Diego, CA). Blood flow (BF) of individual microvessels is calculated from centerline red blood cell velocity (CRBCV) and diameter (D) for each microvessel as:

$$BF = \pi (D/2)^2 \times CRBCV/K$$

where K represents the Baker/Wayland factor [17], considering the parabolic velocity profile of blood in microvessels. Extravasation of fluorescent compounds and flow behaviour of blood cells are analyzed by means of computer-assisted image analysis (CAMAS).

The microcirculation of transplanted islets of Langerhans

Transplanted islets are revascularized completely after a 10- to 14-day period [13,15], revealing a glomerulum-like network of capillaries (Fig. 1), similar to that of pancreatic islets *in situ* [5,6]. In addition, arteriolar supply and capillary/venular drainage of the implanted and revascularized islets are comparable as known for islets *in situ*: Islets are supplied by one or two arterioles, and drained by individual postcapillary venules (Fig. 1) [5]. Beside the venular drainage, the islet implants develop, - in analogy to the

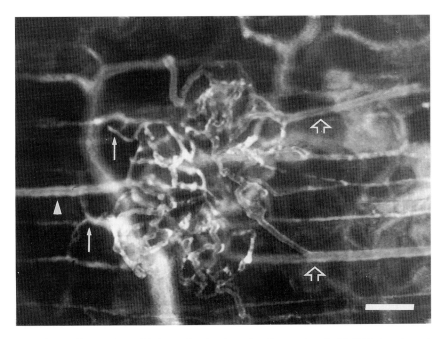

Fig. 1: Islet of Langerhans 10 days after implantation into a dorsal skinfold chamber of a syngeneic animal. Note the arterial supply vessels (⇒), the glomerulum-like network of capillaries and the venular drainage, which is made up by an individual venule (>) and intercapillary anastomoses between islet and striated muscle capillaries (→). Intravital fluorescence microscopy, contrast enhancement by 5 % FITC-dextran 150.000, i.v. (bar represents 100 µm).

insulo-acinar portal system -, with intercapillary anastomoses between islet and striated muscle capillaries

Immunohistochemical analysis of intracellular insulin documents homogeneous staining pattern within the islets [14], and scanning electron microscopic studies reveal normal fine ultra-structure [14,18], indicating morphologically intact islets.

Functional response of the islet's microvasculature

Endothelial integrity of the islet's microvasculature prevents extravasation of the high molecular weight compound FITC-dextran 150.000 (Fig. 1), similar as the endothelial lining of pancreatic islets *in situ* [11]. Furthermore, the islet's microvasculature is freely permeable for low molecular weight fluorescent compounds, such as rhodamine and acridine orange in both, implanted islets [15] and islets *in situ* (Fig. 2) [19].

Beside analysis of the characteristics of endothelial permeability, adequate functional response of the islet's microvasculature may be assessed by investigating microcirculatory responses to metabolic challenges. In several experimental studies, hyperglycemia has been proven to significantly increase microvascular blood perfusion in islets of Langerhans *in situ* [7,8,20,21], probably by dilatory effects of hyperglycemia on the microvasculature [20,21]. Using the fluorescent dye vasoflavine for direct visualization, Hellerström and Hellman [21] have demonstrated in hyperglycemic animals wider and more contorted islet capillaries as well as a larger blood cell content within the islet's microvasculature. Similarly, in the model of islet implantation for *in vivo* microscopy of the islet microcirculation, hyperglycemia enhances blood perfusion, presumably due to the presence of wider capillaries and hence lower resistance to blood flow [18,22]. The capillaries of implanted islet present not only with an increase of diameter, but appear to be more tortuous [18], similar as known for capillaries of pancreatic islets *in situ* [21].

Furthermore, studies on the vasomotor control of the islet circulation have shown that the islet microcirculation is markedly inhibited by sympathomimetic agents, such as epinephrine, which reduces blood flow to almost flow stop [1,2]. Bunnag et al. [2] have demonstrated that epinephrine causes vasoconstriction of both the afferent and efferent vessels of the islets of Langerhans, followed by cessation of the circulation in the intrainsular plexus. In parallel to these findings, in the present model epinephrine induces complete cessation of the islet's blood perfusion due to vasoconstriction of the feeding arterioles (Fig. 3).

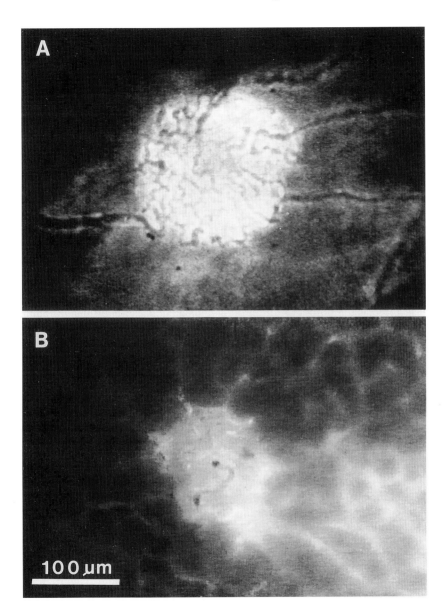

Fig. 2: Islet of Langerhans 10 days after implantation into the dorsal skinfold chamber of a syngeneic animal (Fig. 2a). Extravasation of the low molecular weight fluorescent compound acridine orange from the microvessels of the islet, but not from the microvessels of the striated muscle. Fig. 2b visualizes an islet of Langerhans *in situ* after in vivo staining with rhodamine-6G. Note the marked extravasation of rhodamine from the islet's microvessels as compared to the surrounding exocrine tissue. Intravital fluorescence microscopy, epi-illumination technique (Fig. 2a with permission from 11).

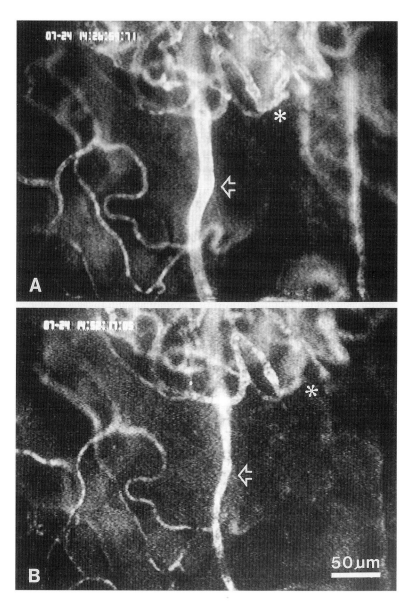

Fig. 3: Part of the microvasculature of an islet of Langerhans (*) 14 days after implantation into a dorsal skinfold chamber of a syngeneic animal. Note the arterial supply (⇒), feeding the glomerulum-like network of capillaries (Fig. 3a, *). Intravenous injection of 0.3 mg/kg body weight epinephrine results in cessation of capillary blood perfusion due to the marked vasoconstriction of the feeding arteriole (Fig. 3b, ⇒). Intravital fluorescence microscopy, contrast enhancement by 5 % FITC-dextran 150.000, i.v..

Summary

In vivo fluorescence microscopy of isolated islets of Langerhans, implanted into the dorsal skinfold chamber of syngeneic Syrian golden hamsters, may represent a useful tool for the study of the microcirculation of pancreatic islets. The model provides excellent visualization of the islet's microvasculature, which allows for quantitation of microhemodynamic parameters, such as functional capillary density, red blood cell velocity, diameters and blood flow of individual microvessels, as well as microvascular permeability and flow behaviour of white blood cells and platelets. Morphologic and microhemodynamic analyses reveal great similarities between islets *in situ* and islets after implantation into the dorsal skinfold chamber, including the capillary angioarchitecture, the islet's vascular supply and drainage, as well as the ultra-fine structure. In addition, functional response of implanted islets is comparable to that of islets *in situ*, including changes of microvascular blood perfusion due to metabolic challenges, such as hyperglycemia, and due to application of sympathomimetic agents, such as epinephrine. Since the implanted islets demonstrate physiologic conditions and function after revascularization as well as high morphologic similarity of the angioarchitecture as compared to pancreatic islets *in situ*, we like to propose that the model can be used for basic analysis of the microangiodynamics of islets of Langerhans.

References

1. ROOTH, P. & I.-B. TÄLJEDAL (1987): Vital microscopy of islet blood flow: catecholamine effects in normal and ob/ob mice. Am. J. Physiol. 252, E130-E135.
2. BUNNAG, S.C., N.E. WARNER & S. BUNNAG (1977): Vasomotor reactions in the islets affecting the blood glucose levels. Bibl. Anat. 16, 445-449.
3. BRUNFELDT, K., K. HUNHAMMER & A.P. SKOUBY (1958): Studies on the vascular system of the islets of Langerhans in mice. Acta Endocrinol. 29, 475-480.
4. FUJITA, T. & T. MURAKAMI (1973): Microcirculation of monkey pancreas with special reference to the insulo-acinar portal system. A scanning electron microscope study of vascular casts. Arch. Histol. Jpn. 35, 255-263.
5. BONNER-WEIR, S. & L. ORCI (1982): New perspectives on the microvasculature of the islets of Langerhans in the rat. Diabetes 31, 883-889.
6. OHTANI, O. (1983): Microcirculation of the pancreas: A correlative study of intravital microscopy with scanning electron microscopy of vascular casts. Arch. Histol. Jpn. 46, 315-325.

7. JANSSON, L. & C. HELLERSTRÖM (1983): Stimulation by glucose of the blood flow to the pancreatic islets of the rat. Diabetologia 25, 45-50.
8. JANSSON, L. & S. SANDLER (1985): Pancreatic islet circulation in relation to the diabetogenic action of streptozotocin in the rat. Endocrinology 116, 896-900.
9. JANSSON, L. & C. HELLERSTRÖM (1986): Glucose-induced changes in pancreatic islet blood flow mediated by central nervous system. Am. J. Physiol. 251, E644-E647.
10. ROOTH, P., K. GRANKVIST & I.-B. TÄLJEDAL (1985): In vivo fluorescence microscopy of blood flow in mouse pancreatic islets: Adrenergic effects in lean and obese-hyperglycemic mice. Microvasc. Res. 30, 176-184.
11. MENGER, M.D., F. HAMMERSEN & K. MESSMER (1990): The microcirculation of the islets of Langerhans: Present state of the art. Prog. Appl. Microcirc. 17, 192-215.
12. LACY, P.E. & M. KOSTIANOVSKY (1967): Method for the isolation of intact islets of Langerhans from the rat pancreas. Diabetes 16, 35-39.
13. MENGER, M.D., S. JÄGER, P. WALTER, G. FEIFEL, F. HAMMERSEN & K. MESSMER (1989): Angiogenesis and hemodynamics of microvasculature of transplanted islets of Langerhans. Diabetes 38/I, 199-201.
14. MENGER, M.D., S. JÄGER, P. WALTER, F. HAMMERSEN & K. MESSMER (1990): A novel technique for studies on the microvasculature of transplanted islets of Langerhans in vivo. Int. J. Microcirc.: Clin. Exp. 9, 103-117.
15. MENGER, M.D. & K. MESSMER (1991): The microvasculature of free pancreatic islet grafts. In: MESSMER, K. & M. STEIN (eds.): Pathways to Applied Immunology. Heidelberg, Berlin, New York, Tokyo: Springer Verlag, pp. 109-126.
16. MENGER, M.D., S. JÄGER, P. WALTER, F. HAMMERSEN & K. MESSMER (1991): Microvascular phenomena during pancreatic islet graft rejection. Langenbecks Arch. Chir. 376, 214-221.
17. BAKER, M. & H. WAYLAND (1974): On-line volume flow rate and velocity profile measurement for blood in microvessels. Microvasc. Res. 7, 131-143.
18. MENGER, M.D., P. VAJKOCZY, R. LEIDERER, S. JÄGER & K. MESSMER (1992): Influence of experimental hyperglycemia on microvascular blood perfusion of pancreatic islet isografts. J. Clin. Invest. 90, 1361-1369.
19. KUSTERER, K., O. BECK, M. ENGHOFER & K.H. USADEL (1992): In-vivo staining of the islets of Langerhans for microcirculatory investigations. Int. J. Microcirc.: Clin. Exp. 11 (Suppl. 1), S201.
20. KRACHT, J., Y.C. LO & J. RALL (1960): Über Beziehungen zwischen Inselkapillaren und B-Zellfunktion. Endokrinologie 39, 35-43.
21. HELLERSTRÖM, C. & B. HELLMAN (1961): The blood circulation of the islets of Langerhans visualized by the fluorescent dye vasoflavine. Acta Soc. Med. Ups. 66, 88-94.
22. MENGER, M.D., S. JÄGER, P. WALTER & K. MESSMER (1990): Influence of hyperglycemia on the process of angiogenesis and revascularization of freely transplanted islets of Langerhans. Transplant. Proc. 22, 821-822.

Arterial blood flow velocity and elasticity in the fetal guinea pig

O. Aedtner, A. Grillhösl, E. Maneck, R. Götz and W. Moll

Institut für Physiologie der Universität Regensburg

Introduction

The blood flow velocity in fetal arteries has gained increasing interest because the velocity can now be measured non-invasively in humans [3]. The blood flow velocity has been found to be related to placental vascularisation [4] and to be changed during fetal growth retardation [9,6]. The form of the blood flow velocity wave is not yet well understood. The scope of the present paper is to describe the blood flow velocity, the arterial dimensions, and the arterial elasticity in the fetal guinea pig. Blood flow velocity and elasticity are related to each other in order to obtain a quantitative understanding of the normal shape of the blood flow velocity wave.

Methods

Outbred pregnant guinea pigs near term (Pirbright white and BFA, ZH, Kißlegg, Dr. Ivanovas, Kißlegg, Allgäu, FRG) were anaesthetized with diazepam (5 mg/kg) and nembutal (60 mg/kg) and ventilated using a Starling pump. Doppler blood flow velocity was recorded using commercial ultrasound (US) equipment (Ultradopp 862, SIR, 91187 Röttenbach) with 4 MHz and 8 MHz US probes (Minhorst, 56414 Meudt) which were adjusted to conical adapters to increase spatial resolution. They were applied at an angle of 45°. Doppler shift was proved to be proportional to the mean flow velocity between 2 cm/s and 50 cm/s. In our study a time lag of around 30 ms, dampening of higher frequencies and artefact waves in the diastolic phase occurred. Fetal ECG was recorded simultaneously. The voltage output of the amplifiers were fed via an ADC into a computer

(Acer 386 SX), where the data were processed. Curves of blood flow velocity and fetal ECG were printed using the program package STATGRAFICS. Arterial diameters were measured *in vitro* using methods previously described [13]. Shortly, the arteries were excised, cannulated, and pressurized to 20, 30 and 40 mmHg while submerged in Tyrode solution at pH = 7.4 and 37 °C. The external diameter was measured using an ocular micrometer or a photometric device [8]. Wall thickness and internal diameter were derived from arterial wet weight per length. From the data on arterial diameter D at different pressures, the pressure elastic modulus E_p (the change in pressure ΔP per distension $\Delta D/D$) was determined.

Results and discussion

Blood flow velocity was registered in the middle of the thoracic and abdominal aorta. Recordings obtained from 6 fetuses in which thoracic flow rate was in the range reported in a previous study [5] were selected. Fig. 1 shows recordings obtained from the aorta and the umbilical artery. Maximum blood flow velocity was (mean ± SD) 36 ± 6 cm/s (n = 6) in the thoracic aorta, 24 ± 11 cm/s in the abdominal aorta and 17 ± 5 cm/s in the umbilical artery near the cord insertion. There was marked diastolic flow in the aorta (6 ± 3 cm/s) and in the umbilical arteries (8 ± 3 cm/s).

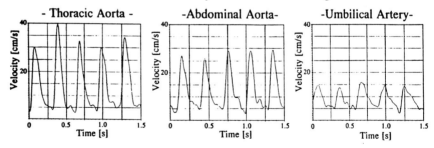

Fig. 1: Arterial blood flow velocity in the guinea pig fetus.

The blood flow velocity wave is conducted through the fetal aorta and the umbilical arteries with the wave velocity c. The wave velocity c was determined from the difference ΔX in distance between the points of observation from the heart over the change $\Delta T_{R-VMAX1/2}$ in time interval between the R wave of the fetal ECG and the time of half maximum flow velocity according to:

$$c = \Delta X / \Delta T_{R - VMAX1/2}.$$

The wave velocity was found to be 4 m/s 2 m/s in the aorta as well in the umbilical artery (Tab. 1). This velocity means that the wave is spread over the combined length of the aorta and the intra-abdominal and extra-abdominal umbilical arteries (120 mm) within 30 ms, a time interval which is 1/5 of the systolic period.

Table 1: Arterial blood flow velocity, arterial dimensions and arterial elasticity in the fetal guinea pig as mean ± SD (n)

	Thoracic aorta	Abdominal aorta	Umbilical artery
Blood flow velocity			
v_{max} (cm/s)	36 ± 6 (6)	27 ± 4 (6)	17 ± 5 (6)
v_{min} (cm/s)	6 ± 2	6 ± 4	8 ± 3
v_{mean} (cm/s)	16 ± 4	13 ± 4	12 ± 4
Internal diameter (mm)	1.7 ± 0.09 (62)	0.17 ± 0.06 (40)	0.13 ± 0.01 (20)
Length (mm)	26 ± 2 (28)	28 ± 14 (21)	37 ± 6 (37)
Wave velocity (meas.) (m/s)	4 ± 2 (14)		4 ± 2 (15)
Pressure elast. modulus (mmHg)	150 ± 40 (56)	350 ± 110 (36)	375 ± 225 (12)
Wave velocity (calc.) (m/s)	3.1	4.7	4.9

Arterial dimensions and elasticity

The data on arterial length measured in situ and the arterial diameters and the pressure elastic modulus measured in vitro are compiled in Table 1. The pressure elastic modulus E_p was around 2.5 mmHg per percent distension in the aorta and 4 mmHg per percent distension in the umbilical artery (Tab. 1). According to the Moens-Korteweg equation [7, 10] wave velocity c is related to the pressure elastic modulus E_P and the specific weight q according to $c = \sqrt{E_P / (2q)}$. As shown in Tab. 1, there is a quantitative agreement between the measured and calculated values of wave velocity in the aorta.

Diastolic blood flow velocity and the distribution of arterial compliances and peripheral resistances

We observed high blood flow velocity in the fetal aorta as well as in the umbilical arteries of the fetal guinea pig. High diastolic velocity has also been found in the human fetus [6] but not in the resting adult [14, 2]. In order to explain the diastolic flow, a windkessel concept discussed for the human fetus [11] shall be applied to the guinea pig fetus making use of the data on arterial diameter, length, and elasticity presented in this paper. In view of the short spreading time of arterial pulse in the guinea pig we may assume that inertial forces in the arterial system vanish rapidly after the ejection period. Viscous resistance in the arteries as described for the sheep fetus [2] is unlikely to occur in the guinea pig fetus according to data on arterial internal diameter [8]. Thus, diastolic flow rate at an arbitrary point of observation in the arterial system is determined by arterial elastance (1/compliance) and peripheral resistance as can be understood on the on the windkessel model presented by Fig. 2. The point of observation divides the arterial system into an upstream compartment and a downstream compartment to which a peripheral resistance R and arterial compliance C is to be

Parameters of Diastolic Flow

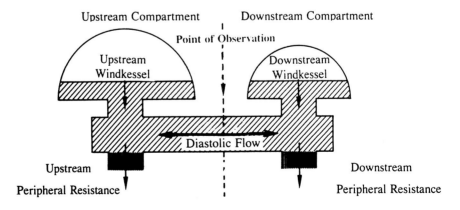

Fig. 2: Schematic diagram illustrating the arterial system composed of an upstream arterial compartment and downstream arterial compartment (modified after Moll 1992).

attributed as indicated by the resistances and windkessels in Fig. 2. In the systolic period both compartments are rapidly filled; in the diastole blood pressure falls at a rate inversely proportionate to the resistance — compliance product (RC product). When the upstream RC product is equal to the downstream RC product the pressure falls in both compartments at the same speed. No intercompartmental pressure gradient and flow occur; in both compartments, peripheral flow is supplied completely and exclusively by the attributed windkessel. If, however, the upstream RC product is higher than the downstream RC product because of large central compliance and/or low downstream resistance, upstream pressure falls slower than downstream pressure. Centripetal pressure gradient and flow occur; part of the downstream peripheral flow is supplied by the upstream windkessel. When the blood flow velocity is observed in the thoracic aorta, the upstream compartment is represented by the arterial system of the upper body, the downstream compartment by the arterial system of the lower body and by the umbilical arteries. As found in a previous study [5] the peripheral resistances are about the same in the upper body, the lower body and the placenta. On the other hand, it can be shown with the present data that the arterial compliance is quite different in these compartments. The compliance C of an artery of cross sectional area A, length l and pressure elastic modulus E_p is given by $C = 2Al/E_p$. Using this equation and the *in vitro* measurements (Tab. 1) C was calculated. C was found to be 0.4, 0.8 and 1.0 µl/mmHg in the aortic arch, the thoracic aorta and the pulmonary artery respectively, i.e. around 2 µl/mmHg for the arteries of the upper body. C was 0.4, 0.05 and 0.15 µl/mmHg in the abdominal aorta, the iliac arteries and the intraabdominal umbilical arteries respectively. In the extraabdominal umbilical arteries C was found to be 0.6 µl/mmHg [8]. Thus, the compliance of the arteries of the lower body and the umbilical arteries was around 1 µl/mmHg. Accordingly, the RC product in the arteries of the upper body is about twice of that of the arteries in the lower body and the umbilical arteries. Thus, diastolic flow in the aorta can be explained by a high upstream - downstream RC product ratio.

Summary

Arterial blood flow velocity and elastance were studied in the fetal guinea pig. In animals with normal thoracic blood flow, maximum flow velocity was found to be around 36 cm/s in the thoracic aorta, 24 cm/s in the abdominal aorta and 15 cm/s in the umbilical artery while end diastolic flow velocity was around 6 cm/s. The velocity wave was spread over the 60 mm long aorta and the 60 mm long umbilical arteries within 30 ms (1/5 of systolic period). Mean wave velocity (4 m/s) was found consistent with the mean pressure elastic modulus in the aorta (2.5 mmHg per percent distension). The rather high diastolic flow velocity in the aorta and in the umbilical artery correlate with the high compliance of the arteries of the upper fetal body and the low placental vascular resistance.

References

1. ADAMSON, S.L., K.J. WHITELEY & B.L. LANGILLE (1992): Pulsatile pressure-flow relations and pulse-wave propagation in the umbilical circulation of fetal sheep. Circ Res 70, 761—772.
2. BUSSE, R., R.D. BAUER, H. KÖRNER, T. PASCH, W. SPERLING & E. WETTERER (1973): Der Einfluß der reaktiven Hyperämie auf die Form der arteriellen Druck- und Strompulse der unteren Extremitäten des Menschen. Verh. dt. Kreisl. Forsch. 39, 228-233.
3. EIK-NES, S.H., A.O. BRUBAKK & M.K. ULSTEIN (1980): Measurement of human fetal blood flow. Brit. Med. J. 280, 283-284.
4. GILES, W.B., B.J. TRUDINGER & P.J. BAIRD (1985): Fetal umbilical artery flow velocity waveforms and placental resistance: pathological correlation. Br.J.Obstet. Gynaecol. 92, 31-38.
5. GIRARD, H., S. KLAPPSTEIN, I. BARTAG & W. MOLL (1983): Blood circulation and oxygen transport in the fetal guinea pig. J. Develop. Physiol. 5, 181-193.
6. GRIFFIN, D., T. COHEN-OVERBEEK & S. CAMPBELL (1983): Fetal and utero-placental blood flow. Clin. Obstet. Gynaecol. 10, 565-601.
7. KORTEWEG, D.J. (1878): Über die Fortpflanzungsgeschwindigkeit des Schalles in elastischen Röhren. Ann. Physik. Chem. 5, 525.
8. GRILLHÖSL, A. (1991): Kontraktilität und Elastizität plazentarer Arterien des Meerschweinchens. Inauguraldissertation, Universität Regensburg.
9. MCCALLUM, W.D., C.S. WILLIAMS, S. NAPEL & R.E. DAIGLE (1978): Fetal blood velocity waveforms. Am.J.Obstet. 132, 425-429.
10. MOENS, A.J. (1878): Die Pulskurve, zit. nach WETTERER E., R.D. BAUER, Th. PASCH: Arteriensystem. In: BAUEREISEN, E. (ed): Physiologie des Kreislaufs. Band 1, Springer Verlag, Heidelberg - New York.
11. MOLL, W. (1990): Modellierung des arteriellen Strompulses im fetalen Kreislauf. Ergebn. exp. Med. 52, 14-27.
12. MOLL, W. (1992): Strömungsgeschwindigkeit und Doppler-Shift in fetalen und maternen Gefäßen. Physiologische Grundlagen. Der Gynäkologe 25, 278-283.
13. MOLL, W. & R. GÖTZ (1985): Pressure-diameter curves of mesometrial arteries of guinea pigs demonstrate a non-muscular, oestrogen-inducible mechanism of lumen regulation. Pflügers Arch. 404, 332-336.

14. SPENCER, M.P. & A.B. DENISON (1963): Pulsatile blood flow in the vascular system. In: HAMILTON, W.F. & P. DOW (eds): Handbook of Physiology, Section II Circulation, Volume II, pp. 839-864, Washington D.C.: Am. Physiol. Soc.
15. VEILLE, J.-C., M. TAVILL, M. SIVAKOFF, I. COHEN, M. BEN-AMI, Y. YUH-CHENG & V. JOVKOSKY (1989): Evaluation of pulsed Doppler echocardiography for measurement of aortic blood flow in the fetal lamb. Am. J. Obstet. Gynecol. 161, 1610-1614.

Smooth muscle contraction kinetics in relation to membrane depolarization and sarcoplasmatic calcium concentration

U. Peiper, J. Dee, S. Klabunde, and K. Schumacher

Physiologisches Institut der Universität Hamburg

Introduction

Sarcoplasmatic calcium concentration plays a key role in controlling contraction. In some smooth muscle types membrane depolarization and release of calcium into the sarcoplasma are strongly coupled. There are two calcium sources: the opening of voltage-operated calcium channels in the cell membrane and the liberation of calcium from intracellular stores. Incubation in calcium-free solution depletes intracellular calcium stores. Subsequent depolarization with a potassium-rich, calcium-free solution may open calcium channels without any subsequent increase in sarcoplasmatic calcium concentration. Under such experimental conditions, the extent of transmembraneous calcium influx depends mainly on the extracellular calcium level. Thus, sarcoplasmic calcium concentration can be varied by changes in the extracellular calcium concentration without any simultaneous change in the membrane potential. Furthermore, the effect of longer intervals between the onset of depolarization and the onset of contraction activation can be tested.

We are interested in both the extent and the rate of force development. The number of attached crossbridges determines the extent of force generation, and the rate of force development reflects actin-myosin interaction kinetics [7]. During tonic activation, rapid length changes increase the detachment rate of crossbridges [3] resulting in a rapid loss of force generation. The rate of post-vibration force recovery after cessation of vibration depends on contraction kinetics.

Methods

Rats of both sexes were slightly anaesthetized with ether and bled by dissecting the carotid artery. The portal vein was prepared and ligated by threads. Both ends of the preparation were connected by loops to a Swema SG-4 force transducer and a Ling 101 vibrator. During incubation in Tyrode solution (NaCl 132.2; KCl 4.8; $CaCl_2$ 2.5; $MgCl_2$ 0.49; $NaHCO_3$ 11.9; NaH_2PO_4 0.36; glucose 5.05; pyruvate 2.0 mM; 37 °C; pH 7.4) the resting tension was adjusted to 2 mN. The mean muscle length of the preparations averaged 4.7 ± 0.3 mm.

Determination of the preparation's contractile behaviour: Spontaneous activity stabilized after 10 min of equilibrium. Just before spontaneous activity occurred, contraction was induced by electrical field stimulation (50 Hz, sinus, 7 volts) applied by platin plate electrodes arranged in parallel to the preparation. After 3 sec stimulation, peak force was reached and a length vibration (100 Hz, sinus, 5 % of the muscle length) was induced for 1 sec. As seen in Fig. 1, there is a rapid loss of force followed by force recovery after the cessation of vibration.

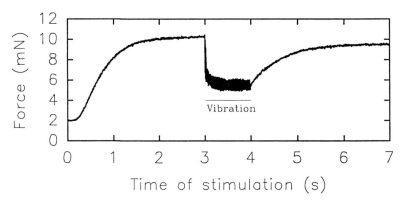

Fig. 1: Force development of the electrically stimulated rat portal vein. 3 s after onset of stimulation, force development was inhibited by length vibration, followed by force recovery after cessation of vibration.

Tonic activation: Depolarization was maintained by a bath solution in which the sodium of the Tyrode solution had been replaced equimolarly by potassium. This depolarization induced tonic contractions which reached their force maximum at about 2 min. Periods of 1 sec vibrations interrupted force generation up to 10 times during 45 min, and each post-vibration force recovery was analyzed.

Calcium depletion: The Tyrode solution was exchanged several times with a calcium-free solution (containing 0.5 mmol/l EGTA). After 10 min of calcium-free incubation, electrical field stimulation was no longer able to induce contractile responses. This was due to depletion of intracellular calcium stores.

Calcium-free depolarization: After calcium-free incubation the preparation was depolarized by a calcium-free, potassium-rich solution (containing potassium instead of sodium as well as 0.5 mmol/l EGTA). After 3 min of depolarization the contractile system was activated by adding $CaCl_2$ to the bath solution. Tonic force generation was interrupted by 1 sec vibrations up to 10 times within 45 min, and each post-vibration force recovery was analyzed.

Analysis of post-vibration force recovery: The data of force recovery were digitized by the DAS16 analogue/digital converter (Keithley Metrabyte Corp.) at a frequency of 40 Hz and stored digitally on floppy disk. By using a digital computer (80286 CPU) we fitted a monoexponential
$$F = F_{ss} - A * \exp(-t/\tau)$$
or a biexponential function
$$F = F_{ss} - A_1 * \exp(-t/\tau_1) - A_2 * \exp(-t/\tau_2)$$
to the data of force (F) and time after cessation of vibration (t). (F_{ss} represents steady state force after complete force recovery; A the amplitude and τ the time constant of force recovery; index 1 the fast and index 2 the slow component of force recovery. Visual evaluation of semilogarithmic plots as shown by [7,8] determined whether a monoexponential or a biexponential function was fitted). F_{ss} was taken as a parameter in relation to the number of attached crossbridges, and $1/\tau$ (or $1/\tau_2$) describes crossbridge kinetics [5,8]. The results are given as mean values ± standard error of the mean. Differences were significant at $p < 0.05$.

Results and discussion

1) Concentration-effect curves

We analyzed the force developed at different extracellular calcium concentrations. After the preparation had been calcium depleted, the smooth muscle was activated either by electrical field stimulation or potassium depolarization, and the calcium concentration was increased stepwise. The EC50 and the EC100 were distinctly lower for contractions induced by electrical field stimulation than for those occurring during potassium depolarization (see Fig. 2). Electrical stimulation may not only induce membrane depolarization and an increase in transmembraneous calcium influx but also an additional release of intracellularly stored calcium and a second messenger effect. We can assume that similar calcium concentrations are required to attain peak force. This maximum-effective sarcoplasmatic calcium concentration may occur at a lower extracellular calcium level during electrical field stimulation than during potassium depolarization. Sarcoplasmatic calcium concentration during longterm depolarization may depend mainly on extracellular calcium, and intracellular stored calcium as well as second messengers are definitely less effectual.

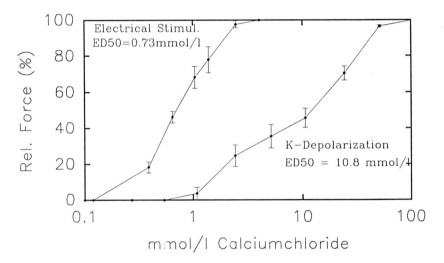

Fig. 2: Cumulative concentration effect curves of the isolated rat portal vein at various extracellular calcium concentrations. Contraction activation was carried out by electrical field stimulation or potassium-depolarization after calcium-free incubation. Data are mean values ± SEM.

2) *Contraction kinetics*

For the time constant of post-vibration force recovery the shortest value calculated was 0.64 ± 0.02 sec during electrical field stimulation (Fig. 3). This rapid force increase was analyzed 4 - 7 sec after onset of stimulation (Fig. 1). During potassium depolarization the time constant was prolonged to 1.54 ± 0.02 sec (Fig. 3) as analyzed 3 - 10 min after the onset of longterm depolarization. This increase in time constants which is typical during tonic smooth muscle activation, would seem to be independent of the activation mode (electrical field stimulation, potassium depolarization, or norepinephrine activation [5] and can be related to the extent of phosphorylation of the myosin light chains [2]. This phenomenon has been termed "down-regulation of crossbridges" by [9].

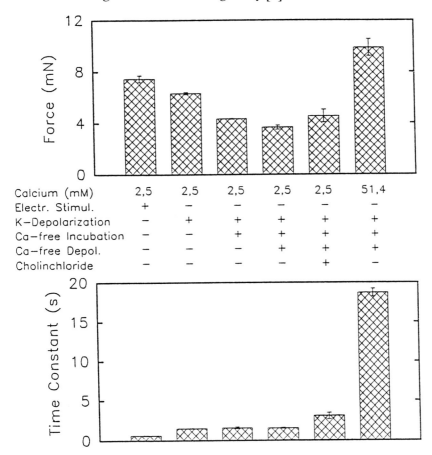

Fig. 3: Extent and rate of post-vibration force recovery of the isolated rat portal vein at different calcium concentrations and different activation modes. The preparation was activated either by electrical field stimulation or by potassium-depolarization. Incubation in calcium-free solution depleted the calcium stores, and the depolarization, induced by a calcium-free, potassium-rich solution opened calcium channels. Cholinchloride was added to produce hyperosmolarity like the addition of 51,4 mmol/l $CaCl_2$. Data are mean values ± SEM.

Retardation in the rate of force increase was explained by the formation of latchbridges i.e. noncycling or very slow cycling crossbridges [2]. As in the catch-state of the molluscan smooth muscle [6], latchbridges should be unable to reattach after detachment by vibration. During tonic contraction induced by potassium depolarization, the extent of post-vibration force recovery is fairly similar to the previbration force level. Such behaviour would argue against the existence of latchbridges. Therefore we should prefer to postulate that graded changes in the extent of phosphorylation of the myosin light chains might induce graded changes in the contraction kinetics [8].

Preceding calcium depletion of the intracellular stores decreased force development from 6.32 ± 0.09 mN to 4.35 ± 0.04 mN without any distinct changes in the time constants of post-vibration force recovery. These remained almost unchanged at 1.62 ± 0.1 sec (Fig. 3). Increasing force with unchanged time constants was also found in the rat portal vein contraction after a resting period ("staircase phenomenon") [4].

A prior 3 min calcium-free depolarization followed by the addition of 2.5 mmol/l $CaCl_2$ did not have any distinct effects on either the extent (3.69 ± 0.16 mN) or the rate ($\tau = 1.58 \pm 0.07$ sec) of post-vibration force recovery (Fig. 3). The same results were obtained after prolonging calcium-free depolarization by up to 10 min. Thus, similar contraction kinetics were calculated after sarcoplasmatic calcium increase whether or not there had been any simultaneous membrane depolarization.

In a hyperosmotic medium (77.1 mmol/l cholinchloride added to the potassium-rich Tyrode solution) force generation is increased distinctly (4.55 ± 0.49 mN) and contraction kinetics retarded ($\tau = 3.08 \pm 0.37$ sec, Fig. 3). Similar effects have been reported with the skinned preparation under dextran-induced osmotic compression [1].

The long-term depolarized portal vein produced peak force only in a Tyrode solution containing about 50 mmol/l $CaCl_2$ (Fig. 2). This high calcium concentration is osmotically effective and should be compared with the relatively slight osmotic effect of cholinchloride as mentioned above. In addition to an increase in force production up to a mean value of 9.87 ± 0.66 mN, the time constant of post-vibration force recovery also increased to 18.72 ± 0.51 sec (Fig. 3) and stabilized after about 45 min. This effect would not seem to result from osmotic compression but from a high sarcoplasmatic calcium concentration with a long-term activation of the contractile smooth muscle system. As steady-state force after complete recovery from vibration is also similar to the pre-vibration force level in these experiments, latchbridges would not seem to be involved in the process of contraction kinetics retardation. Low phosphorylation of the myosin light chains might be responsible for this effect due to low protein kinase activity and/or high phosphatase activity.

Pronounced force development in conjunction with retarded actin-myosin interaction kinetics occurring at high sarcoplasmatic calcium levels improves the efficiency of contraction distinctly. This state of the contractile system should be discussed with respect to smooth muscle spasm.

Summary

The contraction kinetics of the isolated rat portal vein were studied by analyzing the rate of force increase after cessation of force-inhibiting length vibration. The reciprocal of the time constant of post-vibration force recovery was used as a parameter of actin-myosin interaction kinetics.
1) The EC50 was 0.73 mmol/l $CaCl_2$ in the bath solution for the preparation activated by electrical field stimulation and 10.8 mmol/l $CaCl_2$ for the maintained potassium-depolarized preparation.
2) Time constants of post-vibration force recovery averaged 1.6 sec in the preparation depolarized by a potassium-rich solution containing 2.5 mmol/l $CaCl_2$. This value remained almost unchanged after prior depletion of intracellular calcium stores. Even an interval of 10 min between potassium depolarization in calcium-free solution and the subsequent addition of 2.5 mmol/l $CaCl_2$ did not change the time constants distinctly.
3) During tonic contraction induced by the maximum effective calcium-concentration of 50 mmol/l $CaCl_2$, high force development occurred with significantly retarded contraction kinetics (time constant = 18.7 sec). This behaviour was obviously not due to hyperosmolarity but may be caused by low kinase / high phosphatase activity in relation to the myosin light chain phosphorylation.

References

1. ARHEDEN, H., A. ARNER & P. HELLSTRAND (1987): Force-velocity relation and rate of ATP hydrolysis in osmotically compressed skinned smooth muscle of the guinea pig. J. Muscle Res. Cell. Mot. 8, 151-160.
2. AKSOY, M.O., S. MRAS, K.E. KAMM & R.A. MURPHY (1983): Ca^{2+}, cAMP, and changes in myosin phosphorylation during contraction of smooth muscle. Am. J. Physiol. 245, C255-C270.

3. GÜTH, K. & J. JUNGE (1982): Low Ca^{2+} impedes cross-bridge detachment in chemically skinned taenia coli. Nature 300, 775-776.
4. KLEMT, P. & U. PEIPER (1978): The dynamics of cross-bridge movement in vascular smooth muscle estimated from a single isometric contraction of the portal vein: the influence of temperature and calcium. Pflügers Arch. 378, 31-36.
5. KLEMT, P., U. PEIPER, R.N. SPEDEN & F. ZILKER (1981): The kinetics of post-vibration tension recovery of the isolated rat portal vein. J. Physiol. (Lond.) 312, 281-296.
6. LJUNG, B. & P. HALLGREN (1975): On the mechanism of inhibitory action of vibrations as studied in a molluscan catch muscle and in vertebrate smooth muscle. Acta. physiol. scand. 95, 424-430.
7. PEIPER, U. (1983): Alterations in smooth muscle contraction kinetics during tonic activation. Pflügers Arch. 399, 203-207.
8. PEIPER, U., C.F. VAHL & E. DONKER (1984): The time course of changes in contraction kinetics during the tonic activation of the rat tracheal smooth muscle. Pflügers Arch. 402, 83-87.
9. SIEGMAN, M.J., T.M. BUTLER & S.U. MOERS (1986): The use of prestimulation and variable relaxation time to prove the regulation of cross-bridge states in mammalian smooth muscle. J. Muscle Res. Cell. Mot. 7, 379-380.

Carbonic anhydrase III regulation under chronic hypoxia and creatine depletion

G. Gros, H.-W. Müller-Dethard, W. Bruns and W. Zingel

Abteilung Vegetative Physiologie, Zentrum Physiologie, Medizinische Hochschule Hannover

Summary

We present here measurements of the muscle enzymes and proteins citrate synthase, lactate dehydrogenase, myoglobin and carbonic anhydrase III in four selected hindlimb muscles: the fast tibialis anterior and extensor digitorum longus, and the slow vastus intermedius and soleus. The influence of two conditions on these enzymes was studied: severe chronic hypoxia and chronic creatine depletion. The results suggest that a) creatine depletion possibly causes a fast-to-slow fiber transformation which might, although not observed by us, eventually lead to an associated increase in CA III; and b) chronic hypoxia in rats as well as in rabbits constitutes a powerful signal for the upregulation of CA III in slow-oxidative muscle fibers. This latter increase in CA III is independent of any fiber type conversion and may represent a specific adaptation of the muscle to chronic hypoxia.

Introduction

Carbonic anhydrase III (CA III) is a cytosolic form of the carbonic anhydrase isozyme family, whose physiological role so far has eluded any clear-cut definition. It occurs at a very high concentration (up to 0.5 mM) in slow oxidative (SO) fibers of mammals, constituting there about 50 % of the cytosolic proteins, but is practically absent in fast muscles (fast-glycolytic, FG, and fast oxidative-glycolytic, FOG, fibers), as has been shown by

Geers et al. (1992) for rats and rabbits. Thus, it appears to be an unequivocal marker enzyme for SO fibers in skeletal muscles of these species.

What do we know about the possible involvement of CA III in physiological functions and its up- or down-regulation under various physiological or pathophysiological conditions? Regarding its function as an enzyme (see Gros and Dodgson, 1988), it should be noted that CA III has the lowest turn-over number of any CA isozyme known, approx. 1,000 s^{-1} versus 1,000,000 s^{-1} for the red cell isozyme CA II. Thus, its intracellular CA activity in SO muscles is moderate in spite of its extremely high concentration. Other properties are its relative resistance towards the classical sulfonamide inhibitors, and, physiologically perhaps most interesting, its phosphatase activity, which it possesses in addition to its CO_2 hydratase activity and whose presence is unique among all CA isozymes. However, no physiological substrate has so far been described for this phosphatase activity. A physiological function of CA III that has been identified, is its contribution to a facilitated intracellular CO_2 diffusion within SO fibers (Gros and Dodgson, 1988). However, Romanowski et al. (1992) have shown that even in the almost purely SO-type muscle soleus of the rabbit, other intracellular isozymes than CA III contribute to facilitated CO_2 diffusion, and that this process occurs also quite significantly in muscles in which CA III is completely lacking such as heart and the fast extensor digitorum longus (EDL). In view of this observation and the very low specific CO_2 hydratase activity of CA III, it seems doubtful whether a mere catalysis of intracellular CO_2 hydration is the only or major function of this enzyme.

A very impressive regulatory change in CA III content in muscle fibers has been reported by Gros and Dodgson (1988). During chronic electrostimulation of the fast rabbit muscles EDL and tibialis anterior (TA) a continuous increase in CA III was observed in both muscles until after a stimulation time of about 2 months CA III reached a maximum at about the 13-fold activity of that found in the unstimulated TA and EDL. This change occurs in the rabbit, although with some delay, together with increases in the enzymes of oxidative metabolism and decreases in the enzymes of anaerobic glycolysis as well as a change in the myosin pattern from the fast to the slow isoforms. Thus, the increase in CA III seems to be part of a complete program converting the fast FG and FOG fibers to slow SO fibers. Rat muscles exhibit a lesser degree of plasticity. Here, the same electrostimulation causes similar changes in the enzymes of oxidative and anaerobic metabolism but no change in the isomyosin pattern and no change in CA III expression (Jeffery et al., 1990).

The question we are asking here is: under what physiological conditions and by which trigger signals is CA III up- or down-regulated? Is the up-regulation of CA III merely part of rigid program turning a fast into a slow fiber, or can conditions be found under which the regulation of CA III dissociates from the regulation of the other components characterizing fast and slow muscles, respectively? Searching for answers to these questions, we have studied here two situations: 1) we have fed rabbits chronically the creatine analogue β-guanidino-propionic acid (GPA), which causes a decrease in muscle creatine phosphate and ATP, and 2) we have exposed rats and rabbits chronically to simulated high altitude and studied the ensuing changes in metabolic enzymes and CA III of their skeletal muscles. These two experiments aim at elucidating the role of two often-discussed candidates for the induction of muscle fiber-type conversion, i) pO_2 and ii) status of the energy-rich phosphates.

Methods

Creatine analogue feeding

The creatine analogue was synthesized according to Rowley et al. (1971) and recrystallized until pure as judged by thin layer chromatography. Rabbits were fed for 6 weeks on pellets that had been supplemented with 1 % of the creatine analogue β-guanidino-propionic acid, GPA. The effect of GPA feeding was monitored by repeated determination of the plasma level of creatinine, which fell from a control value of 95 µM to 55 µM towards the end of the feeding period. The body weight of the control group (6 rabbits) was 2.20 kg before the feeding period, and 3.08 kg after the feeding period; the body weight of the experimental group (also 6 rabbits) was 2.23 kg before the feeding experiment and 3.05 kg after 6 weeks' GPA feeding. Thus the growth of the animals did not seem to be affected by the GPA feeding. Nevertheless, two parameters indicated that protein biosynthesis was reduced in the treated animals: the relative muscle dry weight was reduced in GPA-fed animals to 22.5 % (S.D. ± 1.0 %) compared to the control value of 24.1 % (± 0.5 %); and hematocrit was reduced to 33.8 % (± 1.2 %) from a control level of 36.5 % (± 1.6 %).

Simulated high altitude in rats

12 Han Wistar rats were exposed for 6 weeks to a simulated altitude of 6000 m in a hypobaric chamber, 12 rats of identical age served as a control group. The average body weight of the rats was 210 (S.D. ± 3) g at the start of the experiment. Every three days the pressure in the chamber was slowly increased until sea level conditions were reached, and the door was opened to clean the cages and supply the animals with fresh water and pellets. Subsequently, the pressure was lowered again within a few hours. After the 6 weeks' experimental period, the control group had gained 8 % in body weight, the hypoxic group only 3.2 %. The relative dry weight of the muscle sartorius was 24.5 % in the control group and 25.6 % in the hypoxic group, possibly indicating some degree of exsiccation in the hypoxic animals. The following acis-base status was observed in the control group: $pH_a = 7.33 \pm 0.04$, B.E. = + 0.7 ± 3.1 mM, and in the hypoxic group after removal from the hypobaric chamber: $pH_a = 7.22 \pm 0.05$, B.E. = - 5.8 ± 2.5 mM. As expected, the blood hemoglobin concentration rose from 14.7 (± 1) g % in the control group to 18 (± 1.3) g % in the hypoxic group.

Simulated high altitude in rabbits

Four New Zealand White rabbits were exposed for six weeks to a simulated high altitude of 6000 m as above, four rabbits served as a control group. At the beginning of the experiment the control group's average body weight was 2.9 kg, after the six weeks experimental period it had risen to 3.3 kg. Before the start of the experiment, the hypoxic group's body weight averaged 2.5 kg, after 6 weeks hypoxia it had fallen to 2.3 kg. The relative dry weight of the muscle peroneus longus was 26.4 % in the control group and 24.7 in the hypoxic group, possibly suggesting a reduced protein synthesis in the hypoxic animals. The B.E. value was - 2.2 mM in the control group and - 8.8 mM in the hypoxic animals. The increase in blood red cells during simulated high altitude was more pronounced than in the identically treated rats: hematocrit rose from 39 % in the control group to 74 % in the hypoxic group.

Preparation of muscle homogenate

Animals were anesthetized and the following muscles removed, cut into small pieces and rapidly frozen in liquid N_2: the two fast muscles consisting essentially of FG and FOG fibers, EDL and TA, and the two slow muscles, soleus (SOL, almost completely SO type) and vastus intermedius (VA, with a high proportion of SO fibers). Homogenisation was achieved by powderizing the frozen muscle pieces in a Mikrodismembrator (Braun, Melsungen, Germany). To half of the powder obtained for each pair of muscles Triton X-100 at a final concentration of 1 % was added, the other half remained without Triton. Both samples were centrifuged for 1 hr. at 100,000 g, and the supernatant containing the cytosolic proteins and representing the nearly undiluted cytosol was removed, frozen in liquid N_2 and stored at -80 °C. The supernatants containing Triton were used for the determination of citrate synthase (CS) and CA, the samples without detergent for the measurement of lactate dehydrogenase (LDH) and myoglobin (Mb).

Biochemical assays

Carbonic anhydrase was measured using Maren's micromethod as modified by Bruns and Gros (1991) with the carbonate-bicarbonate buffer system. CA III was determined by performing the assay in the presence of $5 \cdot 10^{-6}$ M acetazolamide, which inhibits completely all other CA isoforms present in muscle but leaves CA III unaffected. - Citrate synthase CS and lactate dehydrogenase LDH were determined by optically coupled tests as described by Bass et al. (1969). - Myoglobin was determined spectrophotometrically as described by Reynafarje (1963). The wavelengths employed were 538 nm and 568 nm, and [Mb] in mM was obtained from $(A_{538} - A_{568}) \cdot 0.355$. - Protein concentrations of the supernatants were measured by Lowry's method using the Sigma kit including the precipitation step and the use of deoxycholate. - CrP and ATP in muscle tissue were determined as described by Bergmeyer (1985); other details see Geers and Gros (1990).

Table 1: Energy-rich phosphates in rabbit muscles after creatine analogue feeding (in mmoles/kg wet weight)

The muscle tissue concentrations of creatine phosphate, [CrP], and ATP, [ATP], are given for four hindlimb muscles of rabbits. The rabbits had been fed on pellets that contained 1 % of the creatine analogue β-guanidino-propionic acid, GPA, for 6 weeks. Each group, control and GPA-fed, consisted of 6 animals. Given are means ± standard deviation.

	[CrP]		[ATP]	
	Controls	GPA - fed	Controls	GPA - fed
Tibialis anterior, **TA**	**21.9** ± 5.4	**4.4** ± 1.6	**5.6** ± 1.6	**2.9** ± 0.9
Extensor digitorum longus, **EDL**	**27.1** ± 5.2	**4.7** ± 1.6	**6.0** ± 2.5	**2.6** ± 0.6
Vastus intermedius, **VA**	**11.4** ± 2.7	**4.3** ± 1.7	**2.9** ± 1.7	**2.0** ± 0.3
Soleus, **SOL**	**15.9** ± 11.8	**4.4** ± 1.1	**4.3** ± 2.6	**2.3** ± 0.5

Results

Effects of creatine depletion on rabbit muscle enzymes

Table 1 shows the effects of 6 weeks' GPA feeding of rabbits on energy-rich phosphates in four hindlimb muscles. Compared to the respective control muscles, the contents of creatine phosphate, CrP, and ATP are markedly lower in all muscles from treated animals. [CrP] is 1/5 to 1/3 of the control value in both fast and slow muscles after the treatment with GPA. Similarly, [ATP] is reduced to about 1/2 of the control value in all muscles studied. The decrease in CrP is due to the replacement of most of the muscles' creatine with GPA, which is also a substrate of creatine kinase, but whose rate of dephosphorylation is extremely slow so that it is not available as a physiologically accessible energy store (Meyer et al., 1986). The deficiency in CrP appears to be the cause of the decrease in ATP, and this very likely, although not proven by the present data, represents a decrease in the muscle cells' phosphorylation potential.

Table 2: Muscle enzymes in rabbits after 6 weeks creatine analogue feeding

The four hindlimb muscles tibialis anterior, TA, extensor digitorum longus, EDL, Vastus intermedius, VA, and soleus, SOL, were studied. All measurements were done on the undiluted homogenate supernatant from these muscles. Given are, as means ± S.D., the total protein concentration of the supernatants in mg/ml, the activity of carbonic anhydrase III in U (where one unit U is defined as the factor by which the CO_2 hydration reaction is accelerated in the supernatant under the conditions of the assay employed, minus 1), the specific activity of CA III, CA III_{sp} (= activity per protein concentration), the specific activities of lactate dehydrogenase, LDH_{sp}, and citrate synthase, CS_{sp}, and the specific concentration of myoglobin, Mb_{sp}. The latter three were also obtained by dividing the absolute activities or concentrations in the undiluted supernatant, respectively, by the total protein concentration of the supernatant. Statistical significance was tested by the unpaired Student's t-test, levels of significance of differences between experimental and control groups are indicated as follows: * $P < 0.05$, ** $P < 0.02$, *** $P < 0.01$.

	Protein (mg/ml)	CA III (U)	CA III_{sp} (U·ml/mg)	LDH_{sp} (U/mg)	CS_{sp} (U/mg)	$Myogl._{sp}$ (mmol/g) x 10^{-4}
TA, control	88 ± 7	4.6 ± 0.9	0.05 ± 0.02	18 ± 2	0.15 ± 0.02	7.2 ± 0.5
TA, GPA	77 ± 8	5.1 ± 0.4	0.07 ± 0.01	14 ± 2 ***	0.20 ± 0.02 ***	9.1 ± 1.3 **
EDL, control	86 ± 9	7.8 ± 1.7	0.09 ± 0.03	17 ± 2	0.10 ± 0.01	8.0 ± 0.9
EDL, GPA	79 ± 10	7.4 ± 0.3	0.10 ± 0.01	16 ± 2	0.15 ± 0.04 **	7.3 ± 1.6
VA, control	64 ± 12	350 ± 130	5.9 ± 2.6	5.4 ± 2.1	0.19 ± 0.05	35 ± 13
VA, GPA	59 ± 7	360 ± 70	6.2 ± 1.3	5.2 ± 3.9	0.22 ± 0.02	31 ± 6
SOL, control	56 ± 2	390 ± 40	6.9 ± 0.6	3.9 ± 0.6	0.22 ± 0.05	43 ± 6
SOL, GPA	51 ± 2	380 ± 30	7.4 ± 0.4	3.2 ± 0.7	0.21 ± 0.04	43 ± 3

Table 2 shows how the chronic changes in energy-rich phosphates affect a number of muscle enzymes and proteins: 1) in the muscle homogenate supernatants of all GPA-fed rabbits the total protein concentration is about 10 % lower than for the control muscles. This agrees with the suggestion of a reduced protein biosynthesis derived above from the observations of a reduced muscle dry weight and a reduced hematocrit in the treated animals. 2) The activity of CA III shows no significant changes in any of the muscles studied, and this still holds when the specific CA III activity, CA III$_{sp}$, i.e. the CA III activity per total protein concentration, is considered, although the latter seems to show a tendency to increase in all muscles studied (see column 3 of Tab. 2). In some cases the specific activities for the two fast muscles show signs of a shift from an anaerobic to an oxidative state of metabolism: the specific activity of the mitochondrial marker enzyme citrate synthase is significantly increased for both fast muscles, and in the case of TA specific myoglobin concentration is increased while specific LDH activity is significantly reduced. No significant changes are observed in the two slow muscles VA and SOL. In conclusion, creatine depletion does not cause significant changes in the slow rabbit muscles, but it causes a moderate shift from anaerobic to oxidative metabolic properties in the fast rabbit muscles. However, this shift, in contrast to what is observed during chronic electrostimulation, is not associated with a clearcut increase in CA III.

Effects of chronic hypoxia on rat muscle enzymes

The response to simulated high altitude seen in rat muscles is quite different to what has been seen in the muscles of GPA-fed rabbits (Tab. 3). Although in one single muscle, SOL, chronic hypoxia produced a significant increase in the mitochondrial marker CS, no effect was detectable in all other muscles. Myoglobin increased in VA and TA significantly and perhaps shows a tendency to do so in SOL and EDL. Taken together, this may indicate a weak increase in oxidative capacity of the muscles under hypoxia and insofar is comparable to the observations with GPA-fed rabbits (although in the latter all these observations were restricted to fast muscles). The major deviation from the results with GPA-fed rabbits is that the extreme hypoxia applied here produces in SOL, VA and TA a highly significant increase in LDH indicating a clear increase in anaerobic associated with the weaker increase in oxidative capacity. Thus, the response observed here cannot be interpreted as a fast-glycolytic to slow-oxidative fiber transition. It is most remarkable that under these conditions there is a highly significant increase in CA III activity in both slow muscles SOL and VA, by 20 % and 22 %, respectively, but clearly no change in CA III of TA and EDL. Again, this is in contrast to chronic electrostimulation, which causes a drastic increase in CA III in *fast* muscle fibers.

Table 3: Muscle enzymes in rats after 6 weeks simulated high altitude at 6000 m.

The same muscles as in rabbits were investigated for the same proteins and enzymes (see Table 2). Absolute activities and concentrations are given as means ± S.D. Control and hypoxic group consisted of 12 rats each. Levels of significance are indicated as in Table 2.

	CA III (U)	LDH (U/ml)	CS (U/ml)	Myoglobin (mM)
TA, control	84 ± 22	1240 ± 250	13.7 ± 3	0.18 ± 0.02
TA, hypoxia	83 ± 18	1890 ± 290 ***	16 ± 1.3	0.20 ± 0.02 *
EDL, control	40 ± 7	560 ± 150	5.5 ± 2.2	0.12 ± 0.06
EDL, hypoxia	38 ± 6	450 ± 100	4.6 ± 1.3	0.16 ± 0.03
VA, control	322 ± 59	550 ± 230	17.5 ± 3.5	0.27 ± 0.04
VA, hypoxia	392 ± 32 **	1100 ± 250 **	18.7 ± 2.7	0.33 ± 0.04 **
SOL, control	1160 ± 130	144 ± 77	6.8 ± 2.5	0.27 ± 0.07
SOL, hypoxia	1390 ± 160 **	258 ± 100 *	11.8 ± 2.8 **	0.29 ± 0.03

Effects of chronic hypoxia on rabbit muscle enzymes

Since it is known that rabbit muscles show a greater degree of plasticity under chronic electrostimulation than rat muscles (Jeffery et al., 1990; Pette and Vrbova, 1992), it was interesting to compare the effects of chronic hypoxia on rat with those on rabbit skeletal muscles. The results for the latter are summarized in Table 4. 6000 m must be considered an extreme altitude for rabbits, so it was not surprising that this treatment led to a loss of body weight plus to a decrease in muscle dry weight, indicating a pronounced catabolic situation of these animals. This is also reflected in the fact that both fast muscles from hypoxic animals exhibit a lower protein concentration in their homogenate supernatant than control muscles. This is not so in slow muscles, for reasons that will become evident from the discussion of the behaviour of CA III that follows below. Table 4 shows that the metabolic marker enzymes are affected quite differently from what

Table 4: Muscle enzymes in rabbits after 6 weeks simulated high altitude at 6000 m.

The same muscles and the same enzymes and proteins were studied as in Table II. Absolute activities and concentrations are given as means ± S.D. Control and hypoxic group consisted of 4 animals each. Levels of statistical significance are given as explained in Table 2.

	Protein (mg/ml)	CA III (U)	LDH (U/ml)	CS (U/ml)	Myoglobin (mM)
TA, control	101 ± 13	6.8 ± 2.5	1700 ± 200	11 ± 2	0.07 ± 0.01
TA, hypoxia	89 ± 17	12.2 ± 3.1 *	1400 ± 300	7 ± 3	0.05 ± 0.01 *
EDL, control	75 ± 6	6.0 ± 4.5	1800 ± 300	7.6 ± 0.9	0.11 ± 0.02
EDL, hypoxia	67 ± 8	10.9 ± 1.8	1200 ± 300	6.1 ± 2.5	0.09 ± 0.01
VA, control	50 ± 6	390 ± 30	320 ± 100	13 ± 2	0.22 ± 0.04
VA, hypoxia	57 ± 3	470 ± 20 ***	190 ± 40	11 ± 3	0.26 ± 0.04
SOL, control	34 ± 5	330 ± 30	200 ± 60	10 ± 3	0.22 ± 0.05
SOL, hypoxia	40 ± 7	550 ± 30 ***	150 ± 30	7 ± 1	0.26 ± 0.06

we saw for hypoxic rat muscles: although no significant changes of LDH and CS appear in Table 4, it is apparent that in every single muscle LDH as well as CS are lower in the hypoxic animals than in controls. Mb also tends to decrease in the fast muscles, but may rise a little in the slow muscles. Overall, the severely catabolic situation of the hypoxic rabbits appears to lead to a loss of enzymes associated with anaerobic as well as with oxidative metabolism. Quite in contrast to this is the behaviour of CA III: it increases under hypoxia in all muscles studied, by 80 % in TA, 82 % in EDL, 21 % in VA and by 67 % in SOL. However, while the changes observed in the two fast muscles are very small on an absolute scale and by far not comparable to the 13-fold change observed under chronic electrostimulation (Gros and Dodgson, 1988), the changes in the two slow muscles VA and SOL are enormous if it is considered that already under control conditions CA III makes up a fraction of the cytosolic proteins of these muscles which is in the order of 50 %. It is understandable then that in spite of the loss of other proteins total protein concentration increases in these two slow muscles. A likely interpretation of this behaviour of CA III in rabbit muscles seems to be that chronic hypoxia induces CA III markedly in SO fibers, which already have it in high amounts, but not in FOG and FG fibers, which lack this enzyme (Geers et al., 1992). The very small proportion of SO fibers in TA and EDL would then explain the small absolute increase in CA III in these fast muscles, and the dominant presence of SO fibers in rabbit SOL and VA would explain the dramatic absolute increase in CA III in these two slow muscles.

Discussion

What can we conclude from the above data on the effects of creatine depletion and chronic hypoxia with respect to the following two questions? 1) Does either of these two conditions induce a fast-anaerobic to slow-oxidative fiber conversion ? In other words, is creatine depletion and/or hypoxia a trigger signal for fast-to-slow fiber type transition? 2) Does either of these two conditions constitute a trigger signal for induction of CA III? And if so, does CA III change in the context of a general fast-to-slow transformation or is it regulated separately and thus has possibly tasks that do not necessarily coincide with those fulfilled by a slow muscle?

Fast-to-slow fiber transformation

An important criterion for such a transformation is a change in the pattern of isomyosins, which has not been studied here. However, other characteristic features of this transformation, as mentioned above, are an increase in oxidative capacity (and thus CS) and a decrease in anaerobic-glycolytic capacity (and thus LDH), and also a drastic increase in CA III (Gros and Dodgson, 1988). Are any of these latter criteria fulfilled for chronic hypoxia? Let us first consider the *rat muscles* (Table 3). The changes that are significant are i) an increase in CS, ii) an increase in LDH, and iii) an increase in CA III in the slow but not the fast muscles. Since especially the increases in LDH are quite convincing, and since CA III does not increase in fast muscles, these changes cannot be part of a program transforming fast to slow fibers. Rather, the regulation of the two metabolic enzymes CS and LDH can be viewed as a reasonable response of the muscle to a very severe hypoxia, which does not, however, result in a catabolic situation. The rats in these experiments still continued to grow, although at a reduced rate. It may be noted that an increase in mitochondrial density or mitochondrial marker enzymes such as CS under hypoxia has previously been reported by several authors (Tappan et al., 1964; Holm et al., 1972; Holm et al., 1973; Bylund et al., 1976; Gimenez et al., 1977; Hoppeler et al., 1981; Elander at al., 1984, 1985).

Does hypoxia induce a fast-to-slow transformation in *rabbit muscles*? Although hypoxia causes here an increase in CA III in all muscles studied, we do not observe the inverse regulation of CS and LDH that is characteristic for fast-to-slow conversion, but instead both CS and LDH decrease markedly and consistently, if not significantly, in all muscles studied. Rather than of a fiber-type transformation, this seems to be indicative of the catabolic situation of the rabbits, for which the hypoxia employed is extreme. Again, similar combinations of decreases in enzymes of both oxidative and anaerobic metabolism have been observed previously, especially under conditions of simultaneous hypoxia and physical exercise (Green et al., 1989; and decreases of mitochondrial markers alone by Howald et al., 1990; Hoppeler et al., 1990). We conclude that in neither species, rat nor rabbit, the effects of chronic hypoxia observed by us indicate a fast-to-slow fiber transformation. We have no evidence, therefore, that hypoxia is a stimulus for this process.

Does creatine depletion, or the decrease in energy-rich phosphates associated with it, cause a fast-to-slow muscle transformation? In the fast rabbit muscles (Table 2) we find an increase in CS and a decrease in LDH, a pattern compatible with such a transition (it should be noted that an increase in mitochondrial enzymes under GPA treatment has also previously been reported by Shoubridge et al., 1985). That CA III, although it shows a tendency to increase, does so not significantly, may be due to the slower time course of the rise in CA III compared to the changes in CS and LDH. While CA III responds to a transforming stimulus such as electrostimulation with a time delay of about three weeks, CS and LDH have during this time already reached a new final plateau value (Gros and Dodgson, 1988). Thus, it is conceivable that a fiber transformation indeed occurs under creatine depletion, but that the time of exposure of the animals was not sufficient in the present study for the change in CA III to become significant. In line with this is the observation of Kushmerick et al. (1990) of significant shifts in the isomyosin pattern of mice under GPA treatment, e.g. showing an increased expression of slow myosin in soleus. Definite proof of a fiber tranformation in rabbits under creatine depletion has to await studies of the myosin pattern after a perhaps extended GPA exposure. If this were confirmed, it would indicate that the intracellular concentrations of high-energy phosphate compounds, or some other signal dependent on them, constitute a trigger for fiber transformation.

Regulation of CA III

We have tentatively concluded that creatine depletion may lead to an increase in CA III when this condition is maintained for a longer period than the present 6 weeks. If so, however, this would very likely occur in association with a general fast-to-slow fiber transformation. In this process, the up-regulation of CA III is one element of a program by which practically the entire muscle cell is regenerated (Pette and Vrbova, 1992). The present data show another situation which leads to a massive increase in CA III without causing a fast-to-slow fiber transformation: chronic hypoxia. In rats and even much more in rabbits, severe chronic hypoxia causes a clear-cut increase in CA III in slow muscles. It appears likely that this up-regulation of CA III is restricted to SO fibers and does not occur in FG and FOG fibers. Since especially the rabbit soleus consists nearly of 100 % SO fibers, a fast-to-slow fiber transition can clearly not be involved in this up-regulation.

It is tempting to speculate that CA III in some way helps to save energy (and/or oxygen) in these slow fibers. It is entirely unclear how CA III could achieve this. But the idea is supported by the recent observation of Geers et al. (1995) showing that CA inhibitors in concentrations sufficiently high to block CA III cause an increase in O_2 consumption of the rat soleus (which is high in CA III) but not the rat EDL (which nearly lacks CA III). Accordingly, an active CA III would reduce the O_2 consumption of SO fibers. A conceivable basis for such a phenomenon might be the phosphatase activity of CA III possibly dephosphorylating and inactivating some crucial enzyme linked to energy metabolism.

References

1. BASS, A., D. BRDICZKA, P. EYER, S. HOFER & D. PETTE (1969): Metabolic differentiation of distinct muscle types at the level of enzymatic organization. Eur. J. Biochem. 10, 198-206.
2. BERGMEYER, H.U., ed. (1985): Methods of Enzymatic Analysis, VCH, Weinheim.
3. BRUNS, W. & G. GROS. (1991): Modified micromethod for assay of carbonic anhydrase activity. In: The Carbonic Anhydrases: Cellular Physiology and Molecular Genetics, DODGSON, S.J., R.E. TASHIAN, G. GROS & N.D. CARTER, eds. Plenum Publishing, New York, pp. 127-132.
4. BYLUND, A.-C., J. HAMMERSTEN, J. HOLM & T. SCHERSTEN (1976): Enzyme activities in skeletal muscles from patients with peripheral arterial insufficiency. Eur. J. Clin. Invest. 6, 425-429.
5. ELANDER, A., J.-P. IDSTRÖM, S. HOLM, T. SCHERSTEN & A.-C. BYLUND-FELLENIUS (1984): Metabolic adaptation in response to intermittent hypoxia in rat skeletal muscles. Adv. Exp. Med. Biol. 169, 507-513.
6. ELANDER, A., J.-P. IDSTRÖM, T. SCHERSTEN & A.-C. BYLUND-FELLENIUS (1985): Metabolic adaptation to reduced muscle blood flow. I. Enzyme and metabolite alterations. Am. J. Physiol. 249, E63-E69.
7. GEERS, C. & G. GROS (1990): Effects of carbonic anhydrase inhibitors on contraction, intracellular pH and energy-rich phosphates of rat skeletal muscle. J. Physiol. 423, 279-297.
8. GEERS, C., D. KRÜGER, W. SIFFERT, A, SCHMID, W. BRUNS & G. GROS (1992): Carbonic anhydrase in skeletal and cardiac muscle from rabbit and rat. Biochem. J. 282, 165-171.
9. GEERS, C., K. BENZ & G. GROS (1995): Effects of carbonic anhydrase inhibitors on oxygen consumption and lactate accumalation in skeletal muscle. Comp. Biochem. Physiol. in the press.
10. GIMENEZ, M., R.J. SANDERSON, O.K. REISS & N. BANCHERO (1977): Effects of altitude on myoglobin and mitochondrial protein in canine skeletal muscle. Resp. Physiol. 34, 171-176.
11. GREEN, H.J., J.R. SUTTON, A. CYMERMAN, P.M. YOUNG & C.S. HOUSTON (1989): Operation Everest II: adaptation in human skeletal muscle. J. Appl. Physiol. 66, 2454-2461.
12. GROS, G. & S.J. DODGSON (1988): Velocity of CO_2 exchange in muscle and liver. Ann. Rev. Physiol. 50, 669-694.
13. HOLM, J., P. BJÖRNTORP & T. SCHERSTEN (1972): Metabolic activity in human skeletal muscle. Eur. J. Clin. Invest. 2, 321-325.
14. HOLM, J., P. BJÖRNTORP & T. SCHERSTEN (1973): Metabolic activity in rat skeletal muscle. Eur. J. Clin. Invest. 3, 279-283.
15. HOPPELER, H., O. MATHIEU, R. KRAUER, H. CLAASSEN, R.B. ARMSTRONG & E.R. WEIBEL (1981): Design of the mammalian respiratory system. VI. Distribution of mitochondria and capillaries in various muscles. Resp. Physiol. 44, 87-111.
16. HOPPELER, H., E. KLEINERT, C. SCHLEGEL, H. CLAASSEN, H. HOWALD, S.R. KAYAR & P. CERRETELLI (1990): Morphological adaptations of human skeletal muscle to chronic hypoxia. Int. J. Sports Med. 11, S3-S9.
17. HOWALD, H., D. PETTE, J.-A. SIMONEAU, A. UBER, H. HOPPELER & P. CERRETELLI (1990): Effects of chronic hypoxia on muscle enzyme activities. Int. J. Sports Med. 11, S10-S14.

18. JEFFERY, S., C.D. KELLY, N. CARTER, M KAUFMANN, A. TERMIN & D. PETTE (1990): Chronic stimulation-induced effects point to a coordinated expression of carbonic anhydrase III and slow myosin heavy chain in skeletal muscle. FEBS Lett. 262, 225-227.
19. KUSHMERICK, M.J., T.S. MOERLAND & N.G. WOLF (1990): Adaptive changes in myosin isoforms and in energy metabolism in muscles containing analogues of creatine as the phosphagen. In: The Dynamic State of Muscle Fibers, ed. PETTE, D. De Gruyter, Berlin-New York, pp. 551-566.
20. MEYER, R.A., T.R. BROWN, B.L. KRILOWICZ & M.J. KUSHMERICK (1986): Phosphagen and intracellular pH changes during contraction of creatine-depleted rat muscle. Am. J. Physiol. 250, C264-C274.
21. PETTE, D.& G. VRBOVA (1992): Adaptation of mammalian skeletal muscle fibers to chronic electrical stimulation. Rev. Physiol. Biochem. Pharmacol. 120, 115-202.
22. REYNAFARJE, B. (1963): Simplified method for the determination of myoglobin. J. Lab. Clin. Med. 61, 138-145.
23. ROMANOWSKI, F., J. SCHIERENBECK & G. GROS (1992): Facilitated CO_2 diffusion in various striated muscles. In: Quantitative Spectroscopy in Tissue. Eds. K. FRANK & M. KESSLER, Frankfurt/M, pp. 205-211.
24. ROWLEY, G.L., A.L. REENLEAF & G.L. KENYON (1971): On the specificity of creatine kinase. New glycocyamines and glycocyamine analogs related to creatine. J. Am. Chem. Soc. 93, 5542-5551.
25. SHOUBRIDGE, E.A., R.A.J. CHALLISS, D.J. HAYES & G.K. RADDA (1985): Biochemical adaptation in the skeletal muscle of rats depleted of creatine with the substrate analogue β-guanidinopropionic acid. Biochem. J. 232, 125-131.
26. TAPPAN, D.V., B. REYNAFARJE, R. VAN POTTER & A. HURTADO (1957): Alterations in enzymes and metabolites resulting from adaptation to low oxygen tensions. Am. J. Physiol. 190, 93-98.

Quantitation of erythropoietin messenger RNA in organs of the rat

J. Fandrey* and H. F. Bunn*

Department of Physiology, University of Bonn* and Division of Hematology/Oncology Harvard Medical School**

Introduction

The glycoprotein hormone erythropoietin (Epo) regulates the proliferation and terminal differentiation of erythroid progenitors in the bone marrow. For maintenance of normal erythropoiesis low level constitutive Epo production is required. Arterial hypoxia or anemia with decreased tissue oxygen tension induce Epo production in the kidney and liver resulting in enhanced output of erythrocytes from the bone marrow and increased oxygen transport capacity of the blood [1]. Following hypoxic stress Epo mRNA levels in the kidneys rise [2-4] as a result of enhanced Epo gene transcription [5]. For a better understanding of the transduction pathway from low oxygen tension to enhanced Epo gene expression a means of accurately quantitating Epo mRNA is required. Conventional methods of mRNA analysis such as Northern blot and "dot blot" hybridization permit only crude quantitation of mRNA. The sensitivity of these methods is too low to detect Epo mRNA in uninduced cells or a small number of cells. In contrast ribonuclease protection assay has provided specific and accurate quantitation of low levels of Epo mRNA [6].

Because of its high sensitivity the polymerase chain reaction (PCR) has been widely used to amplify cDNA copies of low abundance mRNA [7]. We have adapted competitive PCR for the quantitation of Epo mRNA from rat tissue. Coamplification of a competitive template circumvents the main constraint in obtaining quantitative data inherent in the exponential product increase with PCR [8]. Our accurate measurements of Epo mRNA provide new insights on critical aspects of Epo gene regulation including the tissue distribution of mRNA expression for different degrees of anemia.

Methods

Male Sprague-Dawley rats weighing 200-250 g were purchased from the Charles River Laboratories (Wilmington, MA). Different degrees of anemia were induced by single or repeated i.p. injections of phenylhydrazine (60 mg/kg body weight). Seven hours to four days after the last injection of phenylhydrazine the rats were bled to death from the dorsal aorta under ether anesthesia. Kidneys, liver, spleen, heart and lungs were removed and snap-frozen in liquid nitrogen. Hematocrits were determined in quadruplicate by spinning microcapillaries in a hematocrit centrifuge. Epo protein was measured by a sensitive radioimmunoassay as decribed [9]. The frozen organs were weighed and homogenized in 4 M guanidinium isothiocyanate with 0.1 M β-mercaptoethanol and 10 % N-lauryl-sarcosine using a Polytron homogenizer (Kinematica GmbH, Luzern, Switzerland) at setting 10 for 15 s. Total RNA was isolated by CsCl centrifugation as described [10], redissolved in water and the concentration determined by absorption at 260 nm.

Competitive polymerase chain reaction (PCR) was performed as previously described [11]. In brief, five micrograms of total RNA were reverse transcribed into first strand cDNA using oligo dT [15] as a primer for reverse transcriptase (M-MLRV RT Superscript; Gibco, Eggenstein, FRG). In all experiments the presence of possible contaminating genomic DNA from the cells, cDNA from previous PCRs or plasmid DNA was excluded by control reactions. Amplification was carried out on samples in which 1) reverse transcriptase was omitted from the reverse transcription reaction mixture or 2) no RNA was added to the reaction mixture.

PCR was performed in 1 x PCR-Buffer (10 mM Tris-HCl, pH 8.3; 50 mM KCl; 1.5 mM $MgCl_2$; 0.01 % wt/vol gelatine), 200 μM of each dNTP (Pharmacia, Freiburg, FRG), 30 pmol of each 5' and 3' primer and 5 units/ml of Taq polymerase (Gibco) in a final volume of 100 l. To each tube one microliter of cDNA of unknown concentration and one microliter of a dilution series containing known amounts of a mutant competitor (see below) were added. PCR was then carried out for 35 cycles after an initial denaturation for 3 min at 94 °C. The amplification profile of each cycle consisted of denaturation at 94 °C for 1 min, primer annealing at 58 °C for 1 min 30 s and elongation at 72 °C for 3 min.

The mutant competitor DNA (mutDNA) was prepared by site-directed mutagenesis in the fifth exon of genomic Epo DNA [12]. By introducing 3 base pairs (bp) mutations an AccI restriction site was ablated and a Hind III site a few base pairs upstream created. The same pair of primers amplified cDNA and mutDNA fragments in the PCR in which they competed for available PCR substrates. With an equal efficiency of amplification for the cDNA and the mutDNA the ratio of products remained constant through the amplification process. By titrating an unknown amount of cDNA template against a dilution series of known concentrations of mutDNA an equivalence point was reached where the starting concentration of the mutDNA and the cDNA had been the same [8].

Identification of the amplified products was achieved by digesting the PCR products with restriction enzymes AccI and HindIII (Gibco, Eggenstein, FRG). Whereas the cDNA derived products were cut with AccI, only the mutDNA products were digested by HindIII. The cut DNA-fragments were subsequently separated on a 2 % agarose gel, stained with ethidium bromide (0.5 µg/µl) and visualized under UV-light.

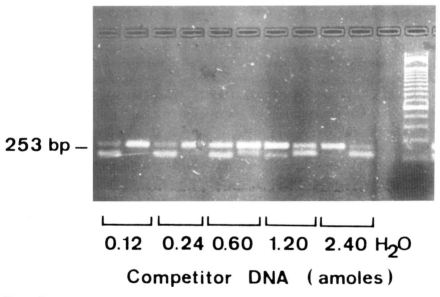

Fig. 1: Example of quantitation of Epo mRNA from 5 µg of total RNA from a kidney of a rat with anemia (hematocrit = 0.18). Lane 1 from right represents a molecular weight marker (100 bp-ladder). The lanes are in pair-wise order, i.e. lane 1 from left shows the PCR product cut with Acc I, lane 2 cut with Hind III from the same PCR reaction with 0.12 amol of competitor DNA added. The equivalence point of this titration is between 0.6 and 1.2 amoles.

Such a gel is shown in Fig. 1. The uncut PCR product appears as a band of 253 base pairs (bp) reflecting the amplified DNA-fragment spanned by the pair of primers. When wild type cDNA in the PCR reaction was in excess it was preferentially amplified. Accordingly most of the product could be cut with AccI. On the ethidium bromide stained gel a 201 bp fragment appeared in the lane loaded with AccI cut DNA (lane 1 from left) whereas the full length 253 bp fragment remained uncut by HindIII (lane 2 from left). With an input excess of competitor mutDNA, however, the opposite pattern was observed: the 253 bp full length fragment in the AccI lane (lane 4 from right) and the cut 215 bp fragment in the HindIII lane (lane 3 from right). If the PCR products were equally cut with AccI and HindIII the amount of input cDNA and mutDNA were the same.

Results and discussion

Quantitation of Epo mRNA from different organs of the rat was achieved by competitive PCR. As shown in Table 1 Epo mRNA was detectable in kidneys, liver and spleens from non-anemic animals.

Table 1: Organ distribution of Epo mRNA

	non-anemic	moderately anemic	severely anemic
Kidneys (amol)	6 ± 3	85.3 ± 15	786 ± 185
Liver (amol)	2.5 ± 1*	26.5 ± 4	151 ± 56
Spleen (amol)	1.2 ± 1	n.d.	2.1 ± 1
Lung (amol)	0	0	0.9
Heart (amol)	0	0	0

n.d. = not determined; values are the mean ± SD

Lowering the hematocrit led to an exponential rise in the Epo mRNA levels in the kidneys as shown in figure 2. In animals with severe anemia (hct 0.15) there was a 300-fold induction compared to non-anemic animals. Tan et al. [6] demonstrated a 150-fold elevation of Epo mRNA in rats exposed to hypoxic hypoxia (7 % O_2). They detected reproducible signals from normoxic control kidneys which they quantified by ribonuclease protection assay. While the sensitivity of their assay was comparable to what we obtained the ribonuclease protection assay requires 50 to 100 fold more RNA than competitive PCR. Moreover the usage of radioactive compounds is not required for competitive PCR and thus beside special precautions in

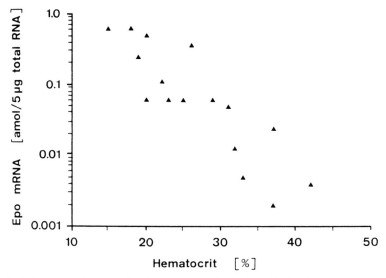

Fig. 2: Relationship between the degree of anemia in phenylhydrazine treated rats and the level of Epo mRNA in the kidney (r = -0.71; P < 0.01; n = 16; r = correlation coefficient; P = level of significance).

handling the reaction products the nonlinearity of autoradiography can be avoided.

Koury et al. [13] have reported a 500-fold increase in Epo mRNA in the kidneys of anemic mice. However, they were unable to detect signals from non-anemic tissue due to the limit of detectability in their ribonuclease protection assay.

The exponential increase in Epo mRNA levels in the kidneys when lowering the hematocrit was closely correlated with the increase in Epo protein levels in the plasma (Figure 3). This was valid for the whole range of hematocrits studied. It provides further evidence that the production of Epo is regulated on the level of mRNA and not markedly influenced by translational mechanisms. The cellular level of Epo mRNA, however, is controlled transcriptionally as well as postranscriptionally [9]. Accurate measurements of the half-life of Epo mRNA from an Epo-producing hepatoma cell line have revealed a hypoxia dependent stabilisation of Epo mRNA. This led to an elongation of the half-life from 2 hours under normoxic conditions to roughly 6 hours hypoxically [9, 11].

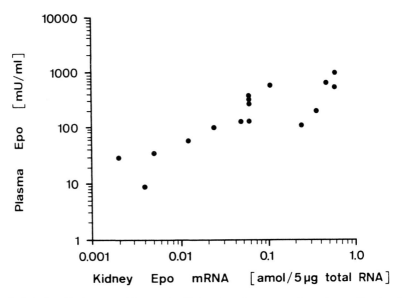

Fig. 3: Relationship between kidney mRNA levels and corresponding plasma Epo levels (r =-0.77; P < 0.01; n = 16; r = correlation coefficient; P = level of significance).

Epo gene expression in the liver was stimulated by anemia as well but to a much lesser degree. However, due to the much higher organ weight the contribution of the liver Epo mRNA to total body Epo mRNA decreased only from 24 % to 16 %. Despite the use of highly sensitive assays [6, 11, 13] uncertainty remains about the contribution of the liver to total Epo production under normoxic circumstances. Tan et al. [6] reported that the liver from hypoxic animals contributes 25 to 50 % of the total. Our results (Table 1) suggest that in anemic rats the liver contributes about 16 to 24 % to the total of the induced Epo mRNA depending on the degree of anemia. Both values are higher than what has been reported so far from studies with mice [2, 13]. The contribution of the liver to the production of Epo under basal and anemic conditions is an issue of considerable pathophysiologic interest. If the contribution of the liver is indeed about 25 % of the total it is hard to understand why this organ cannot compensate for the lack of renal Epo production in chronic renal failure. Further studies are clearly needed to determine whether all the hepatic Epo mRNA can be translated into protein. It has to be elucidated to what extend the hepatic contribution varies among species and possibly as a function of the type of hypoxic stress.

Other organs than kidneys and liver express the Epo gene as well. Small but reproducible signals were observed in lungs from severely anemic rats (hct 0.18 and 0.20). Comparably low but reproducible signals were also obtained from the spleens of rats regardless of whether they were anemic. Our results with competitive PCR are in agreement with ribonuclease protection assay studies [6]. Both methods are sensitive enough to allow the detection of mRNA for Epo in the spleen and lung. Heart tissue served as a negative control where no Epo mRNA was detectable. However, Epo mRNA levels were not significantly stimulated by anemia. Therefore, the physiological significance of Epo gene expression in these two organs remains to be determined

Another organ of interest in this respect is the target for Epo itself, the bone marrow. Local paracrine production of Epo in macrophages [14] or autocrine production in hematopoietic progenitors [15] has been postulated to contribute to steady-state erythropoiesis. In our hands, however, repeated attempts to detect Epo mRNA in bone marrow from hypoxic animals by competitive PCR have been unsuccessful so far.

Summary

The regulation of Epo production in rats was investigated by competitive PCR, a highly sensitive and accurate means of measuring Epo mRNA levels. Coamplification of the test sample with added mutant Epo cDNA template corrects for variability in the efficiency of amplification. Epo mRNA levels were determined in tissues of normal rats and in animals with varying degrees of anemia. Reduction of the hematocrit from 0.40 to 0.15 resulted in a 300-fold increase in kidney Epo mRNA, which comprised 80 % of the total Epo mRNA versus 20 % from the liver. Lowering the hematocrit led to an exponential rise of Epo mRNA in the kidneys. Serum Epo protein levels rose likewise and were closely correlated with Epo mRNA levels. Very low levels of Epo mRNA were detected in the spleen and the lung. Heart and bone marrow were free of Epo mRNA.

References

1. JELKMANN, W. (1992): Erythropoietin: Structure, control of production, and function. Physiol. Rev. 72, 449-489.

2. BONDURANT, M.C. & M.J. KOURY (1986): Anemia induces accumulation of erythropoietin mRNA in the kidney and liver. Mol. Cell. Biol. 6, 2731-2733.
3. BERU N., J. MCDONALD, C. LACOMBE & E. GOLDWASSER (1986): Expression of the erythropoietingene. Mol. Cell. Biol. 6, 2571-2575.
4. SCHUSTER, S.J., J.H. WILSON, A.J. ERSLEV & J. CARO (1987): Physiologic regulation and tissue localization of renal erythropoietin messenger RNA. Blood 70, 316-318.
5. SCHUSTER, S.J., E.V. BADIAVAS, P. COSTA-GIOMI, R. WEINMANN, A.J. ERSLEV & J. CARO (1989): Stimulation of erythropoietin gene transcription during hypoxia and cobalt exposure. Blood 73, 13-16.
6. TAN, C.C., K.-U. ECKARDT & P.J. RATCLIFFE (1991): Organ distribution of erythropoietin messenger RNA in normal and uremic rats. Kidney Int. 40, 69-76.
7. CHELLY, J., J-C. KAPLAN, P. MAIRE, S. GAUTRON & A. KAHN (1988): Transcription of the dystrophin gene in muscle and non-muscle tissues. Nature 333, 858-860.
8. GILLILAND, G., S. PERRIN, K. BLANCHARD & H.F. BUNN (1990): Analysis of cytokine mRNA and DNA: Detection and quantitation by competitive polymerase chain reaction. Proc. Natl. Acad. Sci. U.S.A. 87, 2725-2729.
9. GOLDBERG, M.A., C.C. GAUT & H.F. BUNN (1991): Erythropoietin mRNA levels are governed by both the rate of gene transcription and posttranslational events. Blood 77, 271-277.
10. CHIRGWIN, J.M., A.E. PRYZBYLA, R.J. MACDONALD & W.J. RUTTER (1979): Isolation of biologically active ribonucleic acid from sources enriched with ribonuclease. Biochemistry 18, 5294-5299.
11. FANDREY, J. & H.F. BUNN (1993): In vivo and in vitro regulation of erythropoietin mRNA: Measurements by competitive polymerase chain reaction. Blood 81, 617-623.
12. PERRIN, S. & G. GILLILAND (1991): Site-specific mutagenesis using asymmetric polymerase chain reaction and a single mutant primer. Nucleic Acids Res. 18, 7433-7438.
13. KOURY, M.J., M.C. BONDURANT, S.E. GRABER & S.T. SAWYER (1988): Erythropoietin messenger RNA levels in developing mice and transfer of ^{125}I-erythropoietin by the placenta. J. Clin. Invest. 82, 154-159.
14. RICH, I.N., W. HEIT & B. KUBANEK (1982): Extrarenal erythropoietin production by macrophages. Blood 78, 1007-1018.
15. HERMINE, O., N. BERU, N. PECH & E. GOLDWASSER (1991): An autocrine role for erythropoietin in mouse hemapoietic cell differentiation. Blood 78, 2253-2260.

Protein kinase C is a modulator of erythropoietin formation

K.-U. Eckardt and A. Kurtz

Physiologisches Institut I der Universität Regensburg

The glycoprotein hormone erythropoietin (EPO) is the major humoral regulator of erythropoiesis in mammals and is produced in inverse relation to the oxygen availability of the organism [8]. Liver and kidneys are the physiologically important production sites of the hormone and in both organs the major control of EPO formation has been shown to operate at the level of its mRNA [1,2,14]. Little is known, however, about the intracellular pathways leading to EPO mRNA accumulation in response to hypoxia. This is mainly due to the fact that the cells producing EPO in liver and kidneys have up to now only partially been identified and that consequently neither the hepatic nor the renal cells producing EPO could so far be studied in vitro.

Several tumor cell lines of both renal and hepatic origin, however, have been shown to produce EPO, in part in an oxygen-dependent fashion, and have therefore been used in attempts to elucidate the intracellular pathways stimulating EPO production in response to hypoxia [5,6,8]. Although a consistent scheme of oxygen dependent signal transduction has not yet been elaborated, it has been suggested that several "second messenger" pathways may play a role. Some events, such as e.g. the activation of adenylate cylase, were, however, found to be of variable importance, depending on whether kidney or liver carcinoma cells were investigated [4,15]. Another system of intracellular signal transduction, which, in contrast, appears to be of more general importance for EPO formation, is the activation of protein kinase C (PKC). Using renal carcinoma cell cultures, Hagiwara et al. were to our knowledge the first to point to a role of PKC in EPO formation [7]. More recently, evidence was provided by Jelkmann et al. [9] and by our group [11], that PKC is a potent modulator of EPO formation in the human hepatoma cell line Hep G2, which is known to produce EPO in an oxygen dependent fashion [5]. Elucidation of the role of PKC may therefore be of considerable importance for understanding of EPO regulation. However, interpretation of experimental interference with PKC activity is generally difficult for several reasons. Thus stable activators of PKC, such as phorbol esters, have been shown to exert a dual effect, in that stimulation of PKC activity is followed by proteolytic degradation of the enzyme, a process referrred to as "downregulation". Moreover, protein kinase C has been shown to be heterogenous and at least 8 isoenzymes exist, with different affinities for pharmacological activators and inhibitors and differences in their kinetics of activation and "downregulation" [10, 12]. Finally, although potent inhibitors of PKC are available, these substances lack specificty, making their molecular targets hard to define.

Due to this complexity the precise mechanisms by which PKC acitivity influences EPO formation have not yet been clarified and it may not be surprising that some apparently contradictory findings were made. In this brief article we will try to summarize the current experimental evidence on this aspect of EPO regulation and try to outline different ways by which PKC may modulate EPO formation.

The experimental approach used so far in order to assess the effect of PKC activity on EPO formation is basically twofold and includes study of the effect of known activators of the enzyme, such as different phorbol esters and diacylglycerol analogues, as well as study of the effects of pharmacological inhibitors of PKC. Both the secretion of EPO protein and the formation of EPO mRNA following the application of these substances were determined and under some conditions the subcellular distribution of PKC isozymes was also measured.

Effects of phorbol esters on EPO formation

Tumor-promoting phorbol esters, such as phorbol 12-myristate 13 acetate (PMA) have a structure very similar to diacylglycerol, the product of phosphatidylinositol 4,5-biphosphate. Like this "physiological" stimulator of PKC activity, phorbol esters dramatically increase the affinity of the enzyme for Ca^{++}, resulting in its full activation at physiological Ca^{++} concentrations [12].

Using human renal carcinoma cell cultures it was shown that PMA inhibited secretion of EPO protein into the culture medium in a dose-dependent fashion after 24-96 hours and after 18 days of incubation of confluent cells. In the long term cultures this inhibition of EPO formation was paralleled by a reduction in dome formation of the cells, but no effects on cell growth were observed [7].

In the human hepatoma cells Hep G2, PMA was also found to reduce the daily secretion rate of EPO protein for up to 72 hours of incubation in a dose dependent fashion. As illustrated in Fig. 1, this inhibition was observed at 20 % oxygen [9,11], 1 % oxygen and in the presence of $CoCl_2$, a known stimulator of EPO formation in hepatoma cells and in vivo [8]. Half-maximal inhibition was consistently found at a dose of approximately 10 nM [9,11].

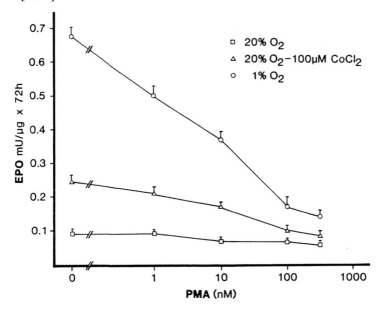

Fig. 1: Effect of phorbol 12-myristate-13 acetate (PMA) on EPO secretion rates in Hep G2 cells grown at 20 % oxygen in the absence or presence of cobalt or at 1 % oxygen (mean ± SE, n=3). Reproduced with permission from [11].

This inhibition of EPO secretion was paralleled by a reduction in EPO mRNA levels in Hep G2 cells, as shown in figure 2. Measurement of EPO mRNA furthermore revealed that the inhibitory effect of PMA (100 nM) on EPO formation occurs rapidly, since a marked reduction in EPO mRNA was found already after 1 hour of incubation (Fig. 2). Moreover, further studies revealed that the effect of PMA was longlasting, because preincubation of Hep G_2 cells with PMA (100 nM) for 24 hours resulted in diminished EPO production for up to three days during subsequent incubation in the absence of the drug.

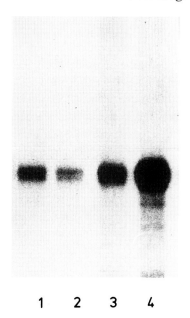

Fig. 2: Autoradiograph of an RNAse protection assay showing the accumulation of EPO mRNA in Hep G2 cells incubated at 1 % oxygen for 1 hour (lanes 1 and 3) or 24 hours (lanes 2 and 4) in the absence (lanes 1 and 2) or presence (lanes 5 and 6) of phorbol 12-myristate-13 acetate (PMA) (100 nM). Note that reduction of EPO mRNA levels in the presence of PMA occured after already 1 hour of incubation and was even more pronounced after 24 hours. Adapted from [11] with permission.

In order to test for the specificty of the effect of PMA on EPO formation another active phorbol ester, phorbol 12, 13 dibutyrate was also tested, and found to reduce EPO formation, whereas the inactive phorbol ester 4-alphaphorbol 12,13 didecanoate was ineffective [11].

To correlate changes in EPO formation with the activation pattern of PKC isozymes, PKC isozymes were determined immunologically by Western Blotting in cytosol and membrane fractions of Hep G_2 cells following treatment with PMA for different time periods. Hep G_2 cells were found to contain mainly the alpha type of PKC [9,11], but small amounts of beta [9], delta, epsilon and zeta were also detected. After PMA treatment for 1 hour, i.e. a time period after which the inhibition of EPO formation was already detectable in these cells, we found a translocation of PKC alpha, epsilon and zeta from cytosol to membrane, which indicates a strong stimulation of these isozymes. After 24 hours of incubation, however, i.e when EPO formation was still inhibited (Fig. 2), downregulation of membrane-bound PKC alpha [9,11], epsilon and zeta was observed.

Effects of diacylglycerol of EPO formation

Analogues of DAG are often used in studies to explore possible roles of PKC in signal transduction, although they are no ideal tools, because both membrane permeability and stability of these substances is variable and may be to small to induce significant biological effects. When testing the effect of the synthetic DAG-analogue 1-oleolyl-2-acetylglycerol (OAG) on EPO formation in renal carcinoma cells, a dose dependent inhibition was observed [7]. In Hep G_2 cells, however, no effect could be seen after 72 hours of incubation in the presence of this or another DAG-analogue (1,2-dioctanoylglycerol) [11].

Effect of kinase inhibitors on EPO formation

Besides attempts to stimulate protein kinase C activity the use of inhibitors of the enzyme is an alternative approach to interfere with its activity. For studies in intact cells basically two different groups of

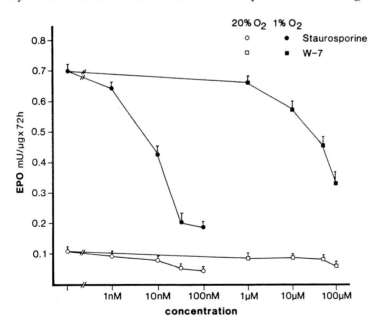

Fig. 3: Effect of the kinase inhibitors staurosporine and 1-(5-isoquinolinylsulfonyl)-2-methylpiperazine (H-7) on EPO production rates in Hep G_2 cells incubated for 72 hours at 1 % or 20 % oxygen; (means ± SE, n=3). Reproduced with permission from [11].

inhibitors are available; the microbial product staurosporine and related substances, characterized by an indole carbazole system and the isoquinolines (e.g. H 7). Assuming that the inhibitory effect of phorbol esters on EPO formation results from stimulation of PKC activity, one could expect, that conversely, inhibition of the enzyme is either ineffective or might even enhance EPO formation. Experimental results, however, showed that staurosporine, a staurosprine analogue (CGP 41 251) and the isoquinoline H 7, have rather the opposite effect and reduce EPO formation (Fig. 3) [9,11]. Moreover, when PMA was added to Hep G_2 cells in the presence of staurosporine or H 7, its inhibitory effect was not attenuated, but additive to that observed with staurosporine and H 7 alone.

Stimulatory or inhibitory effects of protein kinase C on EPO formation?

Although the above observations all seem to indicate that protein kinase C activity modulates EPO formation, it appears difficult to infer the mechanisms of this interference. In fact, at first glance the results appear hardly compatible with each other in several respects. First not only phorbol esters, known stimulators of protein kinase C activity, but also inhibitors of the enzyme led to a reduction in EPO formation. Second, phorbol esters, but not diacylglycerol analogues were found to inhibit EPO formation in hepatoma cells. Third, when correlated with the kinetics of activation and downregulation of PKC isozymes in hepatoma cells an inhibition of EPO formation was seen both during stimulation as well as after downregulation of the predominant subtype of the enzyme in hepatoma cells, PKC alpha. These discrepancies rise the question as to whether PKC does in fact play an essential permissive or even mediating role for EPO formation, so that its inhibition results in reduced EPO production, or whether in contrast the stimulation of the enzyme inhibits EPO production. At present no definite answer seems possible, but in either case different conclusions would result from the experimental findings.

The inhibition of EPO formation in the presence of so-called inhibitors of PKC activity would clearly be compatible with a permissive role of the enzyme for EPO formation. However, since these inhibitors all interfere with the ATP-binding site of PKC, which shows strong homology with ATP binding sites of other serine- and threonine or tyrosine-specific kinases, they are unfortunately rather unselective [13]. The possibility therefore has to be considered that a kinase activity other than that of PKC is required for EPO formation. It is of interest in this respect that in hepatoma cells the oxygen sensor was suggested to be a heme protein [4] and that a bacterial heme protein functioning as a molecular oxygen sensor has recently been found to exert a kinase activity [3].

The lack of an effect of diacylglycerol analogues on EPO formation in hepatoma cells would also undoubtedly be compatible with the assumption that the inhibition and not the stimulation of PKC activity inhibits EPO formation, but as mentioned above, the effectiveness of these substances is uncertain and therefore the negative results may not exclude the possibility that stimulation of PKC inhibits EPO formation, all the more as these substances were found to be effective inhibitors in renal carcinoma cells.

Somewhat more direct conclusions might be drawn from the comparison of the effects of phorbol esters on EPO formation on the one hand and the activity pattern of different isozymes of PKC on the other hand. In case the *inhibition* of one or more isozymes of PKC is responsible for the observed reduction in EPO formation, these isozyme(s) would have to undergo more rapid downregulation than those detected so far, i.e. alpha, beta, epsilon and zeta and in fact its/their activity would have to be significantly reduced after one hour of incubation with PMA (100 nM), when EPO mRNA levels were already found to be suppressed (Fig. 2).

Alternatively, if the *activation* of one or more isozymes of PKC reduces EPO formation, e.g. PKC alpha appears to be a possible candidate. In that case, however, its activation would have to generate a very stable mediator that is inhibitory for EPO formation, because reduced EPO formation was still observed, when PKC alpha displayed a marked downregulation of its membrane-bound form [9,11].

Finally, given the molecular heterogeneity of PKC, it is also possible that different isozymes might exert opposite, i.e. stimulatory and inhibitory effects on EPO production, so that eventually the balance between divergent effects of PKC activity determines EPO production rates. Further clarification of this regulation might not be possible before development of more specific activators and inhibitors of different subtypes of the enzyme. In the meantime it appears essential to verify, if the findings indicative of a role of PKC in EPO regulation obtained in tumor cells are also valid in non malignant renal and hepatic cells, which are physiological production sites of the hormone. Our preliminary findings indicate, that with respect to liver cells this is in fact the case.

References

1. BONDURANT, M.C. & M.J. KOURY (1986): Anemia induces accumulation of erythropoietin mRNA in the kidney and liver. Mol. Cell Biol. 6, 2731-2733.
2. ECKARDT, K.-U., P.J. RATATCLIFFE, C.C. TAN, C. BAUER & A. KURTZ (1992): Age dependent expression of the erythropoietin gene in rat liver and kidneys. J. Clin. Invest. 89, 753-760.
3. GILLES-GONZALES, M.A., G.S. DITTA & D.R. HELSINKI (1991): A haemoprotein with kinase activity encoded by the oxygen sensor of Rhizobium meliloti. Nature 350, 170-172.
4. GOLDBERG, M.A., S.P. DUNNING & H.F. BUNN (1988): Regulation of the erythropoietin gene: evidence that the oxygen sensor is a heme protein. Science 242, 1412-1415.
5. GOLDBERG, M.A., G.A. GLASS, J.M. CUNNINGHAM & H.F. BUNN (1987): The regulated expression of erythropoietin by two human hepatoma cell lines. Proc. Natl. Acad. Sci. USA 84, 7972-7976.
6. HAGIWARA, M., D.B. MCNAMARA, I.-L. CHEN & J.W. FISHER (1984): Role of endogenous prostaglandin E2 in erythropoietin production and dome formation by human renal carcinoma cells in culture. J. Clin. Invest. 74, 1252-1261.
7. HAGIWARA, M., K. NAGAKURA, M. UENO & J.W. FISHER (1987): Inhibitory effects of tetradecanoylphorbol acetate and diacylglycerol on erythropoietin production in human renal carcinoma cell cultures. Exp. Cell. Res. 173, 129-136.
8. JELKMANN, W. (1992): Erythropoietin: Structure, control of production, and function. Physiol. Rev. 72, 449-489.
9. JELKMANN, W., A. HUWILER, J. FANDREY & J. PFEILSCHIFTER (1991): Inhibition of erythropoietin production by phorbol ester is associated with down-regulation of protein kinase C-alpha isoenzyme in hepatoma cells. Biochem. Biophys. Res. Commun. 179, 1441-1448.
10. KIKKAWA, U., A. KISHIMOTO & Y. NISHIZUKA (1989): The protein kinase C family: heterogeniety and its implications. An. Rev. Biochem. 58, 31-44.
11. KURTZ, A., K.-U. ECKARDT, C.W. PUGH, P. CORVOL, D. FABBRO & P.J. RATCLIFFE (1992): Phorbol ester inhibits erythropoietin production in human hepatoma cells (Hep G2). Am. J. Physiol. 262, C1204-C1210.
12. NISHIZUKA, Y. (1988): The molecular heterogeniety of protein kinase C and its implications for cellular regulation. Nature 334, 661-665.
13. RÜEGG, U.T. & G.M. BURGESS (1989): Staurosporine, K-252 and UCN-01: potent but nonspecific inhibitors of protein kinases. TIPS 10, 218-220.
14. SCHUSTER, S.J., J.H. WILSON, A.J. ERSLEV & J. Caro (1987): Physiologic regulation and tissue localization of renal erythropoietin messenger RNA. Blood 70, 316-318.
15. SHERWOOD, J.B., E.R. BURNS & D. SHOUVAL (1987): Stimulation by cAMP of erythropoietin secretion by an established human renal carcinoma cell line. Blood 69, 1053-1057.

Mechanism of action of thyroid hormones (T_3/T_4) on erythropoietin production

W. Jelkmann*, J. Fandrey*, M. Wolff*, S. Frede* and H. Pagel**

Physiologisches Institut der Universität Bonn* und Physiologisches
Institut der Medizinischen Universität zu Lübeck**

Introduction

The renal and hepatic synthesis of the glycoprotein hormone erythropoietin (Epo) is triggered when the blood O_2 availability is lowered. In turn, Epo stimulates the proliferation and differentiation of erythrocytic progenitors thus increasing red cell production. It is thought that several other hormones augment the effect of tissue hypoxia on erythropoiesis, including the thyroid hormones tetra-(T_4) and triiodothyronine (T_3), androgens and catecholamines [1]. The mechanisms of the action of thyroid hormones in control of erythropoiesis are only incompletely understood.

In vitro studies indicate that thyroid hormones stimulate the growth of erythrocytic progenitors synergisticly with Epo [2,3]. In experimental animals T_3 and T_4 appear to stimulate erythropoiesis primarily by enhancing Epo production at renal and extrarenal sites [4-6]. In humans hyperthyroidism is associated with increased red cell mass and plasma Epo, whereas hypothyroidism leads to reduced red cell mass and plasma Epo.

The alleged stimulation of Epo production by thyroid hormones has been generally explained as part of a physiological reaction to the calorigenic effects of T_3 and T_4. Along these lines hyperthyroidism leads to elevated metabolic rate and O_2 consumption thus creating a decrease in tissue O_2 tension. Some investigators have disputed this interpretation and suggested a non-calorigenic mechanism, because the rate of O_2 consumption is not closely correlated with the increase in erythropoiesis in rodents treated with thyroid hormones [8,9].

The present studies show that T_3 and T_4 dose-dependently increase Epo synthesis in isolated perfused rat kidneys and in human hepatoma cell cultures. Measurements of tissue O_2 tension and O_2 consumption revealed that this effect is not due to increased hypoxia. Instead, transcription of the Epo gene appears to be directly stimulated via flanking thyroid hormone receptor DNA recognition elements.

Methods

Kidney perfusion: Kidneys from male Sprague-Dawley rats (240-390 g) were isolated as described earlier [10]. The exstirpated kidneys were perfused at a constant pressure (100 mmHg) and temperature (37 °C) in a recirculation system for 3 h. The perfusion medium was a Krebs-Henseleit solution supplemented with 60 g/l bovine serum albumin, 5 % human erythrocytes, and substrates as specified [10]. The perfusion medium (0.2 l) was continuously dialysed against 5 l of protein free medium equilibrated with 5 % O_2, 5 % CO_2 and 90 % N_2. Thyroid hormones (kindly supplied by Henning, Berlin) were added both to the perfusate and the dialysate.

Perfusion flow rate was recorded continuously. Based on measurements of the PO_2 in samples from arterial and venous bypasses of the perfusion system (Acid-base analyzer Radiometer ABL3, Copenhagen, Denmark) the renal O_2 supply and consumption were calculated according to [11]. Aliquots of the perfusion media were frozen at -20 °C until assayed for Epo.

Cell cultures: HepG2 cells from the American Type Culture Collection (ATCC No. HB 8065) were maintained in medium RPMI 1640 (Flow Laboratories, Meckenheim, Germany) supplemented with 10 % fetal bovine serum (Gibco, Eggenstein, Germany) and sodium bicarbonate (2.2 g/l) in a humidified atmosphere (5 % CO_2 in air) at 37 °C (Heraeus incubators, Hanau, Germany). Experiments were carried out using confluent cultures (5 x 10^5 cells/cm^2) in 24-well polystyrene dishes (Falcon, Becton Dickinson, Heidelberg, Germany). For some studies HepG2 cells were kept in serum-free medium (BioRich 2; Flow Laboratories, Irvine, Ireland). At the start of the experiments the cells received fresh medium (1 ml/2 cm^2 well) with the respective thyroid hormone for 24 h. Then the medium was collected and frozen at -20 °C for the determination of Epo. The cell layer was washed with phosphate buffered saline solution and lysed with SDS-NaOH

(5 g/l sodium dodecylsulfate in 0.1 M NaOH). Total cellular protein was measured by means of a micro determination kit (Sigma Diagnostics, Taufkirchen, Germany). Pericellular O_2 pressure was measured with a polarographic O_2-sensitive solid state catheter probe (Neocath; Biomedical Sensors, High Wycombe Bucks, England) positioned in the monolayer via holes in the culture dish cover. The data were processed on a microcomputer (LICOX PO_2; GMS, Kiel-Mielkendorf, Germany). Microelectrode measurements revealed that the PO_2 in the pericellular space dropped from 142 mmHg to <1 mmHg within 1 h after renewal of the medium when the cells were incubated in an atmosphere of 5 % CO_2 in air. Thus the experiments were carried out under conditions of diffusion-limited O_2 supply.

Normoxic experiments were performed with HepG2 cells grown on culture dishes with a gas permeable bottom (Petriperm; Heraeus, Hanau, Germany). Here, the pericellular PO_2 was similar to the ambient PO_2 of the incubator gas.

Measurement of O_2 consumption in HepG2 cultures: O_2 consumption was measured with an attachment made of non-oxidizable steel which covered the culture dish and contained a polarographic O_2-sensitive electrode (GMS, Kiel-Mielkendorf, Germany). The electric signals from the electrode were processed on a microcomputer (LICOX pO_2; GMS) The experiments were started by replacing the medium with fresh medium pre-warmed to 37 °C and equilibrated with air and 5 % CO_2. The whole measuring device was immersed in a 37 °C temperature controlled water bath. The PO_2 within the chamber was recorded continuously. The O_2 consumption was calculated from the averaged slope of the records taking into account the O_2 content of the medium and the cellular protein.

Quantitation of Epo-mRNA, Epo-protein and α-fetoprotein: Epo-mRNA was assayed exactly as described elsewhere in this monograph [12]. Epo-protein was measured by radioimmunoassay. Human urinary Epo standard was used for the assay of HepG2 culture media [13]. Rat kidney perfusion medium was 5-fold concentrated for the assay (Centricon 10 microconcentrators; Amicon, Witten, Germany) and rat serum Epo served as a standard [10]. The lower detection limit was 5 U/l for human Epo and 2.5 U/l for rat Epo.

For the determination of α-fetoprotein a commercial radioimmunoassay kit was used (Pharmacia, Uppsala, Sweden).

Statistical analysis: Dunnett's test was used to calculate statistical significance. Results are given as mean values ± SD.

Table 1: Effects of thyroid hormones on some functional parameters of isolated perfused rat kidneys (arterial PO_2 35 mmHg, hematocrit 0.05).

Additive	Perfusion flow rate (ml/min/g)	GFR (µl/min/g)	O_2-supply µmol/min/g	O_2-consumption µmol/min/g
None	25 ± 2	474 ± 191	17 ± 4	8 ± 3
T_4 (10^{-7}M)	25 ± 3	340 ± 129	18 ± 4	8 ± 3
T_3 (10^{-8}M)	25 ± 3	303 ± 129	19 ± 4	7 ± 2

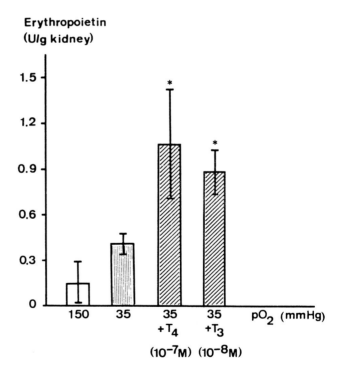

Fig. 1: Effects of thyroid hormones (tetraiodothyronine, T_4; triiodothyronine, T_3) on the production of Epo in the isolated perfused rat kidney. Data are the mean ± SD of 3-6 perfused kidneys per treatment.

Results

Isolated perfused rat kidney: Without thyroid hormones 0.42 ± 0.07 U Epo per g kidney was produced during the 3 h perfusion period (Fig. 1). The addition of T_4 (10^{-7} M) or T_3 (10^{-8} M) to the perfusion medium resulted in a 2-3 fold increase in Epo production. Table 1 shows that thyroid hormones did not alter perfusion flow rate, O_2 supply and O_2 consumption, although they tended to lower glomerular filtration rate (GFR).

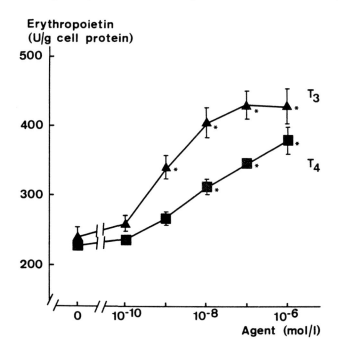

Fig. 2: Effects of thyroid hormones (tetraiodothyronine, T_4; triiodothyronine, T_3) on the production of Epo in HepG2 cells incubated hypoxically for 24 h. Data are the mean ± SD of 8 experiments; *: P <0.05 compared to controls (Dunnett's test). Reproduced with permission from [16].

Hepatoma cell cultures: Due to the diffusion-limited O_2 supply some Epo (200 - 250 U/g cell protein in 24 h) was produced by HepG2 cells maintained in conventional polystyrene culture dishes when incubated in air. T_4 and T_3 stimulated the hypoxically induced Epo production in a dose-dependent manner (Fig. 2). Note that L-reverse-triiodothyronine, L-diiodo-tyrosine and tyrosine were ineffective at concentrations from 10^{-10} to 10^{-6}

M. Epo mRNA was quantitated from HepG2 cells that were either hypoxically incubated without (control) or with thyroid hormones. The level of Epo mRNA in cells stimulated with T_4 or T_3 was 2- to 3-fold higher than in control cells. The influence of T_3 on the production of α-fetoprotein was studied to confirm that the effect of thyroid hormones on Epo synthesis was specific. Basal production of α-fetoprotein was 9.9 ± 0.6 MU/g cell protein in 24 h (n=4). Over the whole dose range tested T_3 did not stimulate α-fetoprotein production (e.g. 8.8 ± 0.4 MU/g at 10^{-8} M and 8.9 ± 0.7 MU/g at 10^{-6} M; n=4). Under serum-free conditions HepG2 cells displayed a reduced basal production rate of Epo (154 ± 18 U/g cellular protein; n=8). However, T_4 and T_3 were still effective in stimulating Epo production (T_4 10^{-7} M: 225 ± 11 U/g protein; T_3 10^{-8} M: 213 ± 14 U/g protein; n=4). To test whether T_3 stimulates Epo production in normoxia as well, HepG2 cells grown on gas-permeable culture dishes were either exposed to O_2 at partial pressures of 142 mmHg (normoxia) or 7 mmHg (hypoxia). The basal 24-h rate of the production of Epo under normoxic conditions was 42.6 ± 5.6 U/g cell protein (n=8). This value was not increased by T_3 in the range 10^{-10} to 10^{-6} M. In the corresponding experiments under hypoxia Epo production increased from 240 ± 32 U/g (n=12) to 363 ± 84 U/g (n=12) and 376 ± 98 U/g (n=12) in presence of T_3 (10^{-8} and 10^{-6} M, respectively). Basal O_2 consumption rate in confluent HepG2 cultures was 6.6 ± 1.2 μmol x min^{-1} x g^{-1} cell protein (21 expts.). Cells treated with T_3 (10^{-6} M for 24 h) consumed 6.5 ± 1.0 μmol x min^{-1} x g^{-1} cell protein (11 expts.).

Discussion

The present studies provide first evidence that Epo producing tissues are directly stimulated by thyroid hormones. This stimulation was demonstrated in isolated perfused rat kidneys and in human hepatoma cultures. In hypoxic hepatoma cells it was furthermore shown that T_3 and T_4 increase the mRNA levels for Epo. Note that thyroid hormone proved to augment the hypoxia-induced synthesis of Epo but it did not induce Epo production in normoxic cells.

Mainly from a teleologic point of view most investigators have explained the increase in red cell mass in hyperthyroidism by means of an increased O_2 demand of the tissue. Increased O_2 consumption has been assumed to cause a sufficiently low PO_2 in the tissue to trigger the production of Epo [5]. However, the present findings clearly show that the effect of thyroid hormones on Epo synthesis in kidney and liver cells is independent of the O_2 consumption.

Thus a novel explanation is warranted with respect to the mechanism by which thyroid hormones enhance Epo gene expression. Genes whose transcription is controlled by thyroid hormones are known to possess DNA recognition sequences to which thyroid hormone receptors bind [14]. Indeed, in a recent study of the flanking sequences of the Epo gene Blanchard et al. [15] have identified DNA elements resembling half-site steroid/thyroid hormone receptor response motifs (Fig. 3). It seems likely that these elements control the activity of the Epo promoter and enhancer DNA sequences thus enabling thyroid hormones to augment the hypoxia-induced stimulation of Epo production.

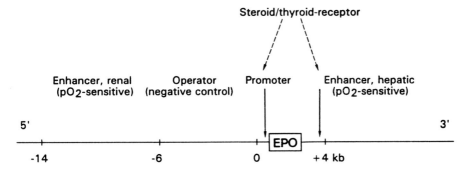

Fig. 3: Scheme of the human Epo gene and surrounding regulatory DNA elements (kb: kilobasepairs) which are thought to be controlled by PO_2 and thyroid hormones [15,17].

Summary

The hypothesis that thyroid hormones stimulate the synthesis of erythropoietin directly at the gene level rather than indirectly by creating tissue hypoxia was tested in isolated perfused rat kidneys and with the Epoproducing hepatoma cell line, HepG2. L-triiodothyronine and L-thyroxine dose-dependently stimulated hypoxia-induced Epo formation both in the kidney and in HepG2 cultures. HepG2 cells treated with thyroid hormones had 2- to 3-fold higher Epo messenger RNA levels. Measurements of O_2 consumption in kidney and HepG2 cells revealed that this effect was not due to increased hypoxia. We conclude that thyroid hormones stimulate Epo production in a non-calorigenic way.

Acknowledgements

Supported by Deutsche Forschungsgemeinschaft (DFG Je 95/6-2).

References

1. JELKMANN, W. (1986): Renal erythropoietin: properties and production. Rev. Physiol. Biochem. Pharmacol. 104, 139-215.
2. GOLDE, D.W., N. BERSCH, I.J. CHOPRA & M.J. CLINE (1977): Thyroid hormones stimulate erythropoiesis in vitro. Br. J. Haematol. 37, 173-177.
3. POPOVIC, W.J., J.E. BROWN & J.W. ADAMSON (1977): The influence of thyroid hormones on in vitro erythropoiesis. J. Clin. Invest. 60, 907-913.
4. FISHER, J.W., B.L. ROH & S. HALVORSEN (1967): Inhibition of erythropoietic effects of hormones by erythropoietin antisera in mildly plethoric mice. Proc. Soc. Exp. Biol. Med. 126, 97-100.
5. PESCHLE, C., G.F. SASSO, G. MASTROBERARDINO & M. CONDORELLI (1971): The mechanism of endocrine influences on erythropoiesis. J. Lab. Clin. Med. 78, 20-29.
6. ZANJANI, E.D. & M. BANISADRE (1979): Hormonal stimulation of erythropoietin production and erythropoiesis in anephric sheep fetuses. J. Clin. Invest. 64, 1181-1187.
7. DAS, K.C., M. MUKKERJEE, T.K. SARKAR, R.J. DASH & G.K. RASTOGI (1975): Erythropoiesis and erythropoietin in hypo- and hyperthyroidism. J. Clin. Endocrinol. Metab. 40, 211-220.
8. DONATI, R.M., M.A. WARNECKE & N.I. GALLAGHER (1964): Effect of triiodothyronine administration on erythrocyte radioiron incorporation in rats. Proc. Soc. exp. Biol. Med. 115, 405-407.
9. MEINEKE, H.A. & R.C. CRAFTS (1964): Evidence for a non-calorigenic effect of thyroxin on erythropoiesis as judged by radioiron utilization. Proc. Soc. Exp. Biol. Med. 117, 520-524.
10. PAGEL, H., W. JELKMANN & C. WEISS (1991): Isolated serum-free perfused rat kidneys release immunoreactive erythropoietin in response to hypoxia. Endocrinology 128, 2633-2638.
11. SIGGAARD-ANDERSEN, O. (1974): The Acid-base Status of the Blood, ed. 4. Copenhagen: Munksgaard.
12. FANDREY, J. & H.F. BUNN: Quantitation of erythropoietin-mRNA in organs of the rat and in Hep3B cells. In: Funktionsanalyse biologischer Systeme (this volume).
13. JELKMANN, W. & G. WIEDEMANN (1990): Serum erythropoietin level: relationship to blood hemoglobin concentration and erythrocytic activity of the bone marrow. Klin. Wochenschr. 68, 403-407.
14. GLASS, C.K., J.M. HOLLOWAY, O.V. DEVARY & M.G. ROSENFELD (1988): The thyroid hormone receptor binds with opposite transcriptional effects to a common sequence motif in thyroid hormone and estrogen response elements. Cell 54, 313-323.
15. BLANCHARD, K.L., A.M. ACQUAVIVA, D.L. GALSON & H.F. BUNN (1992): Hypoxic induction of the human erythropoietin gene: cooperation between the promoter and enhancer, each of which contains steroid receptor response elements. Mol. Cell. Biol. 12, 5373-5385.

16. FANDREY, J., H. PAGEL, S. FREDE, M. WOLFF & W. JELKMANN (1994): Thyroid hormones enhance hypoxia-induced erythropoietin production in vitro. Exp. Hematol. 22, 272-277.
17. SEMENZA, G.L., S.T. KOURY, M.K. NEJFELT, J.D. GEARHART & S.E. ANTONARAKIS (1991): Cell-type-specific and hypoxia-inducible expression of the erythropoietin gene in transgenic mice. Proc. Natl. Acad. Sci. USA 88, 8725-729.

The increased production of erythropoietin by antidiuretic hormone is not mediated by vasoconstriction

H. Pagel and A. Engel

Physiologisches Institut, Medizinische Universität zu Lübeck

Introduction

The principal regulator of erythropoiesis is the renal glycoprotein hormone erythropoietin (Epo). Tissue hypoxia is the main stimulus for its production. In addition, the synthesis of Epo is influenced by several hormones [1].

Hypophysectomy is followed by the development of anemia in rats [2] and reduced plasma levels of Epo in hypoxemic rodents [3]. Subcutaneous injection of antidiuretic hormone (ADH) into polycythemic mice significantly increases incorporation of Fe-59 into erythrocytes as a measure of Epo activity [4]. Panhypopituitaric patients receiving ADH have increased red cell mass and plasma Epo levels [5].

The mechanism of action of ADH in enhancing the production of Epo is not fully understood. Since ADH is a hormone with vasopressor activity [6], it was assumed that the application of ADH lowers renal blood flow resulting in ischemic hypoxia [5, 7, 8].

However, there are experimental findings, which make this explanation improbable. We have earlier shown that even a drastic reduction of renal blood flow in rats to 10 % of normal is followed by an only slight increase in plasma Epo level [9]. Furthermore, infusions of pharmacological amounts of ADH result in only minimal elevation of arterial blood pressure in rats, rabbits, dogs and man [10, 11]. The contraction potential of ADH, which can be demonstrated in isolated perfused blood-vessels [12], aortic strips [13] or vascular smooth muscle cells [14], appears to be offset in vivo by a fall of cardiac output [10]. In contrast to other organs [15], renal circulation appears very insensitive to the acute vasoconstrictor effect of ADH

[16]. Treatment of rats with ADH for a few hours does not affect renal hemodynamics, prolonged administration results even in a 50 % increase in both glomerular filtration rate and renal blood flow [17].

ADH acts through binding to specific membrane-bound receptors present at the surface of the target cells [18]. Renal V2-receptors, through adenylate cyclase activation and generation of cyclic adenosine monophosphate, largely account for the renal antidiuretic effect of ADH [19]. Vascular V1a-receptors mediate the vasoconstrictor actions of ADH through a phosphatidylinositol bisphosphate-dependent system leading to intracellular calcium mobilization [20]. In addition, there is a second V1-receptor subclass, the V1b-receptor mediating the modulation of the adrenocorticotropic hormone secretion from the anterior pituitary by ADH [21]. Specific antagonists of the responses of ADH are powerful pharmacological tools for exploring the physiological importance of the actions of ADH [22].

In the present study the question was raised as to whether the vasopressor potency of ADH via its vascular V1a-receptor is responsible for the Epo stimulating effect.

Methods

Animals

Adult, male Sprague-Dawley rats weighing 300-400 g were studied. Up to the experiments, food and water were provided ad libitum. The experiments were performed on unanesthetized animals in individual study cages.

Study protocol

In a first set of experiments, the Epo response of rats during stimulation by ADH and selective V1a-receptor blockade was studied (cf. Fig. 1, protocol A). Ten animals received subcutaneous injections of ADH (0.4 IU, applicated twice at an interval of 30 min; Pitressin, Parke-Davis, Berlin). Another group of 10 animals received 15 min before the first ADH-injection a V1a-receptor antagonist (1-β-mercapto-β, β-penta-methylene-propionyl, 2-0-Me-Tyr)-ADH (0.1 mg/kg body weight via a lateral caudal vein; "Manning compound", 23; Sigma, Deisenhofen). Nine animals served as controls receiving saline instead of V1a-antagonist or ADH. Four hours after the application of the first subcutaneous injection, a blood sample was taken by heart puncture for the determination of Epo (ELISA, medac, Hamburg).

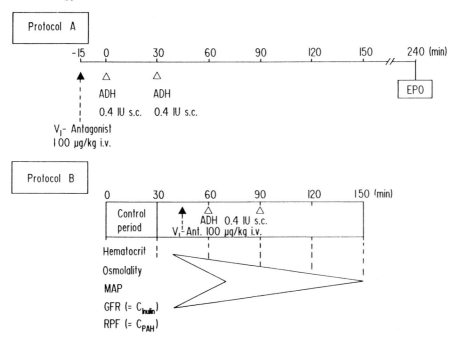

Fig. 1: Scheme of the experimental design. Protocol A: Study of the erythropoietin (EPO) response after subcutaneous (s.c.) application of antidiuretic hormone (ADH) with or without previous intraveneous (i.v.) injection of V1-antagonist. Protocol B: Study of functional parameters under ADH with or without V1-antagonist (V1-Ant.); MAP - mean arterial pressure; GFR - glomerular filtration rate; RPF - renal plasma flow.

In a second set of experiments, renal and systemic functional parameters were determined (cf. Fig. 1, protocol B). Before being transferred into individual study cages, the animals were etherised and PE-50 catheters were inserted into the carotid artery and the jugular vein. The carotid catheter was connected with a pressure transducer; through the jugular catheter a solution containing inulin and p-aminohippuric acid (PAH) was infused. After a control period of 30 min, the ADH injection (0.4 IU twice) with or without previous application of the V1a-receptor antagonist (0.1 mg/kg i.v.) was performed. Every 30 minutes the following parameters were determined: urine osmolality (vapour pressure osmometer Wescor 5100C), mean arterial pressure (MAP), glomerular filtration rate (GFR, on the basis of the clearance of inulin), and renal plasma flow (RPF, on the basis of the clearance of PAH). To avoid superfluous blood losses, the hematocrit was determined only at the beginning and the end of the experiments.

Results and discussion

Fig. 2 shows the Epo-response of the animals after the injection of ADH and the combined application of V1a-antagonists and ADH, respectively. The concentration of Epo in plasma was doubled following the injection of ADH. This is in agreement with earlier studies [5].

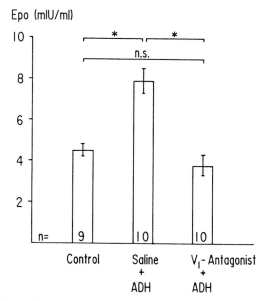

Fig. 2: Erythropoietin (Epo) response in rats after application of ADH or V1-antagonist plus ADH (means ± SEM; n.s.: P>0.05, *: P<0.05, Dunnett's test).

After blockade of the V1a-receptor the Epo-concentration in plasma was not different in comparison to that of the controls. Thus, the V1a-blockade completely abolished the Epo-stimulating effect of ADH.

The hematocrit - being the most important parameter determining the oxygen content of the blood [24] and, consequently, the rate of the synthesis of Epo [1] - did not change during the experiments. The respective values were 41.8 ± 0.7 % at the beginning and 41.1 ± 1.1 % at the end of the experiments in the group of animals receiving ADH. In the rats receiving V1a-antagonists plus ADH the values amounted to 42.8 ± 0.4 % and 42.9 ± 0.7 %, respectively.

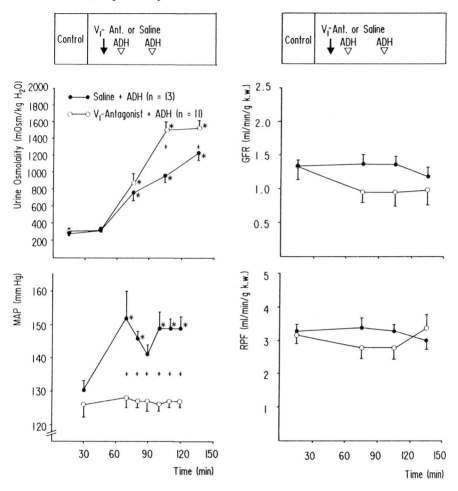

Fig. 3: Functional parameters in rats after application of ADH or V1 antagonist plus ADH (means ± SEM; *: P<0.05 vs. control value, Dunnett's test; +: P<0.05 between groups, Student's t-test; MAP - mean arterial pressure, GFR - glomerular filtration rate, RPF - renal plasma flow, k.w. - kidney weight).

Fig. 3 shows the behaviour of the functional parameters in respect to time after application of ADH with or without presence of the V1a-antagonist. In the lower left-hand corner of Fig. 3 the mean arterial pressure (MAP) is depicted. MAP increased significantly after application of ADH and remained on the raised level after the second dose of ADH. After blockade of the V1a-receptor MAP persisted in the control level. As shown in the upper left-hand corner of Fig. 3, urine osmolality increased in both groups. These results show that the V1a-antagonist completely obviated an increase of MAP [cf. 25, 26]. However, it did not prevent the antidiuretic action of ADH, which is mediated by the renal V2-receptor [19].

The right half of Fig. 3 shows the results of the measurements of the glomerular filtration rate (GFR) and the renal plasma flow (RPF). Neither ADH alone nor the combined giving of V1a-antagonist and ADH had an influence on GFR or RPF.

From these results it can be concluded that a constriction of renal vessels is not suitable for an explanation of the enhancement of the Epo-synthesis by ADH. There is rather a direct stimulation of the Epo-synthesis by ADH via its V1a-receptor.

The vascular V1a-receptor stimulates a G protein coupled phospholipase C [27] leading to the hydrolysis of polyphosphoinositides and, in turn, the production of inositol 1,4,5-triphosphate and 1,2-diacylglycerol [28]. The formation of inositol 1,4,5-triphosphate is responsible for calcium mobilization [14] and, consequently, for vascular smooth muscle cell contraction [29]. 1,2-Diacylglycerol activates a protein kinase C [30], which initiates an increased gene expression and protein synthesis [31].

The ADH-induced increase in mRNA levels is markedly reduced by cytochrome P-450 inhibitors [31]. Recently published theoretical considerations [32] and experimental findings [33] strongly support the idea that microsomal cytochrome P-450 oxidases also play an important role in the control of Epo synthesis. Therefore, it is suggested that the enhanced production of Epo by ADH is mediated by a cytochrome P-450 oxidase. Reminding the fact that this stimulation only occurs, when a relatively high dose of ADH is applied, further investigations remain to be done, whether this is of physiological importance.

References

1. JELKMANN, W. (1992): Erythropoietin: structure, control of production, and function. Physiol. Rev. 72, 449-489.
2. BERLIN, N.I., D.C. VANDYKE, W.E. SIRI & C.P. WILLIAMS (1950): The effect of hypophysectomy on the total circulating red cell volume of the rat. Endocrinology 47, 429-435.

3. HALVORSEN, S., B.L. ROH & J.W. FISHER (1968): Erythropoietin production in nephrectomized and hypophysectomized animals. Am. J. Physiol. 215, 349-352.
4. JEPSON, J. & L. LOWENSTEIN (1966): The effect of vasopressin, testosterone and erythropoietin on erythropoiesis. Clin. Res. 14, 483 (abstr.).
5. JEPSON, J., E.E. MCGARRY & L. LOWENSTEIN (1968): Erythropoietin excretion in a hypopituitary patient. Arch. Int. Med. 122, 265-270.
6. OLIVER, G. & E.A. SCHÄFER (1895): On the physiological action of extracts of pituitary blood and certain other glandular organs. J. Physiol. 18, 277-279.
7. FISHER, J.W., & D.M. GROSS (1977): Hormonal influences on erythropoiesis: anterior pituitary, adrenocortical, thyroid, growth and other hormones. In: FISHER, J.W. (ed.): Kidney Hormones, Vol. II, pp. 415-435, London, Academic Press.
8. FISHER, J.W. (1988): Pharmacologic modulation of erythropoietin production. Ann. Rev. Pharmacol. Toxicol. 28, 101-122.
9. PAGEL, H., W. JELKMANN & C. WEISS (1988): A comparison of the effects of renal artery constriction and anemia on the production of erythropoietin. Pflügers Arch. 413, 62-66.
10. COWLEY, A.M., J.F. LIARD, M.M. SKELTON, E.W. QUILLEN, J.W. OSBORN & R.L. WEBB (1985): Vasopression-neural interactions in the control of cardiovascular function. In: SCHRIER, R.W. (ed.): Vasopressin, pp. 1-10, New York, Raven Press.
11. ABBOUD, F.M., J.S. FLORAS, P.E. AYLWARD, G.B. GUO, B.N. GUPTA & P.G. SCHMID (1990): Role of vasopressin in cardiovascular and blood pressure regulation. Blood Vessels 27, 106-115.
12. EDWARDS, R.M., W. TRIZNA & L.B. KINTER (1989): Renal microvascular effects of vasopressin and vasopressin antagonists. Am. J. Physiol. 256, F274-F278.
13. TAKKAR, A.P.S. & C.J. KIRK (1981): Stimulation of inorganic phosphate incorporation into phosphatidylinositol in rat thoracic aorta mediated through V1-vasopressin receptors. Biochem. J. 194, 167-172.
14. OKADA, K., S. ISHIKAWA & T. SAITO (1991): Mechanisms of vasopressin-induced increase in intracellular sodium in vascular smooth muscle cells. Am. J. Physiol. 261, F1007-F1012.
15. LIARD, J.F., O. DERIAZ, P. SCHELLING & M. THIBONNIER (1982): Cardiac output distribution during vasopressin infusions or dehydration in conscious dogs. Am. J. Physiol. 243, H663-H669.
16. STEIN, J.H. (1990): Regulation of the renal circulation. Kidney Int. 38, 571-576.
17. GELLAI, M., J.H. SILVERSTEIN, J.C. HWANG, F.T. LA-ROCHELLE & H. VALTIN (1984): Influence of vasopressin on renal hemodynamics in conscious Brattleboro rats. Am. J. Physiol. 246, F819-F827.
18. MICHELL, R.H., J.C. KIRK & M.M. BILLAH (1979): Hormonal stimulation of phosphatidylinositol breakdown with particular reference to the hepatic effects of vasopressin. Biochem. Soc. Trans. 7, 861-865.
19. MOREL, F., M. IMBERT-TEBOUL & D. CHABARDES (1987): Receptors to vasopressin and other hormones in the mammalian kidney. Kidney Int. 31, 512-520.
20. THIBONNIER, M. (1988): Vasopressin and blood pressure. Kidney Int. 34, Suppl. 25, S52-S56.
21. JARD, S., R.C. GAILLARD, G. GUILLON, J. MARIE, P. SCHONENBERG, A.F. MULLER & M. MANNING, W.H. SAWYER (1986): Vasopressin antagonists allow demonstration of a novel type of vasopressin receptor in the rat adenohypophysis. Mol. Pharmacol. 30, 171-177.

23. KRUSZYNSKI, M., B. LAMMEK, M. MANNING, J. SETO, J. HALDAR & W.H. SAWYER (1980): (1- (β-mercapto-β, β-cyclopentamethylenepropionic acid), 2-(O-methyl) tyrosine) arginine-vasopressin and (1-(β-mercapto-β, β-cyclopentamethylenepropionic acid)) arginine-vasopressin, two highly potent antagonists of the vasopressor response to arginine-vasopressin. J. Med. Chem. 23, 364-368.
22. LIARD, J.F. (1988): Vasopressin antagonists and their use in animal studies. Kidney Int., 34, Suppl. 26, S43-S47.
24. FAN, F.C., R.Y.Z. CHEN, G.B. SCHUESSLER & S. CHIEN (1980): Effects of hematocrit variations on regional hemodynamics and oxygen transport in the dog. Am. J. Physiol. 238, H545-H552.
25. MANNING, M., S. STOEV, K. BANKOWSKI, A. MISICKA, B. LAMMEK, N.C. WO & W.H. SAWYER (1992): Synthesis and some pharmacological properties of potent and selective antagonists of the vasopressor (V1-receptor) response to arginine-vasopressin. J. Med. Chem. 35, 382-388.
26. ERVIN, M.G., M.G. ROSS, R.D. LEAKE & D.A. FISHER (1992): V1- and V2-receptor contributions to ovine fetal renal and cardiovascular responses to vasopressin. Am. J. Physiol. 262, R636-R643.
27. GOPALAKRISHNAN, V., Y. XU, P.V. SULAKHE, C.R. TRIGGLE & J.R. MCNEILL (1991): Vasopressin (V1) receptor characteristics in rat aortic smooth muscle cells. Am. J. Physiol. 261, H1927-H1936.
28. THIBONNIER, M., A.L. BAYER, M.S. SIMONSON & KESTER (1991): Multiple signaling pathways of V1-vascular AVP receptors of A7r5 cells. Endocrinology 129, 2845-2856.
29. HAJJAR, R.J. & J.V. BONVENTRE (1991): Oscillations of intracellular calcium induced by vasopressin in individual fura-2-loaded mesangial cells. J. Biol. Chem. 266, 21589-21594.
30. TANG, E.K.Y. & M.D. HOUSLAY (1992): Glucagon, vasopressin and angiotensin all elicit a rapid, transient increase in hepatocyte protein kinase C activity. Biochem. J. 283, 341-346.
31. THIBONNIER, M. (1992): Signal transduction of V1-vascular vasopressin receptors. Regulatory Peptides 38, 1-11.
32. GOLDBERG, M.A., S.P. DUNNING & H.F. BUNN (1988): Regulation of the erythropoietin gene: evidence that the oxygen sensor is a heme protein. Science 242, 1412-1415.
33. FANDREY, J., F.P. SEYDEL, C.P. SIEGERS & W. JELKMANN (1990): Role of cytochrome P-450 in the control of the production of erythropoietin. Life Sciences 47: 127-134.

Energy-dependent injury to hepatic endothelial cells in organ preservation solutions

U. Rauen*, W. Lauchart**, H.D. Becker** and H. de Groot*

Institut für Physiologische Chemie, Universitätsklinikum Essen* und
Abteilung für Allgemeine Chirurgie, Chirurgische Universitätsklinik der
Universität Tübingen**

Introduction

Transplantation invariably includes a period of ischemia for the organ being transplanted. The predominant injury during this period is thought to be due to hypoxia [1]. In order to minimize this hypoxic injury, the organ is stored at low temperature (0-5 °C). However, although cold slows down metabolism and thereby delays energy depletion, it also aggravates electrolyte imbalances by inhibiting the Na^+/K^+-ATPase and thus promotes cell oedema [1-3]. To minimize the negative effects of cold ischemia, most solutions used for flushing and cold storage, the socalled preservation solutions, are based on high potassium and low sodium concentrations and on more or less impermeable substances to counteract the osmotic pressure exerted by intracellular proteins [2]. Solutions used for preservation of the liver are University of Wisconsin (UW) solution, Histidine-Tryptophan-Ketoglutarate (HTK) solution and Euro-Collins solution, of which HTK and the most widely used UW solution have been shown to give the best results [4,5].

Although cold in combination with these preservation solutions allows up to 3-days-storage of kidneys, liver preservation is limited to about 24 hrs [1,5]. Surprisingly, not the metabolically very active hepatocytes but the endothelial cells are damaged first [6-9]. This preferential endothelial cell damage during cold preservation of the liver is difficult to explain as liver endothelial cells are very resistant to hypoxia at 37 °C (unpublished results).

To assess the role of energy-depletion in the pathogenesis of this endothelial cell injury we studied cultured endothelial cells from rat liver under preservation conditions (i.e. preservation solutions, cold, hypoxia).

Methods

Endothelial cells were isolated from the livers of male Wistar rats (200-240 g) by collagenase perfusion, differential centrifugation and selective adherence [10]. Cells were cultured in RPMI 1640 medium (Boehringer, Mannheim, Germany) with 20 % fetal calf serum (Biospa, Wedel, Germany), supplemented with L-glutamine (2 mM), dexamethasone (1 µM), gentamycin (100 µg/ml), cefotaxime (10 µg/ml) and amphotericine B (5 µg/ml). Culture flasks were coated with collagen (collagen R, Serva, Heidelberg, Germany; diluted 1:10 with aqua bidest. before use). Subcultures were obtained by trypsinization (0.25 % trypsin in citrate saline for 6-8 min).

Confluent 2nd to 6th passage cultures in 5.5 cm^2 culture tubes (Nunc, Roskilde, Denmark) were used for experiments: cells were rinsed three times with warm HBSS (37 °C), covered with 2 ml of cold (4 °C) UW solution, HTK solution, Euro-Collins solution or Krebs-Henseleit buffer and incubated at 4 °C. UW solution (DuPont, Bad Homburg, Germany) contains 20 mM Na^+, 140 mM K^+, 5 mM Mg^{2+}, 5 mM SO_4^{2-}, 25 mM $H_2PO_4^-$, 100 mM lactobionate, 30 mM raffinose, 50 g/l hydroxyethylstarch, 1 mM allopurinol, 5 mM adenosine and 3 mM glutathione (pH 7.4); this solution was supplemented with benzylpenicillin 200 000 IU/l, insulin 40 IU/l and dexamethasone 16 mg/l. HTK solution (Köhler, Alsbach, Germany) contains 15 mM Na^+, 10 mM K^+, 4 mM Mg^{2+}, 50 mM Cl^-, 2 mM tryptophan, 1 mM ketoglutarate, 180/18 mM histidine/histidine HCl and 30 mM mannitol (pH 7.2.); Euro-Collins solution (Fresenius, Bad Homburg, Germany) contains 10 mM Na^+, 115 mM K^+, 15 mM Cl^-, 15 mM $H_2PO_4^-$, 43 mM HPO_4^{2-}, 10 mM HCO_3^- and 198 mM glucose (pH 7.3) and the modified Krebs-Henseleit buffer we used contained 144 mM Na^+, 6 mM K^+, 1.2 mM Mg^{2+}, 2.5 mM Ca^{2+}, 128 mM Cl^- 25 mM HCO_3^-, 1.2 mM SO_4^{2-}, 1.2 mM $H_2PO_4^-$ and 20 mM HEPES (pH 7.4).

Hypoxic conditions were simulated by the addition of the respiratory chain inhibitor KCN (1 mM) or other inhibitors of mitochondrial ATP formation (antimycin A, 1 µM; rotenone, 1 µM; oligomycin, 10 µM; carbonylcyanide-m-chlorophenylhydrazone 1 µM; all from Sigma, Deisenhofen, Germany). Viability was assessed by the uptake of the vital dyes trypan blue and propidium iodide and the release of cytosolic lactate dehydrogenase (LDH). LDH was measured using a standard assay [11]. ATP was determined enzymatically using a 3-phosphoglycerate kinase assay [12] and a two-wavelength spectrophotometer; lactate was determined as described in [10]. For inhibition of pinocytosis cells were preincubated with cytochalasin B (2-50 µg/ml) or colchizine (5 and 20 µg/ml) for 2 hrs or with monensin (0.1-10 µM) for 4 hrs in culture medium at 37 °C; for the subsequent cold incubations these inhibitors were added to UW solution in the same concentrations. In one set of experiments non-confluent cultures were used.

Data are expressed as means ± SE. Comparisons among multiple groups were performed using an analysis of variance with Student-Newman-Keuls post hoc comparisons [13]. A p value of < 0.05 was considered significant.

Results and Discussion

During cold incubation in UW solution liver endothelial cells in confluent monolayer cultures were injured rapidly under aerobic control conditions: after 12 hrs of incubation the release of cytosolic LDH was already 46 % and after 24 hrs of incubation 71 %. Simulation of hypoxic conditions by blockade of the mitochondrial respiratory chain with KCN (1 mM) did surprisingly not aggravate but ameliorate the injury (Fig. 1); even after 72 hrs LDH release was only 44 ± 12 %. This "paradoxical" protection by cyanide was confirmed when other parameters of viability, i.e. the uptake of the vital dyes tryphan blue and propidium iodide, or other inhibitors of oxidative phosphorylation such as antimycin A, rotenone, oligomycin and carbonylcyanide-m-chlorophenylhydrazone were used (data not shown).

Addition of glucose (10 mM) allowed anaerobic glycolysis to proceed at a rate of 5-6 nmol lactate/10^6 cells per hour and thus allowed energy formation in the presence of cyanide. The addition of glucose did not significantly alter the injury under aerobic control conditions but caused a marked increase of the injury in cyanide-containing UW solution (Fig. 1).

The "paradoxical" protective effect of cyanide and the partial abolishment of this protection by the addition of glucose suggest an energy-dependence of the injury ocurring to cultured liver endothelial cells in cold UW solution. ATP determinations confirmed high energy levels of the cells in cyanide-free UW solution, i.e. of the cells that subsequently died first, and low energy levels in the presence of UW + KCN, i.e. of those cells that survived best (Tab. 1).

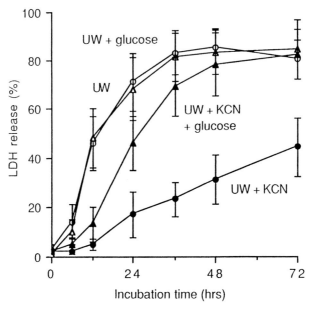

Fig. 1: Injury to cultured liver endothelial cells during cold (4 °C) incubation in University of Wisconsin solution (UW) in the absence and in the presence of 1 mM KCN and 10 mM glucose. Injury was assessed by the release of cytosolic lactate dehydrogenase (LDH). Values shown represent means ± SE of 8 experiments.

During cold incubation of liver endothelial cells in HTK solution similar results were obtained: cells died rapidly under aerobic control conditions, the addition of cyanide protected the cells and the addition of glucose was damaging (Tab. 1). Again, injury occurred first in those incubations with the highest ATP levels during the first few hours of incubation. Thus, the injury occurring to cultured liver endothelial cells during cold incubation in HTK solution appears to be energy-dependent as the injury occurring in UW solution.

In cold Krebs-Henseleit buffer, in contrast, cells were damaged by the addition of cyanide and protected by the addition of glucose (Tab. 1). Similarly, the addition of cyanide to Euro-Collins solution had a damaging effect. Thus, in Krebs-Henseleit buffer and in Euro-Collins solution injury to cultured liver endothelial cells was increased when energy levels were low and decreased when energy levels were high; these results are in line with current concepts of hypoxia-induced preservation injury [1,3].

Tab. 1: ATP levels and LDH release of liver endothelial cells during incubation in UW, HTK and Euro-Collins solutions and in Krebs-Henseleit buffer at 4°C in the absence and in the presence of glucose (10 mM) and KCN (1 mM). Values shown represent means ± S.E. of 4 experiments. Initial ATP levels, i.e. ATP levels before the start of cold incubation, were 15.1 ± 1.6 nmol/10^6 cells.

Incubation medium	ATP (nmol/10^6 cells) 4 hrs	LDH release 12 hrs	24 hrs
UW	17.8 ± 3.6	46 ± 11	71 ± 12
UW + glucose	14.9 ± 3.9	48 ± 12	68 ± 13
UW + KCN	2.2 ± 1.8	5 ± 2	17 ± 9
UW + KCN + glucose	6.6 ± 2.1	13 ± 7	46 ± 11
HTK	10.8 ± 2.2	87 ± 13	85 ± 10
HTK + glucose	10.9 ± 2.5	89 ± 8	86 ± 7
HTK + KCN	1.9 ± 0.8	28 ± 1	63 ± 15
HTK + KCN + glucose	4.3 ± 0.3	59 ± 13	87 ± 6
Euro-Collins	13.1 ± 1.6	25 ± 15	48 ± 20
Euro-Collins + KCN	9.4 ± 1.2	40 ± 16	68 ± 12
Krebs-Henseleit	13.8 ± 2.8	10 ± 4	32 ± 9
Krebs-Henseleit + glucose	13.1 ± 1.4	9 ± 5	13 ± 3
Krebs-Henseleit + KCN	2.5 ± 0.7	25 ± 12	63 ± 14
Krebs-Henseleit + KCN + glucose	4.3 ± 1.0	19 ± 7	42 ± 8

In contrast to these current concepts of preservation injury, UW and HTK solution - offering good protection against hypoxic injury - damage cultured liver endothelial cells in an energy-dependent way (Fig. 2). Endothelial cell toxicity of organ preservation solutions has been described using macrovascular endothelial cells [14]; in this study, however, the injury was not investigated under hypoxic conditions. Endothelial cell toxicity of cardioplegic solutions has been attributed to a high potassium concentration [15] and Ca^{2+}-free solutions have been shown to be toxic to hepatocytes under aerobic conditions [16,17]. With regard to the results in Euro-Collins solution neither the absence of Ca^{2+} nor the presence of a high potassium or a low sodium concentration can account for the injury occurring in UW and HTK solution; likewise, omission of Mg^{2+} from these two solutions did not prohibit the paradoxical cyanide effect (data not shown). Besides these electrolytes, UW and HTK solution do not possess a common substance that might provoke the injury. Preincubation with and addition of cytochalasine B, colchizine and monensin did not abolish the paradoxical cyanide effect (data not shown), thereby suggesting that the energy-dependent injury observed is not due to (energy-dependent) pinocytosis of the unphysiologic solutions by the liver endothelial cells which are characterized by a high pinocytotic activity [18].

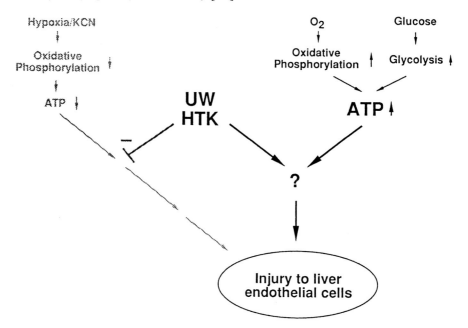

Fig. 2: Injury to cultured liver endothelial cells during cold incubation in UW and HTK solutions. Although the solutions protect the cells very efficiently against hypoxic injury, in the presence of high ATP levels the cells are damaged in a so far unknown way.

The energy-dependent injury only occurred in confluent, but not in non-confluent cultures. In non-confluent cultures the injury occurring under aerobic control conditions was largely decreased whereas the injury occurring in the presence of cyanide was largely increased - leading to an overall damaging, i.e. "normal", cyanide effect. This different behaviour of non-confluent cells could not be attributed to a decreased cell/medium ratio, it rather appeared to be related to a different "state" of the confluent, quiescent cells. Whether this "state" is related to differences in metabolism or differentiation is currently as unclear as is the mechanism of the energy-dependent injury occurring in confluent cultures.

In summary, our experiments showed that rat liver endothelial cells in confluent monolayer culture are damaged in UW and HTK solutions in an energy-dependent way. The mechanism of this injury, that is in contrast to current concepts of preservation injury and that only occurs in confluent but not in non-confluent cultures, is unclear.

References

1. BLANKENSTEIJN, J.D. & O.T. TERPSTRA (1991): Liver preservation: the past and the future. Hepatology 13, 1235-1250.
2. BELZER, F.O. & J.H. SOUTHARD (1988): Principles of solid-organ preservation by cold storage. Transplantation 45, 673-676.
3. HOCHACHKA, P.W. (1986): Defense stategies against hypoxia and hypothermia: Science 231, 234-241.
4. GUBERNATIS, G., R. PICHLMAYR, P. LAMESCH, H. GROSSE, A. BORNSCHEUER, H.J. MEYER, B. RINGE, M. FARLE & H.J. BRETSCHNEIDER (1990): HTK-solution (Bretschneider) for human liver transplantation. First clinical experiences. Langenbecks Arch. Chir. 375, 66-70.
5. KALAYOGLU, M., R.M. HOFFMANN, A.M. D'ALLESSANDRO, J.D. PIRSCH, H.W. SOLLINGER & F.O. BELZER (1989): Results of extended preservation of the liver for clinical transplantation. Transplant. Proc. 21, 3487-3488.
6. CALDWELL-KENKEL, J.C., R.T. CURRIN, Y. TANAKA, R.G. THURMAN & J.J. LEMASTERS (1991): Kupffer cell activation and endothelial cell damage after storage of rat livers: Effects of reperfusion. Hepatology 13, 83-95.
7. MCKEOWN, C.M.B., V. EDWARDS, M.J. PHILLIPS, P.R.C. HARVEY, C.N. PETRUNKA & S.M. STRASBERG (1988): Sinusoidal lining cell damage: the critical injury in cold preservation of liver allografts in the rat. Transplantation 46, 178-191.
8. FRATTE, S., J.L. GENDRAULT, A.M. STEFFAN & A. KIRN (1991): Comparative ultrastructural study of rat livers preserved in Euro-Collins or University of Wisconsin solution. Hepatology 13, 1173-1180.
9. MOMII, S. & A. KOGA (1990): Time-related morphological changes in cold-stored rat livers: a comparison of Euro-Collins solution with UW solution. Transplantation 50, 745-750.
10. RAUEN, U., M. HANßEN, W. LAUCHART, H.D. BECKER & H. DE GROOT (1993): Energy-dependent injury to cultured sinusoidal endothelial cells of the rat liver in UW solution. Transplantation 55, 469-473.
11. BERGMEYER, H.U. & E. BERNT (1974): Lactat-Dehydrogenase: UV-Test mit Pyruvat und NADH. In: BERGMEYER, H.W. (ed): Methoden der enzymatischen Analyse. pp. 607-612, Weinheim: Verlag Chemie.
12. JAWOREK, D., W. GRUBER & H.U. BERGMEYER (1974): Adenosin-5'-triphosphat: Bestimmung mit 3-Phosphoglycerat-Kinase. In: BERGMEYER, H.W. (ed): Methoden der enzymatischen Analyse. pp. 2147-2151, Weinheim: Verlag Chemie.
13. ZIVIN, J.A. & J.J. BARTKO (1976): Statistics for disinterested scientists. Life Sciences 18, 15-26.

14. OPPELL, U.O. VON, S. PFEIFFER, P. PREISS, T. DUNNE, P. ZILLA & B. REICHART (1990): Endothelial cell toxicity of solid-organ preservation solutions. Ann. Thorac. Surg. 50, 902-910.
15. MANKAD, P.S., A.H. CHESTER & M.H. YACOUB (1991): Role of potassium concentration in cardioplegic solutions in mediating endothelial damage. Ann. Thorac. Surg., 51, 89-93.
16. BRECHT, M., C. BRECHT & H. DE GROOT (1992): Late steady increase in cytosolic Ca^{2+} preceding hypoxic injury in hepatocytes. Biochem. J. 283, 399-402.
17. LINDELL, S., M. AMETANI, F.O. BELZER & J.H. SOUTHARD (1989): Hypothermic perfusion of rabbit livers: effect of perfusate composition (Ca and lactobionate) on enzyme release and tissue swelling. Cryobiology 26, 407-412.
18. BLOUIN, A., R.P. BOLENDER & E.R. WEIBEL (1977): Distribution of organelles and membranes between hepatocytes and nonhepatocytes in the rat liver parenchyma: a stereological study. J. Cell. Biol. 72, 441-455.

Modulation of oxygen deprivation-induced cellular dysfunction by glycine and alanine

G. Gronow, O. Jung and M. Mályusz

Department of Physiology, University of Kiel

Introduction

A high rate of oxygen delivery to the kidney and a low arteriovenous difference of oxygen concentration have contributed to the widespread contention of a relatively high tolerance of the kidney to ischemia and anoxia. Time intervals between 25 and 60 minutes of ischemic tolerance are reported in the literature [8]. This variation may have originated from imponderables like preexisting organ insufficiency, cooling by room temperature, blood supply by undetected vascular collaterales, diffusion of atmospheric oxygen through the organ surface, or different availability of metabolic energy by anaerobic substrates. Under controlled experimental conditions of extreme hypoxia (PO_2 < 1 mmHg) and no substrate supply, however, 10 minutes of normothermic oxygen deprivation were suffcient to induce irreversible functional and structural defects in isolated tubular segments of the rat kidney cortex [5].

Recent experiments indicate that the hypoxic tolerance of the kidney may by modified by certain amino acids. In studies on the protective role of glutathione (GSH) in renal reoxygenation damage Weinberg and co-workers [13] detected in 1987 that not the tripeptide GSH, but one of its components, the amino acid glycine suppressed hypoxic alterations in isolated tubular segments of rabbit renal cortex. Later experiments confirmed the cytoprotective role of glycine [4, 12, 14]. Alanine, the chain-elongated C-3-derivative of glycine induced less pronounced effevts in isolated renal tubules of the rabbit [13], but it markedly reduced hypoxic damage in the isolated perfused rat kidney [1]. Therefore the aim of the present study was to compare in reoxygenated tubular segments of rat kidney cortex structure-related cytoprotection by glycine and ist derivatives L-alanine (=α-methyl-glycine), L-serine (=β-hydroxy-alanine) and pyruvate (=desaminated alanine). Posthypoxic cellular viability was checked by monitoring mitochondrial respiratory function and the ability of the cells for lactate gluconeogenesis. Intactness of cellular membranes was judged by the loss of cell constituents into the incubation medium.

Methods

Tubular segments from rat renal cortex were isolated by collagenase treatment. Details of this method have been reported elsewhere [7]. Isolated tubular segments (ITS) were incubated at 37 °C in a modified Krebs-Ringer-bicarbonate (KRB) medium containing 0.5 $g \cdot dl^{-1}$ bovine albumine and 10 $mmol \cdot l^{-1}$ lactate. KRB-media contained additionally isomolar (5 $mmol\ l^{-1}$) either glycine, alanine, serine or pyruvate. Extreme hypoxia (PO_2 30 min < 1 mmHg) was introduced by gassing the surface of the suspension with water saturated 95 % N_2: 5 % CO_2. After variable periods of hypoxia (10 to 90 min) ITS were subsequently reoxygenated (60 min) by gassing the surface with 95 % O_2: 5 % CO_2. All probes were immediately withdrawn, centrifuged and analyzed for protein, glucose, enzymes, and mitochondrial respiration.

Isolation of renal mitochondria from posthypoxic ITS was performed according to the method described by Goldstein [3]. The mitochondrial respiratory control ratio (RCR = state 3 over state 4 respiration) was calculated in 5 $mmol \cdot l^{-1}$ malate and 5 $mmol \cdot l^{-1}$ glutamate as the ratio of 0.5 $mmol \cdot l^{-1}$ ADP-stimulated oxygen consumption over mitochondrial respiration after the ADP-effect had worn off. Tubular and mitochondrial protein was measured colorimetrically by the method of Lowry [8]. Measurements of enzyme activitiy (LDH = lactate dehydrogenase, EC 1.1.27; GlDH = glutamate dehydrogenase, EC 1.4.1.3) and of glucose in the supernatant of centrifuged cell suspensions were performed according to standard procedures and previously described methods [5, 6]. All values are expressed per mg tubular protein and are means ± SD. Statistical analysis was employed as paired t-Test. A P-value of 0.05 or less was assumed to indicate a significant difference.

Results and discussion

Persistent change of posthypoxic mitochondrial function indicates an intimate relationship between the loss of renal cellular viability following long lasting respiratory arrest [15]. In a first series of experiments we studied the recovery of tubular cell function like mitochondrial respiratory control rate (RCR, state 3 over state 4 respiration) and ATP-dependent gluconeogenesis in isolated tubular segments of rat kidney cortex. We have reported previously that in the isolated rat kidney even after 40 min of anoxic perfusion mitochondrial RCR was supported by an amino acid mixture containing among others glycine and alanine [6].

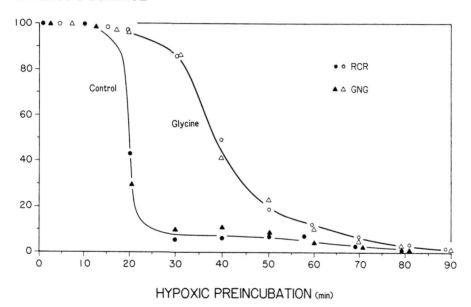

Fig. 1: Recovery (% of aerobic control) of posthypoxic mitochondrial respiratory control rate (RCR, circles) and of gluconeogenetic activity (GNG, triangles) as a function of preceeding intervals (0-90 min) of extreme hypoxia (PO_2 < 1 mmHg, 37 °C) in isolated tubular segments of rat kidney cortex. Aerobic 100 % control = 4.92 ± 0.87 (RCR) and 4.5 ± 1.1 nmol glucose mg^{-1} min^{-1} (GNG). Symbols represent means of 5 observations (closed = hypoxic control, open = 5 mmol l^{-1} glycine added).

In the present experiments RCR of mitochondria isolated from tubules suspended without amino acids remained stable for 10 min at a PO_2 < 1 mmHg (Fig. 1, closed circles, RCR = 4.92 ± 0.87). However, after 20 minutes of extreme hypoxia RCR fell steeply to about 50 % of control values. Mitochondria from ITS maintained for more than 30 min at that low oxygen tension exposed virtually no ADP-stimulated respiration. Glycine in the incubation medium, however (Fig. 1, open circles), supported mitochondrial respiratory function dramatically. The posthypoxic decline in RCR was less steep, 50 % reduction of RCR occurred not until 40 min of oxygen deprivation. Thus, the observed improvement in posthypoxic mitochondrial function in the presence of glycine may also contribute substantially to the reversibility of active metabolic function like gluconeogenesis in reoxygenated renal cortical cells.

Gluconeogenesis (GNG) is highly dependent on the provision of metabolic energy. Untreated isolated tubules produced 4.5 ± 1.1 nmol glucose ·mg protein^{-1}·min^{-1} in the presence of 10 mmol·l^{-1} lactate. Posthypoxic mitochondrial dysfunction and the preceeding hypoxic depletion of ATP-stores reduced GNG during reoxygenation (Fig. 1, triangles). GNG fell in close relationship to the observed decrease in RCR. A 50 % reduction of GNG occurred after about 20 min of hypoxic preincubation, and nearly no posthypoxic glucose formation was observed after 30 min of oxygen deprivation. Similar observations of GNG-sensivity against hypoxia have been reported earlier [5]. The close relationship between GNG and RCR was also observed in the presence of glycine, but the flattened decline of GNG as a function of preceeding hypoxia was markedly shifted to the right. 50 % reduction of GNG occurred after about 40 min of oxygen deprivation. Thus, the time interval necessary to induce a 50 % reduction in RCR and GNG had doubled in the presence of glycine.

Insufficient supply with oxygen and lack of anaerobic substrates reduces transmembraneous ion pumping, induces cellular swelling, and disrupts cellular membranes [10]. A sensitive parameter of membrane leakiness is the liberation of cell constituents into the extracellular compartment [5]. In order to evaluate a suitable marker enzyme we tested in the next series of experiments at extreme low oxygen tension the liberation of 4 celluar marker enzymes (Fig. 2): With respect to normoxic controls the activities of cytoplasmatic lactatedehydrogenase (LDH, closed circles) and of gamma-glutamyltransferase (GGT, triangles) were significantly elevated after 10 min of hypoxic incubation. LDH indicated unphysiological cellular membrane permeability, GGT monitored the disruptive swelling of renal tubular microvilli. LDH-liberation was more sensitive to oxygen deprivation than GGT, 50 % of its final release was observed after about 20 min, GGT-leakage reached the 50 % loss 10 min later.

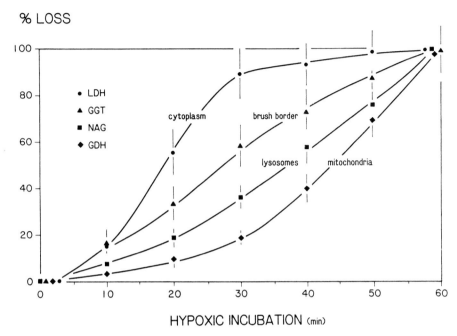

Fig. 2: Hypoxic loss (% of maximal release) of cell constituents, as indicated by the appearence of 4 marker enzymes in the incubation medium (LDH = lactate dehydrogenase, EC 1.1.27; GGT = gamma-glutamyltransferase, EC 2.3.2.2; GIDH = glutamate dehydrogenase, EC 1.4.1.3; NAG = N-acetyl-β-D-glucosaminidase) of isolated tubular segments of rat kidney cortex (PO_2 < 1 mmHg, 37 °C, n = 14).

The liberation of marker enzymes enclosed in cellular organelles was delayed, 50 % activity of the lysosomal N-acetyl-ß-D-Glucosaminidase (NAG, squares) was liberated after about 40 min, and 50 % of mitochondrial glutamate dehydrogenase (GLDH, rhombs) after about 45 min. Obviously, the unphysiological leakage of cytoplasm (LDH) advanced other cell components (NAG and GLDH). LDH was more sensitive to hypoxia than the liberation of structurally bound GGT (Fig. 2). LDH-leakage as a function of preceeding hypoxia paralleled inversely the steep reduction of the functional parameters RCR and GNG (Fig. 1). After an only short period of hypoxia (10 min) LDH-loss was even more sensitive to oxygen deprivation than the functional parameters RCR and GNG. Posthypoxic RCR and GNG were still unchanged after 10 min of hypoxia when LDH-activity in the incubation medium was already significantly elevated.

The last series of experiments was performed in order to gain additional information about the structural requirements for renal cytoprotection by amino acids during hypoxia. LDH-release was chosen as a sensitive parameter for comparing the cytoprotective effect of glycine with the structurally related derivatives a) chain-elongated glycine = L-alanine, b) β-hydroxylated L-alanine = L-serine, and c) desaminated alanine = pyruvate. In this series isolated tubuli were incubated for 30 minutes at extreme low oxygen tension (PO_2 < 1 mmHg), a time period sufficient to suppress RCR and GNG irreversibly without the protection by amino acids.

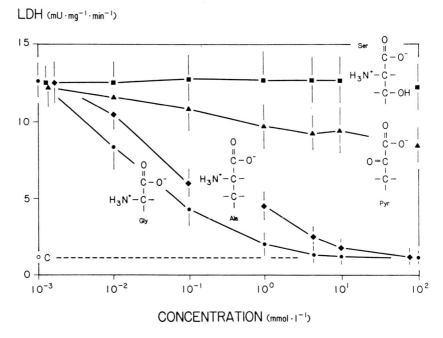

Fig. 3: Hypoxic loss (PO_2 < 1 mmHg, 37 °C) of lactate dehydrogenase (EC 1.1.27, in mU mg^{-1} min^{-1}) from isolated tubular segments of rat kidney cortex at variable concentrations of glycine (gly), L-alanine (ala), L-serine (ser), or pyruvate (pyr), n = 14.

L-serine ((Fig. 3, squares), which is synthetized in the kidney from glycine, exerted no protective effect, the LDH-leakage remained high (about 13 mU·mg^{-1}·min^{-1}) within the range of tested concentrations (0.001 - 100 mmol·l^{-1}). In contrast, glycine (closed circles) suppressed LDH-leakage with increasing concentrations. A marked reduction could already be observed in the presence of glycine at 0.01 mmol·l^{-1}. At 5 mmol·l^{-1} glycine, no significant difference could be detected between aerobic control values (Fig. 3, dashed line) and the hypoxic liberation of LDH. The cytoprotective effect of alanine (rhombs) was to some extent smaller, but significantly more pronounced then in the presence of pyruvate or serine.

In the presence of L-alanine (Fig. 3, rhombs) the LDH-leakage of isolated tubules, expressed as a function of preceeding hypoxia, was shifted to fhe right. A maximal suppression was achieved at a concentration of 10 mmol·l^{-1}. Pyruvate (triangles) also reduced LDH-leakage significantly, but the cytoprotective effect was much smaller than observed with glycine or L-alanine. From the present experiments it could not be deduced whether this pyruvate effect originated in part from alanine (by transamination of pyruvate) or whether pyruvate was converted to lactate and improved hypoxic cell function by a decrease of the cytoplasmatic redox potential, i.e. the NADH/NAD$^+$-ratio. Thus, a structural prerequisite for maximal cytoprotection was the molecular configuration of glycine, or a chain-elongated glycine (L-alanine), whereas β-hydroxylation of L-alanine to L-serine obliterated any cytoprotective effect.

L-alanine was nearly effective as glycine in protecting isolated tubules from rat renal cortex. The less effective L-alanine protection in rabbit kidney tubules reported by other investigators [14] may have originated from species differences or the fact that during the preincubation of rabbit tubuli the basic medium already contained 1 mmol·l^{-1} L-alanine, a concentration sufficient to suppress in the present experiments the LDH-leakage by about 60 % (Fig. 1). The protective effect glycine and L-alanine is not related to an improvement in hypoxic cellular energetics [1,2,12]. The exact mechanism of cytoprotection remains still to be clarified [7]. The observed concentration dependent and structure-related protection indeed suggests that glycine and L-alanine may have interacted with receptors involved in degradative processes of cell membranes responsibele for lethal cell injury. One intracellular site of degradation may be in lysolomes. Stabilization of the lysosomal membrane would reduce the liberation of lysosomal enzymes and thus also the risk of mitochondrial damage [6,11]. According to this hypothesis in the present experiments mitochondrial respiratory control rate was significantly supported in the presence of glycine (Fig. 1).

Another location of structure-related interaction with glycine or alanine may be the outer cell membrane. Stabilization of the plasmalemm by direct physico-chemical effects of protective amino acids [1], by a receptor mediated process [7] and/or a reduced activation of degradative enzymes

[6] are in accordance with the reported improvement of hypoxic cellular volume regulation in the presence of glycine [4]. This effect was indicated in the present experiments by a markedly reduced loss of cytoplasmatic LDH (Fig. 3). The improvement in cellular volume regulation may then not only have supported the maintenance of an internal milieu for mitochondrial respiratory function but also the ATP-driven gluconeogenetic activity of reoxygenated renal cortical cells (Fig. 1).

References

1. BAINES, A.D., N. SHAIK & P. HO (1990): Mechanism of perfused kidney protection by alanine and glycine . Am. J. Physiol. 259, F80-F87.
2. GARZA-QUINTERO, R., J. ORTEGA-LOPEZ, J. H. STEIN & M.A. VENKATA-CHALAM (1990): Alanine protects rabbit proximal tubules against anoxic injury in vitro. Am. J. Physiol. 258, F1075-F1083.
3. GOLDSTEIN, L. (1975): Glutamine transport by mitochondria isolated from normal and acidotic rats. Am. J. Physiol. 229, 1027-1037.
4. GRONOW. G., N. KLAUSE & M. MALYUSZ (1990): Support of hypoxic renal cell volume regulation by glycine. Adv. Epx. Med. Biol. 277, 705-712.
5. GRONOW, G., F. MEYA & C. WEISS (1984): Studies on the ability of renal cells to recover after periods of anoxia. Adv. Exp. Med. Biol. 169, 589-595.
6. GRONOW, G., CH. SKREZEK & H. KOSSMANN (1986): Correlation between mitochondrial respiratory dysfunction and Na^+-reabsorption in the reoxygenated rat kidney. Adv. Exp. Med. Biol. 200, 515-522.
7. HEYMAN, S.N., S. ROSEN, P. SILVA, K. SPOKES, M. EGORIN & F.H. EPSTEIN (1991): Protective action of glycine in cisplatin nephrotoxicity. Kidney Int. 40, 273-279.
8. JONES, D.P. (1986): Renal metabolism during normoxia, hypoxia, and ischemic injury. Ann. Rev. Physiol. 48, 33-50.
9. LOWRY, O.H., N.J. ROSEBROUGH, A.L. FARR & R.J. RANDALL (1951): Protein measurement with the folin phenol reagent. J. Biol. Chem. 193, 265-275.
10. MCKNIGHT, A.D.C. & A. LEAF (1977): Regulation of cellular volume. Physiol. Rev. 57, 510-573.
11. MELLORS, A.L., E.L. TAPPEL, P.L. SAVANT & I.D. DESAI (1967): Mitochondrial swelling and uncoupling of oxidative phosphorylation by lysosomes. Biochem. Biophys. Acta 143, 299-315.
12. WEINBERG, J.M., J.A. DAVIS, D.J.A. ABARZUA & T. KIANI (1989): Relationship between cell adenosine. Triphosphate and glutathione content and protection by glycine against hypoxic proximal tubular cell injury. J. Lab. Clin. Med. 113, 612-622.
13. WEINBERG, J.M., J.A. DAVIS, D.J.A. ABARZUA & T. RAJAN (1987): Cytoprotective effect of glycine and gluthathione against hypoxic injury in renal tubules. J. Clin. Invest. 80, 1446-1454.

14. WEINBERG, J.M., M.A..VENKATCHALAM, M. GARZA-QUINTERO, M.F. ROESER & J.A. DAVIS (1990): Structural requirements for protection by small amino acids against hypoxic injury in kidney proximal tubules. FASEB J. 4. 3347-3354.
15. WILSON, D.R., P.E. ARNOLD, T.J. BURKE & R.W. SCHRIER (1984): Mitochondrial calcium accumulation and respiration in ischemic acute renal failure in the rat. Kidney Int. 25, 519-527.

Modulation of the baroreflex by central neuropeptides is due to the route of administration

A. Brattström, E. Appenrodt, M. Sonntag, H. Listing,
A. Brattström jr., R. Miller, W. DeJong, E. Simeonova and L. Pharow

Physiologisches Institut, Medizinische Akademie Magdeburg

Introduction

Neuropeptides in information processing may serve in an autocrine, paracrine as well as endocrine manner. Considering central control on the cardiovascular system not only distinguishable sites of action but also different routes to transmit information have to be kept in mind [7]. Local presence of a neuropeptide may be either the result of being formed locally or only released locally after transportation. Such transportation might be related to both axonal and volume transport [2,10,18,20,21,35]. In additon, blood borne neuropeptides as well as neuropeptides which use the cerebrospinal-fluid (CSF) route might also influence the central control on cardiovascular system. This way may be of particular interest because degradation enzyme activity within CSF is very low [14,30], a separate secretion mode seems to exist [19,21,26] and, moreover neurons have been described which border the CSF space [22,32,33].

It can be speculated that neuropeptides administered into the CSF space may create similar cardiovascular effects as when administered locally into circumscript brain areas which are particularly involved in the central control on the cardiovascular system. In such a case it can be argued that independently from the route of administration the underlying brain areas which mediate the effects observed may be identical. On the other hand if neuropeptides induce different effects when applied either intracerebroventriculary (i.c.v.) or locally this will indicate that rather distinct ways or sites of action might be concerned due to the route of administration.

Therefore experiments were performed to check whether or not neuropeptides when administered either i.c.v. or locally into the nucleus tractus solitarii (NTS) in the lower brainstem will induce similar or rather qualitatively different actions on blood pressure (BP), heart period (inter-beat-interval: IBI) and the barorecptor-heart-reflex (BHR) [11,13].

Methods

The experiments were performed in male Wistar rats either anaesthetized with urethane (1.35 g/kg; microinjection experiments - NTS) or under conscious condition with the animals being chronically instrumend 24-28 h before under hexobarbital anaesthesia (150 mg/kg; i.p. administration). BP was recorded via an indwelling cannula in the femoral artery. In addition, the signal was fed into a computer which calculated, for each pulse, the diastolic, the systolic and the mean blood pressure value together with the IBI [3]. Another catheter was inserted into a femoral vein to allow intravenous (i.v.) injection of either phenylephedrine (PHE) or sodiumnitroprusside (NP) to increase or respective decrease BP entraining either prolongation or shortening of the IBI. By plotting the responding IBI values against the corresponding BP values a linear correlation function was obtained [7,8] and its slope reflects the sensitivity of the BHR (ms/mmHg) [13].

For the experiments in the conscious animals, to permit i.c.v. injection a cannula was inserted into the left lateral ventricle and fixed to the skull with dental cement 7-9 days before the cardiovascular experiments. In the acute experiment after 30-60 min of rest following connection of the different catheters for either BP recording or i.v. and respective i.c.v. administration the experiments were started. First of all BHRs were induced by i.v. injection of PHE (1 µg in 10 µl) and NP (10 µg in 10 µl), respectively, with a delay of 3 min between. After another period of rest (20-30 min) arteficial cerebro-spinal-fluid (aCSF) with or without neuropeptides was i.c.v. administered. The BHR's were repeated several times (2-5 and 15-20 min) after i.c.v. administration.

For the microinjection experiments a small glass cannula was inserted into the NTS by means of a stereotaxic apparatus following exposure of the lower brain stem by incision of the atlanto-occipital membrane. The head of the rat was flexed to 45° and the caudal tip of the area postrema in the midline was used as a rostro-caudal zero. The correct position of the tip of the cannula was verified histologically at the end of the experiment.

After 15 min of rest following the positioning of the cannula, the experiments were started. First of all a BHR was induced by i.v. injection of PHE (1-1.5 μg) dissolved in saline (10-15 μl, given within 10-15 sec) by which the BP was elevated by about 30-40 mmHg. After another 5 min period of rest bilateral NTS microinjections of aCSF with or without neuropeptides were made. Since the micropipette was not removed from the injection site until the pressure within the microinjection system had again reached the baseline indicating the drug release had been completed, there was a delay of about 2 min between the two injections. The BHR was repeated several times after the second injection.

Data were represented as means ± SE. For statical analyses, Student's t-test for paired samples was used, p values of less than 0.05 being considered to indicate significant differences.

Results and discussion

1. CSF - route

In the conscious animals, i.c.v. administration of angiotensin II (AN II) in those amounts as used by other [23,24] (20,200 ng) confirmed the reported results, i.e. increase in BP and prolongation in IBI (Fig. 1, upper part). In the case of 200 ng AN II, the sensitivity of the BHR was found significantly impaired for both the PHE- and the NP-test. This impairment was already present 3-5 min after i.c.v. administration and lasted still 15-20 min later (Fig. 1, lower part). The 20 ng AN II dosage increased BP and prolonged IBI as the 200 ng AN II dosage did but failed in changing the BHR sensitivity. When the amount of AN II was further reduced to 100 pg, which rather may reflect natural circumstances [17,23,24,29)] the resting values of BP and IBI remained completely unchanged but, surprisingly, now a long lasting augmentation in the BHR sensitivity was recognized. No changes at all in the resting values of BP and IBI were obtained, however, a remarkable augmentation in the BHR sensitivity was seen after i.c.v.administraion of 100 pg AN III (Fig 1, lower part). This may be of interest considering the discussion which of the compounds is more important for information processing via the CSF route [1,15,34]. An antagonist to AN III did not change any of the values monitored, indicating there is no tonic influences by AN III from the CSF space under the control conditions.

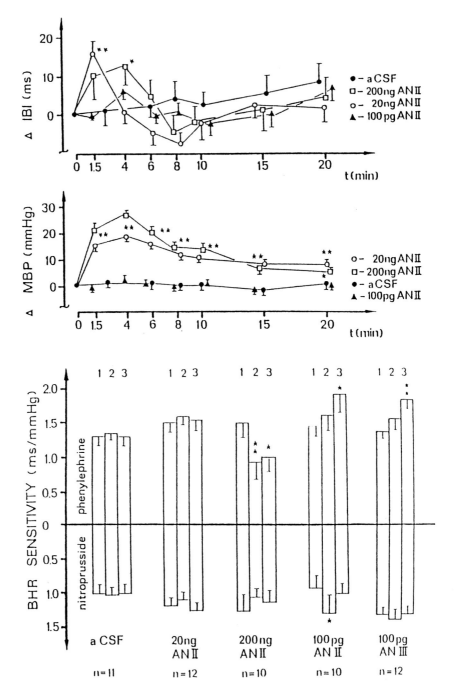

Substance P (SP) i.c.v. administered in those amounts as reported in the literatur (1 and 10 µg) induced an BP increase and a biphasic reaction in IBI with an initial shortening which is followed either by returning to baseline (1 µg SP) or even prolongation of IBI (10 µg SP) at the end of the observation period (20 min). Considering BHR within the 3-5 min period after i.c.v. administration, there was a significant impairment in sensitivity either in both tests (1 µg SP), i.e. PHE and NP test, or only in the PHE test (10 µg SP) whilst the NP test remained unaltered. 15-20 min after that i.c.v. administration the sensitivity of the BHR was at the control level even if the resting values of BP were still elevated (data not shown). The fact, no changes in the BHR sensitivity 15-20 min after i.c.v. administration, was also found in the anaesthetized rats [9]. In the conscious state, the rats demonstrated specific behaviour which includes motor activity (e.g. scratching and biting) in that particular period 3-5 min after i.c.v. treatment with SP when the BHR sensitivity was found reduced. Since motor activity is also capable or changing the BR sensitivity by itself [28] it can not be distinguished whether or not this effect of i.c.v. SP on the BHR seen immediately after i.c.v. administration is simple related to that behaviour or has rather to be considered as a specific action of SP on the cardiovascular control process.

Arginine vasopressin (AVP) when i.c.v. administered in an amount exceeding 5-20 ng into conscious rats elevates BP and change IBI [24] whilst the BHR sensitivity is found increased (31). However, the detectable amount of AVP in the CSF of the rat ranged between 10-60 pg/ml [19,26]. When therefore the i.c.v. applied amount of AVP was reduced to 30 pg or even 10 pg no detectable changes in the resting values of BP and IBI were seen but the BHR sensitivity was significantly impaired [6].

This impairment was observed in a time period of about 30-90 min after that i.c.v. administration. By applying 1 pg of an V_1 antagonist $D(CH_2)_5Tyr(Me)$-AVP the opposite effect on the BHR sensitivity was obtained indicating a longlasting influence of CSF-routed AVP on the BHR sensitivity which is already present under original condition. This reflex impairment caused by i.c.v. AVP in the low pg range is in contrast to that reflex augmentation recognized after peripheral [12] or local administration of AVP into the NTS (see below).

Fig. 1: Responses of IBI and MBP to i.c.v. administration of different amounts of AN II in conscious rats (upper part) and the BHR sensitivity (in ms/mmHg) proved before (1) and 3-5 min (2) as well as 15-17 min (3) after i.c.v. treatment with or without different amounts of AN II and AN III, respectively (lower part). NB. in relation the amount of AN applied, the BHR sensitivity changed qualitatively particularly when the bradycardia response is considered.

Oxytocin (OT) is another hypophyseal neuropeptide which has been reported to act in many aspects inversely to AVP. I.c.v. administration of OT in the ug range increased heart rate without affecting BP [16]. Smaller amounts of OT (0,05-10 ng) failed to elicit any changes of the resting values, however, the 10 ng dose reduced the BHR sensitivity 15-30 min after administration. The detectable amount of OT within CSF of the rat, however, ranged only between 10-60 pg/ml (19) with a half-time of 28 min (blood 1-2 min). Therefore, experiments were performed to check whether OT in the low pg range (10, 40 and 100 pg) may influence the cardiovascular control process similar as AVP does. OT in this low amount when i.c.v. administered did not change the resting values of BP and IBI but the BHR sensitivity was remarkably increased, an example is given for the 100 pg dosage of OT (Fig. 2).

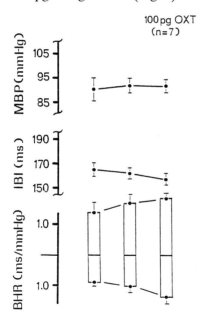

Fig. 2: Responses of IBI, MBP and BHR sensitivity alter i.c.v. administration of 100 pg Oxytocin. N.B. the longlasting improvement of the BHR sensitivity without changes in the resting values of IBI and MBP.

2. Local administration - Nucleus tractus solitarii (NTS)

AN II microinjected into the NTS in the low pg range (10, 40 or 100 pg) reduced BP and prolonged IBI. Saralafsin (SAR; 10, 40 od 100 pg) an antagonist to AN II with some agonistic acitivity at AN II receptors, elicited similar effects as AN II, except that the 10 pg dose of SAR was inactive in this respect. Both of the compounds, i.e. AN II and SAR, augmented the

BHR sensivity with the exception of the 10 pg dose of SAR. AN III in the same low picogram range (10, 40 or 100 pg) caused similar reactions of the resting values of BP and IBI as AN II did, i.e. BP reduction and IBI prolongation. But in contrast to AN II the BHR sensitivity was remarkably impaired after AN III [8]. Those results suggest it has to be distinguished between influences on basal tone and BHR performances. Furthermore, it seems noteworthy to remind, that CSF routed AN II as well as AN III (100 pg dose) created uniform effects on BHR sensitivity (enhancement) without affecting BP or IBI. These differences in the results considering the routes of administration suggest both of the pathways may be activated separately.

AVP microinjected into the NTS in the low pg range (1-100 pg) decreased BP and prolonged IBI [4]. Smaller fragments of AVP share these effects, however, the evoked hypotension and bradycardia were less marked [5]. The sensitivity of the BHR was clearly enhanced (approx. 40 %) when checked 10 min after bilateral microinjection of 100 pg AVP. Spontaneously hypertensive rats (SHR) responded to 100 pg AVP microinjection into the NTS with a pronounced bradycardia without changes in BP together with an enormous augmentation in BHR sensitivity (nearly 80 % vs. 40 % in the WKY controls) (Fig. 3) which lasted longer than in the normal Wistar-rats or the Wistar Kyoto-rats (WKY). Considering WKY they behaved similarly as the normal Wistar did, i.e. BP decrease (although less pronounced) and prolongation of the IBI together with an increase in BHR sensitivity of about 40 % occured. Therefore, the differences between normotensive and hypertensive animals may point to differences in the accessibility for AVP and/or the metabolism of AVP within the lower brainstem of the hypertensive rats. Despite this it should be kept in mind, CSF routed small amounts of AVP never influenced baseline values of BP or IBI but impaired the BHR. These results again may support the idea that both of the routes may be activated separately.

Local administration of small amounts of endothelins (ET-1; ET-3) into the NTS (unilateral microinfusion: 0.11 µl/min, 1-500 pg/min) elicited reductions in BP and heart rate (HR). The overall dose-response curve could be described as bell shaped with the 10 pg dose (ET-3) and the 50 pg Dose (ET-1) being most effective, respectively. Responses generally reached a maximum towards the end of the infusion and both BP and HR returned to pre-infusion level within the next 10 (ET-1) or 20 (ET-3) min of observation. These effects on BP and HR were repeatable [8]. When 10 pg ET-3 was infused into the NTS the BHR sensitivity was found to be reduced by about 25 % and this effect lasted for at least 20 min (Fig. 4).

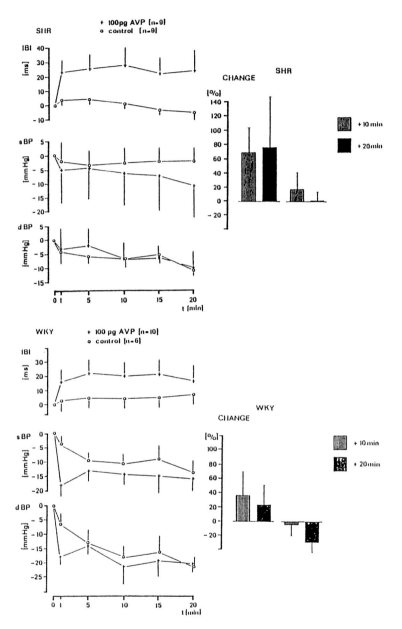

Fig. 3: Changes in IBI and systolic as well as diastolic BP after bilateral microinjection of 100 pg AVP into the NTS of spontaneously hypertensive rats (SHR) and their related controls (WKY).
N.B. the remarkable prolongation of IBI in the SHR and, particularly, the longlasting increase of the BHR sensitivity.

General considerations

Neuropeptides within CSF might belong to distinct control mechanisms. Not only their releasing into the CSF, which may happen either directly or rather indirectly, e.g. by volumen transmission [10,18,20], follows obviously specific rules but also their metabolism, including cleavages into active fragments and degradation, possesses kinetics distinct from those in the brain tissue or blood. It may be of interest that neuropeptides as AN II, AN III, AVP and OT in the low picogram range which might be considered physiological range when given i.c.v. changed the BHR sensitivity long-lasting without influencing the baseline values of BP and IBI.

Cardiovascular changes induced by CSF routed neuropeptides in the low picogram range were distinct from those evoked by neuropeptide microinjections into the NTS indicating distinct pathways and, moreover, the possibility for being activated separately as well as together.

The neuropeptides which are known to increase BP by peripheral actions (AN II, AVP, ET-1) caused generally in the low picogram range a BP decrease and an IBI prolongation after microinjection into the NTS. In this way their central actions oppose their peripheral actions to some degree. It may be of interest that the area postrema which is adjacent to th NTS [27] is capable of sensing the plasma level of the vasoactive neuropeptides [23] and may serve to adjust baroreflex control at different circumstances or challenges. In addition, the concentration of the neuropeptides reported here was in any case subthreshold to their considered direct vasoconstrictor activity. Therefore the cardiovascular effects caused by NTS microinjection of these neuropeptides have to be related to specific actions rather than to local ischemia caused by local vasoconstrictor effects.

In conclusion, central neuropeptides may use different routes including the CSF space to modulate differentially the cardiovascular control process.

References

1. ABHOLD, R.H., J.M. HANESWORTH & J.W. HARDING (1988): Comparison of ^{125}I-Angiotensin III and ^{125}I-Angiotensin II binding to rat brain membranes. J. Neurochem. 50, 831-838.
2. BLOOM, F.E. (1991): An integrative view of information handling in the CNS. In: Volume transmissions in the brain: novel mechanisms for neural transmission (FUXE, K. & L.F. AGNATI, eds.), pp. 11-23, Raven Press, Ltd. New York.
3. BRATTSTRÖM, A., W. SCHÄLIKE, G. ORLOW & C. KREHER (1988a): Mikrorechnereinsatz in Kreislaufexperimenten. Z.Klin.Med. 43, 379-382.

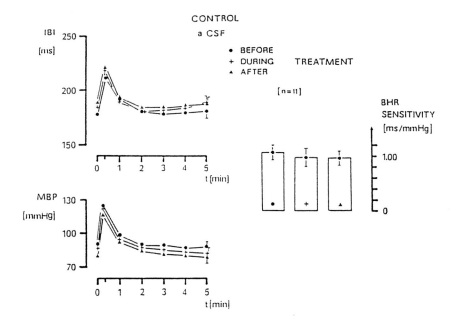
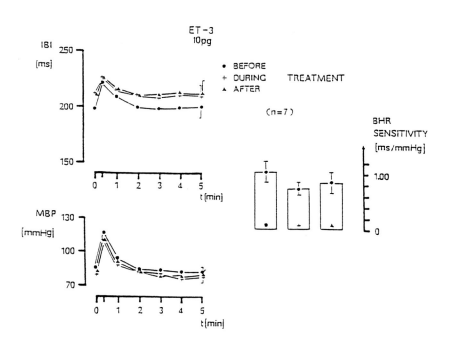

4. BRATTSTRÖM, A., W. DEJONG & D. DEWIED (1989b): Vasopressin microinjections into the nucleus tractus solitarii decrease heart rate and blood pressure in anaesthetized rat. J. Hypertension 6, 5521-5524.
5. BRATTSTRÖM, A., W. DEJONG, J.P.H. BURBACH & D. DEWIED (1989): Vasopressin, vasopressin fragments and a C-terminal peptide of the vasopressin precursor share cardiovascular effects when microinjected into the nucleus tractus solitarii. Psychoneuroendocrinology 14, 461-467.
6. BRATTSTRÖM, A., W. DEJONG & D. DEWIED (1990): Central vasopressin impairs the baroreceptor heart rate reflex in conscious rats. J. Cardiovas. Pharmacol. 15, 114-117.
7. BRATTSTRÖM, A., M. SONNTAG, E. APPENRODT, T. SEIDENBECHER, S. MANUTSCHAROW, A. BRATTSTRÖM JR., W. SCHÄLIKE & C. BLUMENSTEIN (1992a): Rapid Resetting of the Baroflex is Part of Behavioral Changes in Cardiovascular Parameters. In: Psychoneuroimmunology (SCHMOLL, H.-J., U. TEWES & N.P. PLOTNIKOFF, eds.), pp. 148-157, Hogrefe & Huber Publisher, Lewiston, NY, Toronto, Bern, Göttingen.
8. BRATTSTRÖM, A., M. SONNTAG, H. LISTING, R. MILLER & W. DEJONG (1992b): Neuropeptides within the nucleus tractus solitarii modulate the central cardiovascular controll process. Progr. Brain Res. 91, 75-79.
9. BRATTSTRÖM, A. & T. SEIDENBECHER (1992c): Central substances P increased blood pressure, heart rate and splanchnic nerve activity in anaesthetized rats without impairment of the baroreflex regulation. Neuropeptides 23, 81-86.
10. BUNNEMANN, B., K. FUXE, B. BJELKE & D. GANTEN (1991): The brain renin-angiotensin system and its possible involvement in volume transmission. In Volume transmission in the brain: novel mechanisms for neural transmission (FUXE, K. & L.F. AGNATI, eds.), pp. 131-158), Raven Press, Ltd., New York.
11. CHAPLEAU, M.W., G. HAJDUCZOK & F.M. ABBOUD (1989): Peripheral and central mechanisms of baroreflex resetting. Clin. Exp. Pharmcol. Physio. 15, 31-43.
12. COWLEY JR. A.W., D. MERRILL, J. OSBORN & B.J. BARBER (1984): Influence of vasopressin and angiotensin on baroreflexes in the dog. Cir. Res. 54, 163-172.
13. DORWARD, P.K. & P.I. KORNER (1987): Does the brain "remember" the absolute blood pressure? NIPS 2, 10-13.
14. DURDEN, D.A., T.V. NGUYEN & A.A. BOULTON (1988): Kinetics of intraventricularly injected trace amines and their deuterated isotopomers, Neurochem. Res. 13, 943-950.
15. FERRARIO, C.M., K.L. BARNES, C.H. BLOCK, K.B. BROSNIHAN, D.I. DIZ, M.C. KHOSLA & P.A.S. SANTOS (1990): Pathways of angiotensin formation and function in the brain. Hypertension 15, Suppl. I, I13-119
16. FEUERSTEION, G., R.L. ZERBE & A.I. FADEN (1984): Central cardiovascular effects of vasotocin, oxytocin and vasopressin in conscious rats. J. Pharmacol. Exp. Therap. 228, 348-353.
17. HARDING, J.W., L.L. JENSEN, J.M. HANESWORTH, K.A.ROBERTS, T.A. PAGE & J.W. WRIGHT (1992): Release of angiotensins in paraventricular nucleus of rat in response to physiological and chemical stimuli. Am. J. Physiol. 262, F17-F23.
18. HERKENHAM, M. (1991): Mismatches between neurotransmitter and receptor localiza-

Fig. 4: Responses of IBI and MBP to i.v. administration of a phenylephrin-bolus and the calculated BHR sensitivity before, during (10 min period of infusion) and after (10 min after cessation) an unilateral infusion of 10 pg ET-3 into the NTS.
N.B. the impairment of the BHR sensitivity.

tions: Implications for endocrine functions in brain. In: Volume transmission in the brain: novel mechanisms for neutral transmission (FUXE, K. & L.F. AGNATI, eds.), pp. 63-87, Raven Press, Ltd. New York.
19. IVANYI, T., V.M. WIEGANT & D.DEWIED (1991): Differential effects of emotional and physical stress on the central and peripheral secretion of neurohypophysial hormones in male rats. Life Sciences 48, 1309-1316.
20. NILSSON, D., M. LINDVALL-AXELSSON & C. OWMAN (1991): Role of the cerebrospinal cluid in volume transmission involving the choroid plexus. In: Volume transmission in the brain: novel mechanisms for neutral transmission (FUXE, K. & L.F. AGNATI, eds.), pp. 307-315, Raven Press, Ltd. New York.
NILSSON, C., M. LINDVALL-AXELSSON & C. OWMAN (1992): Neuroendocrine regulatory mechanisms in the chorid plexus-cerebrospinal fluid system. Brain Res. Rev. 17, 109-138.
21. MCKINLEY, M.J. (1987): An important region for osmoregulation: the anterior wall of the third ventricle. NIPS 2, 13-16.
22. PAPAS, S., P. SMITH & A.V. FERGUSON (1990): Electrophysiological evidence that systemic angiotensin influences rat area postrema neurons. Am. J. Physiol. 258, R70-R76.
23. PHILIPPU, A. (1988): Regulation of blood pressure by central neurotrensmitters and neuropeptides. Rev. Physiol. Biochem. Pharmacol. 111, 1-115.
24. PHILLIPS, M.I. (1987): Functions of angiotensin in the central nervous system. Ann. Rev. Physiol. 49, 413-415.
25. REPPERT, S.M., W.J. SCHWARTZ & G.R. UHL (1987): Arginine vasopressin: a noval peptide rhythm in cerebrospinal fluid. TINS 10, 76-80.
26. SHAPIRO, R.E. & R.R. MISELIS (1985): The central neural connections of the area postrema of the rat. J. Comp. Neurol., 234, 344-364.
27. STEVENSON, R.B. (1984): Modification of reflex regulation of blood pressure by behavior. Ann. Rev. Physiol. 40, 133-142.
28. SUZUKI, H., C.M. FERRARIO, R.C. SPETH, K.B. BROSNIHAN, R.R. SMEBY & P. DESILVA (1983): Alternations in plasma and cerebrospinal fluid norepinephrine and angiotensin II during the development of renal hypertension in conscious dogs. Hypertension 5 (Supp. I), l139-l148.
29. TERENIUS, L. & F. NYBERG (1988): Neuropeptide-processing, -converting, and -inactivating enzymes in human cerebrospinal fluid. Int. Rev. Neurobiol. 30, 101-121.
30. UNGER, T., P. ROHMEISS, G. DEMMERT, D. GANTEN, R.E. LANG & F. LUFT (1987): Opposing cardiovascular effects of brain and plasma AVP: role of V1- and V2-AVP receptors. In Brain, peptides and catecholamines in cardiovascular regulation (BUCKLEY, J.P. & C.M. FERRARIO, eds.), pp. 393-401, Raven Press, New York.
31. VAN DER KOOY, D. & L.Y. KODA (1983): Organization of the projections of a circumventricular organ: the area postrema in the rat. J. Comp. Neurol. 219, 328-338.
32. VIGH-TEICHMANN, I. & B. VIGH (1983): The system of cerebrospinal fluid-contacting neurons. Arch. histol. japonicum 46, 427-468.
33. WRIGHT, J.W., K.R. ROBERTS, V.I. COOK, C.E. MURRAY, M.F. SARDINA & J.W. HARDING (1990): Intracerebroventricularly infused (D-Arg^1)angiotensin III, is superior to (D-Asp^1)angiotensin II, as a pressor agent in rats. Brain Res. 514, 5-10
34. ZIEGLGÄNSBERGER, W., H.U. DODT, R. DEISZ & H. PAWELZIK (1991): Peptides in Neurotransmission. In Volume transmission in the brain: novel mechanisms for neural transmission (FUXE, K. & L.F. AGNATI, eds.), pp. 371-380, Raven Press Ltd. New York.

Cardiorespiratory reactions to hyperoxia in young caucasian men with different blood platelet Na^+/H^+ - antiporter activity

J. Lüdemann*, H. Brauer*, A. Gens*, J. Exner*, S. Wussow*,
D. Rosskopf**, W. Siffert** and A. Honig*

Department of Physiology, University of Greifswald*, and Department of Pharmacology, University of Essen**

Introduction

The Na^+/H^+-antiport of the cell membranes is an important mechanism of intracellular pH regulation in a wide variety of mammalien cells [2]. The existence of such an Na^+/H^+-exchanger has also been demonstrated for human platelets [1,2]. It is assumed that the activity of this transport system might be one of the determinants of the reactivity of vascular smooth muscle cells contractile stimuli [2]. Moreover, accumulating evidence suggests an enhanced activity of the Na^+/H^+-exchanger in different cells (erythrocytes, lymphocytes, platelets, and vascular smooth muscle cells) of humans and animals suffering from primary systemic hypertension [1,2,7]. It has been also documented that the activity of the peripheral arterial chemoreceptors during breathing normal air (the so-called "resting drive") and the response to oxygen breathing is already enhanced in young border-line hypertensive men and in young people with a family backround of primary systemic hypertension [5, 6, 8, 9]. An enhanced Na^+/H^+-exchanger activity in Type I cells of peripheral arterial chemoreceptors would support an increase of $[Ca^{2+}]_i$ resulting in the activation of the exocytotic dopamine release of these cells and so in a higher resting drive and/or in stronger and faster reactions of these receptors to hyperoxic, hypoxic or acidic stimuli [3].

The activity of the Na^+/H^+-exchange of human blood platelets as an index of the activity of this transporter in other cells of the organism, can easily be assessed by a recently developed optical swelling test [7] whereas the activity of the peripheral arterial chemoreceptors can be determined by checking the cardiorespiratory reactions to breathing air enriched with oxygen [6, 8].

The aim of our study was to find out if young men with high Na^+/H^+-exchanger activities show faster and/or stronger responses in cardiorespiratory parameters to oxygen breathing and whether these two tests, when applied simultaneously in clinically healthy young men, detect the same subjects as beeing potentially hypertensive.

Materials and methods

The measurements were carried out in 57 healthy male subjects free of any medication and physical or psychological stress. To obtain their own and their family medical history the subjects completed a form containing relevant questions. During the time of the experiments, subjects rested in supine position on a comfortable bed. Systemic arterial blood pressure (noninvasive, oscillometric method) in the brachial artery as well as heart rate were taken using the Component Monitoring System of Hewlett Packard (Palo Alto, USA). Breathing rate, and tidal volume were measured using the respiratory gas monitor system RGM 5250 (Ohmeda, Louisville, USA). All parameters were automatically recorded as means over 30 s intervals.

Measurements of cardiorespiratory parameters started after a resting period of 20-30 min in which the subjects breathed room air at sea-level conditions. Recordings for determinations of the normoxic baselines lasted for 20 min during breathing normal air. In the next period for 10 min during breathing 65 % oxygen in nitrogen the cardiorespiratory reactions to hyperoxia were measured followed by a normoxic post-control for 20 min during normal air breathing.

Blood samples were drawn from a cannula in the cubital vein between 09.00 and 10.00 a.m. or between 01.00 and 02.00 p.m., respectively, i.e. before the beginning of the cardiorespiratory measurements. Details of blood sampling and data processing were as previously described [7]. In the optical swelling test used in our experiments a "rate constant" (RC) is determined that expresses the Na^+/H^+-antiporter activity of the blood platelets [3, 7]; i.e. a high RC indicates a high activity of the Na^+/H^+-exchanger.

To be able to compare the cardiorespiratory parameters as well as their responses to oxygen between probands having low rate constants and those with high rate constants, we simply decided to take those 20 subjects together that had the lowest rate constants and to include the other 20 subjects with the highest rate constants in another group.

The statistical significance of the responses or differences obtained were calculated using a two-way Anova with repeated measures on one factor [4].

Results

The rate constants ranged from 22.2 to 31.9; this is in good agreement with previous reports by other laboratories using the same method [7]. Group 1 consisted of 20 subjects who had the lowest rate constants (range 22.2 - 27.8) and group 2 included 20 subjects with the highest rate constants (range 28.3 - 31.9). 13 other young men exhibiting rate constants ranging from 27.9 to 28.2 were excluded from any further evaluation and their data are not presented in this paper.

No significant differences were found between the subjects with high and low rate constants with respect to age, height, weight, body surface, body mass index and cardiorespiratory baseline values (Tab. 1). Regression analysis failed to reveal any significant relationships between rate constants and cardiorespiratory baseline values. When the values of cardiorespiratory parameters were averaged in half-minute intervals, there was a clear decrease in heart rate in both groups over the full time of hyperoxia (Fig. 1). No significant differences with respect to heart rate responses between the two groups were obtained. In both populations heart rate returned to baseline within 2-3 minutes after finishing the oxygen breathing. In response to oxygen breathing, both groups showed only negligible differences to baseline of both systolic and diastolic blood pressure but the diastolic blood pressure in subjects with high Na^+/H^+-exchanger activities was statistically significant higher. During the first two minutes of oxygen breathing, only a weak response of breathing rate was obtained, and there were also no significant differences in the reaction of these parameters between the two groups of subjects. Breathing rate showed a suppression in both groups at the beginning of the hyperoxic period but returned to baseline after 2-4 minutes. No differences in the half-minute averages of breathing rate reactions of the two groups studied could be observed.

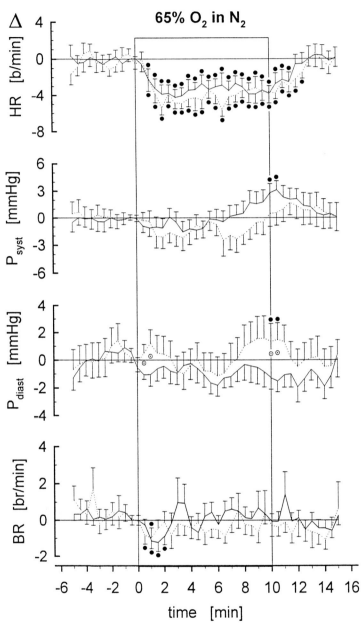

Fig. 1: Reactions of heart rate (HR), systolic (P_{syst}) and diastolic (P_{diast}) blood pressure and breathing rate (BR) in response to oxygen breathing (65 % O_2 in N_2) in men with low (solid line) or with high (dotted line) Na^+/H^+-exchanger activities (Δ, differences to baseline). (● 2p<0.05 vs. baseline; ⊙2p<0.05 between the two groups).

Table 1: Cardiorespiratory baselines (means ± SEM) of BMI (body mass index), HR (heart rate), P_{syst} (systolic blood pressure), P_{diast} (diastolic blood pressure), PP (pulse pressure), MAP (mean systemic arterial blood pressure), BR (breathing rate); V_t (tidal volume), V_E (minute ventilation) and RC (rate constant). These data were determined in the last 20 minutes before oxygen breathing. There were no significant differences between the two groups.

PARAMETER	Group 1 RC< 27.8 n=20	ANOVA	Group 2 RC>28.3 n=20
rate constant [0.0001 s]	26.5 ± 0.06	2p< 0.01	29.5 ± 0.06
age [years]	22.2 ± 0.25	n.s.	22.2 ± 0.23
height [cm]	177 ± 1	n.s.	182 ± 2
weight [kg]	70 ± 2	n.s.	75 ± 2
body surface [m^2]	1.86 ± 0.03	n.s.	1.97 ± 0.03
BMI [kg/m^2]	22 ± 0.40	n.s.	23 ± 0.40
HR [b/min]	69 ± 2	n.s.	69 ± 2
P_{syst} [mmHg]	123 ± 1	n.s.	122 ± 2
P_{diast} [mmHg]	56 ± 1	n.s.	58 ± 2
PP [mmHg]	67 ± 2	n.s.	64 ± 2
MAP [mmHg]	79 ± 1	n.s.	80 ± 2
BR [br/min]	12 ± 1	n.s.	12 ± 1
V_t [ml]	722 ± 66	n.s.	657 ± 44
V_E [l/min]	7.75 ± 0.28	n.s.	7.88 ± 0.25

Supported by the grant 07NBL02 of the Bundesminister für Forschung und Technologie der Bundesrepublik Deutschland.

Figure 2 presents the maximum responses to oxygen and the times in which these maximum responses occured for both groups. All maximum reactions appeared within the first 3 min of oxygen breathing. The maximum heart rate responses of the two groups studied were statistically significant to baseline but not different with respect to either amplitude or time of appeareance. But both systolic and diastolic blood pressures reacted differently to oxygen in the two groups of subjects compared; the maximum re-

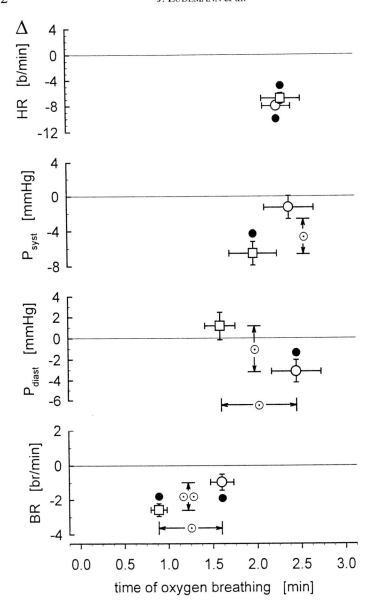

Fig. 2: Maximum responses to hyperoxia (65 % O_2 in N_2) of heart rate (HR), systolic (P_{syst}) and diastolic (P_{diast}) blood pressure and breathing rate (BR) in 20 men with high Na^+/H^+-antiporter activities (RC>28.3 ± 0.06, open squares) and in 20 men with low Na^+/H^+-antiporter activities (RC<27.8 ± 0.06, open circles). Presented are both the averages (± SEM) of the maximum responses and of the times of their appearance (Δ, differences to baseline). (● 2p<0.05 vs. baseline ; ⊙ 2p<0.05 and ⊙⊙ 2p<0.01 between the two groups).

sponses occured earlier in the subjects with high rate constants but only the time difference for the diastolic blood pressures was statistically significant. Moreover, in the subjects having high rate constants during oxygen breathing a larger drop of systolic blood pressure could be observed. In contrast, in response to oxygen diastolic blood pressure rose in the group with high rate constants and fell in the group having low rate constants.

The subjects with high rate constants reacted to oxygen faster and with a more clearly pronounced depression of breathing rate.

Discussion

In the experiments presented here we measured both the activity of the Na^+/H^+-antiporter activity of the blood platelets and noninvasively the cardiorespiratory responses to 10 min breathing of 65 % O_2 in N_2 in the same subject and at the same time. The differences in the reactions to hyperoxia were more distinctly in maximum response analysis. Maximum responses (amplitude) to oxygen of systolic and diastolic blood pressures as well as breathing rate were significantly different between the two groups compared (Fig. 2). Moreover, the time between starting the oxygen breathing and occurence of the maximum reactions in the first three minutes was shorter in the subjects with high Na^+/H^+-exchanger activity. These time differences between the two groups were statistical significant for diastolic blood pressure and breathing rate. At present, one can only speculate about the mechanisms of this phenomenon. Assuming that platelet Na^+/H^+-antiporter activity really reflects the activity of this transport system in all cells of the body the question arises whether the different responses to oxygen (Fig. 2) result from reflex mechanisms or from an effect of the high oxygen pressure elsewhere in the body. As the maximum responses of heart rate and blood pressure occured after a relatively long latency of 60-150 sec it seems to be unlikely that they result solely from reflex effects of the peripheral arterial chemoreceptors, but there is no direct evidence for this assumption. For instance, oxygen breathing might also change arterial and tissue carbon dioxide tensions suggesting a possible involvement of the so-called central CO_2 - and/or - pH-sensitive chemoreceptors in the induction of the responses shown in Fig. 2. These problems remain to be examined experimentally.

The differences of the maximum responses of systolic and diastolic pressures might be also caused by a direct effect of oxygen on vascular and/or cardiac muscle cells. If so, this could mean that the Na^+/H^+-antiporter activity is one of the determinants of the reactivity of the cardiovascular system to oxygen. It has been speculated that perfusion and oxygen supply of the tissue might influence the reactivity of the microcirculation and thus peripheral resistance [8]. If so, our finding that the Na^+/H^+-exchanger determines the reactivity of the cardiovascular system to oxygen would be another mechanism by which the Na^+/H^+-antiporter could be connected with hypertensive diseases.

References

1. AVIV, A. & A. LIVNE (1988): The Na^+/H^+-antiport, cytosolic free Ca^{2+} and essential hypertension: A hypothesis. Am. J. Hypertens. 1, 410-413.
2. DÜSING, R., B.O. GÖBEL, G. HOFFMANN, H. VETTER & W. SIFFERT (1992): Zur klinischen Bedeutung des Na^+/H^+-Antiports. Med. Klin. 87, 378-384.
3. GONZALEZ, C., L. ALMARAZ, A. OBESO & R. RIGUAL (1992): TINS, 15(4), 146-153.
4. HINZE, J.L. (1987): Number Cruncher Statistical System. Kaysville: Selbstverlag.
5. HONIG, A. (1989): Peripheral arterial chemoreceptors and reflex control of sodium and water homeostasis. Am. J. Physiol. 257, R1282-R1302.
6. QUIES, W., T. CLAUS & A. HONIG (1983): Die Hyperventilation der Hypertoniker - eine Pilotstudie zum Verhalten der Reflexe der arteriellen Chemorezeptoren bei hypertensiven Erkrankungen. Dt. Gesundh. Wesen 38, 612-617.
7. ROßKOPF, D., E. MORGENSTERN, W. SCHOLZ, U. OSSWALD & W. SIFFERT (1991): Rapid determination of the elevated Na^+/H^+-exchange in platelets of patients with essential hypertension using an optical swelling test. J. Hypertens. 9, 231-238.
8. TAFIL-KLAWE, MALGORZATA, A. TRZEBSKI, J. KLAWE & T. PALKO (1985): Augmented chemo-receptor reflex tonic drive in early human hypertension and in normotensive subjects with family backround of hypertension. Acta Physiol. Pol. 36, 51-58.
9. TRZEBSKI A. (1992): Arterial chemoreceptor reflex and hypertension. Hypertension 6, 262-266.

A feedforward control of vital compensation of hypoxic-acidotic effects in piglets

U. Zwiener, R. Bauer, H. Witte, W. Buchenau and D. Hoyer

Department of Pathophysiology, University of Jena

Introduction

Hyperventilatory reaction of newborns has been estimated as moderate, transient and not essential [reviews in 6, 16]. But especially in neonatally mature species, this reaction to severe hypoxia has been examined experimentally almost only during pronounced general anaesthesia or under conditions of inconstant body temperature. In addition, in these experiments, reductions of respiratory control sensitivity could not be excluded. In hypoxic human neonates, following hypoxic episodes an impairment of respiratory control caused by the hypoxic-acidotic sequelae can be observed.

Up to now, the role of hyperventilatoric reactions upon severe hypoxia of non-anaesthetized or only slightly anaesthetized newborn animals are not sufficiently known. Possibly, the main effect of hyperventilation during hypoxic hypoxia is a quicker removal of CO_2 molecules [10], but not a significant reduction of hypoxia itself. The amount and pattern of the hypoxia induced hyperventilation in neonates could depend on differences in ontogenetic maturation of vegetative and emergency reactions of different species [6] and on the species themselves [11]. To get results comparable to man, the domestic pig, a perinatal brain developer like man with similar autonomous and cardiovascular reactions [4, 5, 8], was studied. To separate possible metabolic, cardiovascular and cerebral effects of hyperventilatoric hypocapnia interfering with severe hypoxia, we investigated spontaneously breathing as well as artificially ventilated newborn piglets during hypoxic hypoxia.

Methods

In 25 newborn piglets (2nd day of life, 1200-1700 g), slightly anaesthetized with Halan (0.5 Vol %) and N_2O_2 (3:1), catheters were introduced into the A. femoralis (arterial pressure and blood samples), retrogradually in the A. lingualis (for ^{133}Xe-bolus injection into the A. carotis interna while simultaneously occluding the A. carotis externa for cerebral blood flow (CBF) clearance measurements), into the right V. jugularis interna up to the base of the skull with ligation of all extracranial branches (cerebral venous blood samples). After frontoparietal removal of the skin, bilateral frontal [AP-20 (bregma is AP-O), 18], precentral (AP-10, L 10), and occipital Ag-AgCl-surface electrodes for EEG measurement were inserted into the skull bone. Sixteen piglets were paralyzed [d-Tubocurarin; 0.5 mg/kg] and artificially ventilated (11.7-16.7 ml/s, 0.7-1.0 l/min, pressure controlled: 10-13 cm H_2O); 9 piglets breathed spontaneously. When an α-β-EEG appeared few minutes after general anaesthesia, a 1-h hypoxic hypoxia was started (FiO_2= 0.08 ± 0.01 to get a P_aO_2 = 20-24 mmHg). Respiratory movements (impedance respirography [12], subcutaneous Ag-AgCl-electrodes), EEG, arterial pressure and heart rate were (almost continuously) recorded, while P_aO_2, P_aCO_2, arterial pH (pH_a), base excess, CBF (^{133}Xe clearance) were discontinuously recorded according to the time sequence of parameters in Figs. 2 and 3. In control experiments (without hypoxia) all parameters studied were stable at least for 5 h. Further experimental details are given in [15].

The intracranial pressure was continuously recorded via a parietal trephine hole, the body temperature was measured by a rectal thermoelement and kept constant (38-39 °C). At the end of the experiments the surviving animals were killed by a barbiturate and the brain vitally fixed by formalin solution (4 %) for morphological analysis. The computerisation of CBF was performed by a 2-compartment-model with peeling and fitting (mean squares) of the 2 exponentials for the quicker and lower compartments [9] corresponding well in 98 % of data ($p < 0.01$).

Nonparametric statistical tests (Wilcoxon, U-test [13]) were used to assess data differences. The cerebral O_2-supply for the grey or white matter was evaluated by $[O_2]_a$ · CBF calculated from the fast or slow part of the ^{133}Xe clearance curves, the O_2-demand from cerebral $AVDO_2$ · CBF (fast and slow compartment) and the cerebrovascular resistance (R_c) by the quotient of cerebral perfusion pressure to CBF (fast or slow compartment). The cerebral perfusion pressure was calculated by P_a - P_{cv} (central venous pressure), the cerebral $AVDO_2$ by P_aO_2 - P_vO_2 (V. jugularis interna). The quick compartment calculated from the ^{133}Xe-clearance curve corresponds closely to the grey matter, the slow one to the white matter [9; 15].

Results and Discussion

In all 9 spontaneously breathing piglets, a pronounced hyperventilation upon severe hypoxia was observed lasting 40-60 min (especially with a two to threefold increase of the respiratory frequency, Fig. 1) causing hypocapnia P_aCO_2 = 20-22 mmHg (Fig. 2). The hyperventilation already during the early beginning of hypoxia leads to a respiratory alkalosis (pH$_a$: 7.43 ± 0.02; Fig. 2). Thus, respiratory control acts as a feedforward control upon acid-base-homeostasis. Before severe hypoxia effects as a disturbance within the acid-base-control, hyperventilation causes an alkalotic overcompensation (Fig. 2). Subsequently a decrease of the pH$_a$ starts with almost the same velocity (0.1 /20 min), but on a level permanently 0.2 higher than in ventilated animals (Fig. 2). Eight out of 9 spontaneously breathing piglets survived the hypoxic and posthypoxic intervals, but all ventilated animals decompensated vitally, i. e. they showed a mean arterial pressure ≤ 35 mmHg (normal: 70-80 mmHg) and quasi isoelectric EEG before they died (3 piglets did so during the hypoxia, 13 later).

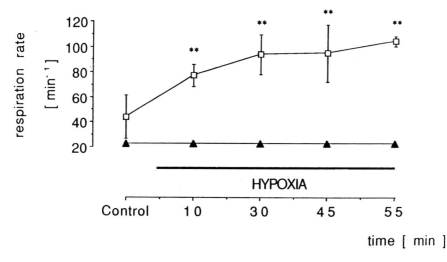

Fig. 1: Respiratory rates of 9 spontaneously breathing (squares) and 16 ventilated (triangles) newborn piglets before (control) and during 1h severe atmosphaeric hypoxia. (No change or increase of tidal volume, relative measurements; in all figures: asterisks = significant differences in comparison to controls; two: $P < 0.01$; one: $P < 0.05$)

The reason for the survival of spontaneously breathing piglets is very likely the weaker systemic acidosis caused by the hyperventilatoric feed-forward control of the acid-base homeostasis. The constantly higher arterial pH during severe hypoxia despite almost the same velocity of pH-decrease is the only permanent difference within the investigated metabolic, cardiovascular, and cerebral parameters (Figs. 2 and 3). Presumably, the state of quickly removed intracellular CO_2 molecules during the hypoxia of spontaneously breathing piglets allows a more sufficient myocardial activity [10]. The mainly cardial cause of vital decompensation in ventilated animals is confirmed by the following: In almost all cases, critical decrease of mean arterial pressure precedes pronounced decrease of CBF and an isoelectric EEG. Moreover, in parallel experiments infusing 1 m HCl into newborn piglets, at the same decrease of pH_a as during the end of hypoxia in ventilated animals (to 7.0-7.1) the cardiac output was reduced to 50 % [14]. In another hypoxia study in ventilated piglets of the same age, the decrease of cardiac output was effected by a decrease of myocardial contractility (dp/dt_{max}), while centralization was maintained (permanent increase of total peripheral resistance [2]. The long lasting decrease in cardiac output during severe hypoxia and direct hypoxic effects on the cerebral circulation might contribute to the vital decompensation of the ventilated animals. In 2 cases CBF-decrease below critical levels and depressed EEG shortly precede critical arterial pressure drop. In addition during the 70th and 90th min a significant increase of R_c of the grey matter (quick compartment) was observed (Fig. 3). In most cases of decompensation of ventilated animals, a delayed summation effect of hypoxia and acidosis must be assumed, due to the frequent decompensation during the posthypoxic phase. The findings can explain the different outcome of both investigated groups because the ventilated animals were stressed by a longer interval of pronounced hypoxia *and* acidosis.

In the artificially ventilated and spontaneously breathing piglets surviving hypoxia, we observed characteristic cerebrovascular and metabolic dynamics (Fig. 3a, b): In both groups an increase in CBF (and no increase, but partly a decrease of cerebrovascular resistance) were observed. But only in spontaneously breathing animals a significant increase of O_2-demand within the quick compartment was seen. The permanent increase of CBF of ventilated piglets during hypoxia and the absence of CBF decrease in the posthypoxic period (Fig. 3b) also confirm a mainly non cerebral, i. e. a cardiac origin of vital decompensation. The insignificantly stronger posthypoxic pH_a decrease of spontaneously breathing ani-

Control of vital compensation hypoxic-acidotic effects 269

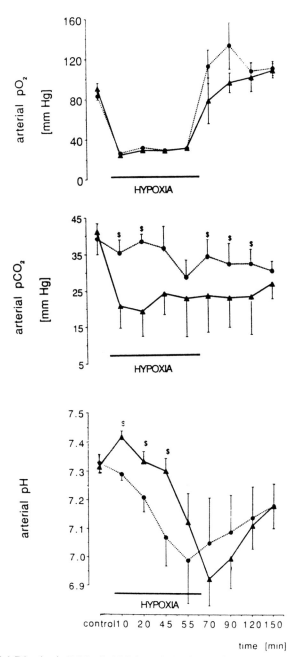

Fig. 2: Arterial PO$_2$ (top), PCO$_2$ (middle), and pH (bottom) of 8 spontaneously breathing (full lines) and 9 ventilated piglets (dotted lines) during and after severe atmosphaeric hypoxia (S: significant differences between the 2 animal groups (P < 0.05)).

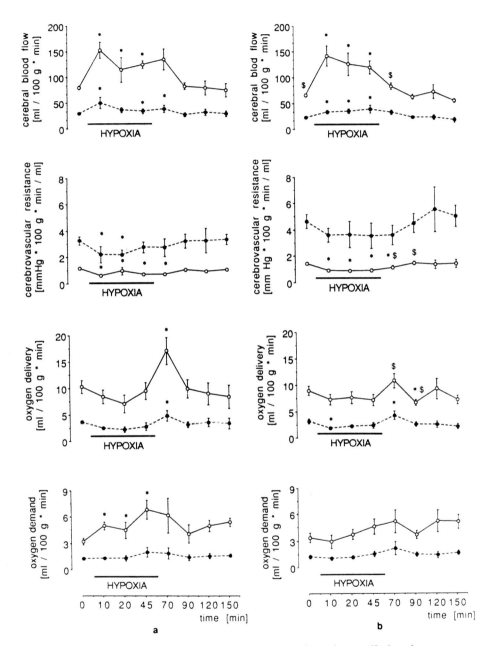

Fig. 3: Cerebral blood flow (CBF, upper row), cerebrovascular resistance (2nd row), oxygen delivery (3nd row), and oxygen demand (last row) of a. 8 spontaneously breathing and b. 9 ventilated piglets (full lines: quick compartment of CBF, dotted lines: slow compartment of CBF; S: significant differences between the 2 animal groups ($P < 0.05$)).

mals as compared to the ventilated ones can not be explained conclusively. Surprisingly, during the hyperventilatoric hypocapnia the spontaneously breathing piglets did not show a decrease of CBF as expected due to the influence of pH increase on the R_c (Fig. 3a), as always observed in hypocapnia in adults. This can be explained by the dilatating effect of severe hypoxia on the smaller brain vessels [7] but also by ontogenetical features, like a lower sensitivity of brain vessels upon hypocapnia [5].

The fact that no decrease of CBF could be found in the spontaneously breathing piglets during hypoxia when using the ^{133}Xe-clearance technique does not exclude the existence of local hypoxaemias as observed when applying the microsphere techniques during mild hypoxia [17]. In addition, already one to one and a half hours after inducing hypoxia, the spontaneously breathing and surviving piglets showed local neuronal necroses within the forebrain [3, 15, 18].

Summarizing, in newborn piglets a feedforward control of the acid-base-state by spontaneous hyperventilation during severe hypoxia can prevent vital decompensation but not local brain damages. These results are not species specific, because hypoxia in newborn rabbits (4 Vol % O_2) induced a similar long lasting hyperventilatoric reaction [1]. A sustained hyperventilation was also observed under hypoxic conditions in lambs [11].

References

1. BAUER, R. (1985): Akute zerebral-vegetative Auswirkungen normobarer hypoxischer Hypoxie beim zwei Wochen alten Kaninchen und deren Folgen auf die Postnatalperiode. Prom. A., Med. Fakultät Friedrich-Schiller-Universität Jena.
2. BAUER, R., W. BUCHENAU, G. BECHER, U. ZWIENER, D. HOYER, A. ODDOY, H. WITTE & G. MERKER (1987): Ventilatorische und kardiovaskuläre Auswirkungen systemischer Hypoxiebelastung in der Neonatalperiode. Ergebn. Exp.Med. 48, 234-246.
3. BAUER, R., U. ZWIENER, W. BUCHENAU, D. HOYER, H. WITTE, V. LAMPE, K. BURGHOLD & M. ZIEGER (1989): Reduced cardiovascular and cerebral compensatory ability of intra-uterine growth retarded newborn piglets in severe hypoxic load. Int. J. Feto-Matern. Med. 2, 98-108.
4. FLECKNELL, P.A., R. WOOTTON & M. JOHN (1982): Accurate measurement of cerebral metabolism in the conscious, unrestrained neonatal pig. II. Glucose and oxygen utilization. Biol. Neonate 41, 221 226.
5. Hansen, N.B., A.M. BRUBAKK, D. BRATLID, W.OH & B.S. STONESTREET (1984): The effects of variations in P_aCO_2 on brain blood flow and cardiac ouput in the newborn piglet. Pediat. Res. 18, 1132- 1136.
6. JANSEN, A.H. & V. CHERNICK (1983): Development of respiratory control. Physiol. Rev. 63, 437-483.

7. KONTOS, H.A., E.P. WEI & A.J. RAPER (1978): Role of tissue hypoxia in local regulation of cerebral microcirculation. Am. J. Physiol 234, H 582-591.
8. KRASNEY, J.A. & R.C. KOEHLER (1980): Neural control of the circulation during hypoxia. In: HUGHERS, M.J., S.C. Barnes (eds.): Research Topics in Physiology, Vol. II: Neural Control of Circulation., pp 123-147, Acad. Press. New York.
9. LASSEN, N.A. & D.H. INGVAR (1972): Radioisotopic assessment of regional cerebral blood flow. In: POTCHEN E.I. & V.R. MCCREADY (eds.): Progr. Nuclear Med., Vol. 1., pp 376-409, Karger Basel.
10. POOLE-WILSON, P.A. (1980): Effects of acidosis and weak acids on the normal, hypoxic, and ischaemic myocardium. In: MORET, P.R., J. WEBER. J.CH. HAISSLY & H. DEMALIN (eds.): Lactat, pp. 197-206, Springer Berlin-Heidelberg-New York.
11. PURVES, M. (1966): The effects of hypoxia in the newborn lamb before and after denervation of the carotid chemoreceptors. J. Physiol., London 185, 60-77.
12. RIHA, M. (1976): Estimation of ventilatory parameters in newborn infants with respiratory disease. Techn. Report Nr. 70, Chalmers Univ. of Techn. Göteborg.
13. WEBER, E. (1980): Grundriß der biologischen Statistik. 8th ed. Gustav Fischer, Jena.
14. ZWIENER, U., R. BAUER, W. BUCHENAU, J. FRENZEL, M. ROTHER & M. EISELT (1986): Correlations between cardiovascular, cerebrovascular and EEG dynamics in hypoxic-ischaemic disorders in neonates - pathogenetic lines and some clinical aspects. In GRAUEL, E.L., I. SYLLM-RAPOPORT & R.R. WAUER: Research in Perinatal Medicine, pp. 196-207, Georg Thieme Leipzig.
15. ZWIENER, U., R. BAUER, W. BUCHENAU, D. HOYER, M. ZIEGER & H. WAGNER (1986): Vascular resistance, metabolism, and EEG within cerebral grey and white matter during hypoxia in neonatal piglets. Biol. Res. Pregnancy 7, 23-29.
16. ZWIENER, U., H.P. LUDIN & H. PETSCHE (1990): Neuropathophysiologie. Gustav Fischer, Jena.
17. ZWIENER, U., R. BAUER, R. BERGMANN & M. EISELT (1991): Experimental and clinical main forms of hypoxic-ischaemic brain damage and their monitoring. Exp. Pathol. 42, 187-196.
18. ZWIENER, U., R. BAUER, M. EISELT, M. ROTHER, H. WITTE & D. HOYER (1991): Implications and consequences from the experimental research for diagnostics and early therapy of brain damages in neonates. Z. Klin. Med. 41, 37-42.

Influence of blood transfusion on fractionation of stable oxygen isotopes under the condition of severe anemia

H. Heller*, K.-D. Schuster*, and B.O. Göbel**

Physiologisches Institut* und Medizinische Poliklinik**
der Universität Bonn

Introduction

Previous studies have demonstrated that the stable, isotopic oxygen molecules $^{16}O_2$ and $^{16}O^{18}O$ are an appropriate tool for investigating entire oxygen transport system under varying conditions [3, 4, 8]. In healthy humans it could be shown that at rest $^{16}O_2$ is transported 0.9 % or 0.72 % more rapidly from inspiratory gas to tissues than its heavier isotopic species $^{16}O^{18}O$ [8, 3], leading to a change in the isotopic composition of oxygen. This so-called overall fractionation effect of respiration, given as δ-value, is defined as percentage deviation of $^{16}O^{18}O$-abundance between inspired (I) and utilized (U) oxygen ($δ_{IU}$).

For interpretation, above given data was compared with the fractionation effects of the different pathways of respiration, which are diffusion, O_2-utilization, and convective processes. The δ-values of these pathways are known to amount to 3 %, 1.3 % [8, 2], and 0 %, respectively. From this it has been concluded that at rest entire oxygen transport is far more limited by metabolism and convective processes, such as ventilation and blood flow, than by diffusion.

In order to assess the contribution of particular processes of respiration to the resistance of the entire oxygen transport system, conditions have to be choosen under which the whole transport system is mostly affected by one of its components. In case of a limitation of respiration by one of these processes, its fractionation effect will contribute most to overall fractionation effect, so that determinations of $δ_{IU}$ would give the opportunity to detect such a limitation.

The aim of the present study was to estimate the influence of alterations in oxygen carrying capacity of blood on the overall fractionation effect of respiration at rest. Measuring δ_{IU} during severe anemia and following blood substitution could help to answer the question as to in which degree a decrease in hemoglobin concentration can be compensated without a detectable limitation of oxygen transport by blood flow.

Methods

Experimental protocol and isotopic analysis

Experiments were carried out on 5 patients suffering from chronic anemia and on 5 healthy humans. Red cell transfusions had to be performed periodically on all patients. During the investigations the test subjects breathed room air in a sitting position. After attaining steady state conditions, up to 40 l of expired gas were sampled into a bag. Respiratory and circulatory conditions during the gas sampling period were quantified by measurements of volume expired, sampling time, heart frequency and alveolar and mixed-expiratory partial pressures of oxygen and carbon dioxide (respiratory mass spectrometry). The experiments were performed shortly before and after transfusion. Using a respiratory mass spectrometer (M3, Varian MAT, Bremen, FRG) which had been adapted for direct measurements of small quantities of oxygen isotopes [6, 7], the $^{16}O^{18}O/^{16}O_2$-ratios of inspired room air as well as of expiratory gas mixtures were determined. The isotopic analysis was operated by detecting the ions $^{16}O_2^+$ and $^{16}O^{18}O^+$ simultaneously at two different collectors.

Calculations

The overall fractionation effect δ_{IU} is given as

$$\delta_{IU} = \frac{X_I - X_U}{X_I} \cdot 100 \quad (\%) \qquad (1)$$

X_I and X_U are the $^{16}O^{18}O/^{16}O_2$-ratios of inspired and utilized oxygen. Since X_U cannot be determined, δ_{IU} has to be derived from

$$\delta_{IU} = \frac{V_E O_2}{\dot{V} O_2} \cdot \delta_{IE} \quad (\%) \qquad (2)$$

where $V_EO_2/\dot{V}O_2$ is the ratio of expiratory oxygen flow to oxygen uptake and δ_{IE} is the measured fractionation effect between inspired (I) and expired (E) oxygen.

Results

In order to exclude the influence of ventilation on the overall fractionation effect [4], all δ_{IU}-values were normalized to δ_{IU}^n referring to a constant alveolar partial pressure of oxygen of $P_AO_2 = 100$ mmHg. The relationship between the normalized values δ_{IU}^n and the hemoglobin concentration of blood ([Hb]) is plotted in Fig. 1. δ_{IU}^n increases from 0.59 % to 0.71 % with

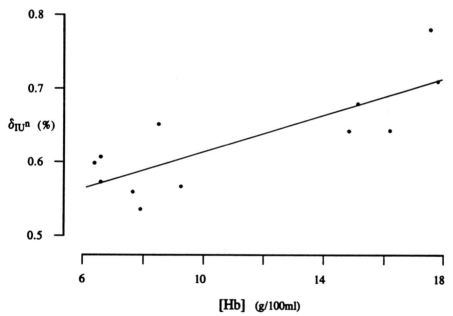

Fig. 1: Linear regression of normalized values of overall fractionation effect of respiration (δ_{IU}^n) on values of hemoglobin content within blood ([Hb]) obtained from patients before transfusion and from healthy humans: $r = 0.814$, $n = 12$.

rising [Hb]-values from 6.4 to 17.8 g/100 ml. Applying linear regression analysis, the relationship between both parameters is given as

$$\delta_{IU}^n = 0{,}489 + 1.25 \cdot 10^{-2} \cdot [Hb] \qquad (\%) \qquad (3)$$

The correlation coefficient r = 0.814 of n = 12 independent measurements is significantly different from zero as is the regression coefficient (P < 0.01, P < 0.002). With regard to the rise of δ_{IU}^n due to an increase in [Hb] caused by transfusion, for 4 patients one can calculate a mean δ_{IU}^n-increase of $4 \cdot 10^{-2}$ %·100 ml/g, which is significantly greater than the slope of regression line (p < 0.005) according to eq. (3), as shown in Fig. 2.

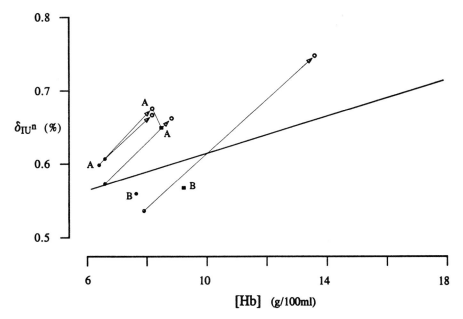

Fig. 2: δ_{IU}^n-values of 5 patients obtained before transfusion (dots), of 4 patients obtained shortly after transfusion (open circles), and of 2 patients (A, B) obtained not earlier than 3 days after transfusion (rectangles). The increase of δ_{IU}^n due to transfusion (arrows) is compared to the slope of regression line transferred from Fig. 1. Patient A underwent experiments 3 times and patient B twice.

Discussion

A resistance model as a basis for interpreting results

On first glance at eq. (1), overall fractionation of oxygen isotopes occurs during a single step of oxygen transport between inspiratory gas and oxygen utilizing tissues. But in fact oxygen transport has to overcome more than a single resistance interposed between room air and tissues. As mentioned above, overall fractionation effect can be split into fractionation effects of the included pathways, which are ventilation (δ_V), O_2-diffusion within lungs (δ_{DL}), blood flow (δ_B), O_2-diffusion within tissues (δ_{DT}) and O_2-utilization (δ_U). Each of these pathways exerts its own resistance on oxygen transport (R_V, R_{DL}, R_B, R_{DT}, R_U). Since total resistance of entire oxygen transport (R_{IU}) is additively connected to these resistances and assuming steady state conditions, δ_{IU} is given as

$$\tag{4}$$

In eq. (4) the different fractionation effects are to be weighted by the ratio of resistance according to each pathway to the total resistance R_{IU}.

Using eq. (4) the contribution of the resistance R_B to R_{IU} can be assessed in anemic patients who received blood transfusion. Since ventilation and blood flow are known (δ_V and $\delta_B = 0$), eq. (4) can be reduced to

$$\tag{5}$$

Moreover, R_{IU} is assumed to be constant under steady state conditions at rest as is the resistance of ventilation R_V due to the normalization of δ_{IU}-values. Taking all this into account, it can be concluded that in the case of a limitation of oxygen transport by convective processes in anemic patients only R_B will increase. Consequently, one or more of the remaining resistances of eq. (5) have to be diminished, so that one or more of the fractionation effects δ_{DL}, δ_{DT} and δ_U will be weighted to a lower extent, and δ_{IU}^n therefore has to decrease.

Dependence of δ_{IU}^n on hemoglobin concentration of blood

According to Fick's principle and Ohm's law, R_B is proportional to the partial pressure difference of oxygen in arterial and venous blood ($P_{av}O_2$) and is in inverse proportion to [Hb] and cardiac output (Q) as

$$\tag{6}$$

The observed decrease of δ_{IU}^n in anemic patients seems to be caused by the increase in R_B with decreasing [Hb]. Heart frequency of the anemic patients (102 ± 10 min^{-1}, mean $\pm$ SD) was significantly greater ($P < 0.025$) than that of the healthy humans (82 ± 6 min^{-1}), supposing an enlarged cardiac output. As δ_{IU}^n of the anemic patients was diminished, the rise in cardiac output was not sufficient to compensate the drop of [Hb]. Although, in anemia above the [Hb]-range of 7 to 8 g / 100 ml the rise in 2,3-DPG content of red blood cells and the decrease in blood viscosity should be able to avoid an increase in cardiac output [1, 5, 9]. However, the decrease in δ_{IU}^n was already observed at a [Hb]-value above this level. The low correlation coefficient of 0.814 of the relationship between δ_{IU}^n and [Hb] indicates a high mean variation of δ_{IU}^n-values, despite the exclusion of the influence of ventilation on δ_{IU}^n by normalization.

Influence of blood transfusion on δ_{IU}^n in anemic patients

In the case of sufficient red cell transfusion, one would expect that decreased δ_{IU}^n-values should be raised in proportion to the increase in [Hb]. Contrary to this assumption, the mean rise in δ_{IU}^n of $4 \cdot 10^{-2}$ following transfusion is more than three times as large as the regression coefficient of the δ_{IU}^n-[Hb]-relationship (eq. (3)). As a result of transfusion, the δ_{IU}^n-values rose overproportionally. This would be in line with a decrease of R_B expected due to the increase in hemoglobin content.

Experiments were performed not later than 1.5 hours after transfusion. Since the reduction in the 2,3-DPG content of stored red blood cells does not rise until 6 to 12 hours after transfusion [9], low 2,3-DPG levels and an impeded oxygen release from blood to tissues have to be expected during the measurements. Consequently, $P_{av}O_2$ and the resistance R_B would have been increased (see eq. (6)). Simultaneously, an increase in cardiac output should have been caused by the increase in blood volume. Suming up, it seems reasonable to suppose that the increase of R_B due to the fall of 2,3-DPG level is covered up by a reduction of R_B brought about by a rise in cardiac output.

The [Hb]-data as shown in Fig. 1 is obviously obtained by a nonrandom sampling of a population. This derives from the aim of the study to investigate the effect of blood transfusion on δ_{IU}^n of patients suffering from severe anemia, and to compare the results to the corresponding data from healthy subjects. Thus, the [Hb]-values were selected, but not randomly sampled.

Above given interpretation of the influence of blood transfusion on δ_{IU}^n is, however, confirmed by the data of the patient A and B.

Another way to interpret results is to compare the sample averages for [Hb] and δ_{IU}^n according to the patients before and after transfusion with those obtained from healthy humans. For the anemic patients, blood transfusion caused an increase of the mean value of δ_{IU}^n from 0.58 ± 0.03 % to 0.69 ± 0.04 %. The latter value is no different to the sample average in the δ_{IU}^n-values of controls which amounted to 0.69 ± 0.06 % (n = 5). The sample averages of [Hb] were 6.88, 9.7 and 16.3 g / 100 ml. The δ_{IU}^n-values of controls were attained shortly after transfusion already at a hemoglobin concentration of 9.7 g / 100 ml. Asssuming this as a final result and rejecting the thesis of further adaptation, this would indicate a strong nonlinear relationship between δ_{IU}^n and [Hb] with a steep δ_{IU}^n-increase within the [Hb]-range of 6.88 to 9.7 g / 100 ml which would be similar to that due to transfusion. Such a relationship is in contrast to the data of patient A and B which covers a similar [Hb]-range. In both patient δ_{IU}^n increases inside the confidence interval of the regression coefficient of eq. (3). Furthermore, all changes of δ_{IU}^n-data due to transfusion are very similar, however they cover a [Hb]-range from 6.4 to 13.6 g/100 ml. Therefore a strong nonlinear dependence of δ_{IU}^n on [Hb] seems to be unlikely within this [Hb]-range.

References

1. BEGEMANN, H. (1986): Anämien. In: BEGEMANN, H. & J. RASTETTER (eds.): Klinische Hämatologie, pp. 216-218, Stuttgart, New York: Thieme Verlag.
2. FELDMAN, D.E., H.T.JR. YOST & B.B. BENSON (1959): Oxygen isotope fractionation in reactions catalyzed by enzymes. Science 129, 146-147.
3. HELLER, H. & K.-D. SCHUSTER (1990): Investigation of oxygen transport to tissues during rest and ergometer work by using oxygen isotopes. Pflügers Arch. 415, R67.
4. HELLER, H., M. KÖNEN & K.-D. SCHUSTER (1993): Dependence of overall fractionation effect of respiration on ventilation at rest. Isotopenpraxis 28, 133-141.
5. ROSSI, E.C. (1991): Pathophysiology of anemia. In: ROSSI, E.C., T.L. SIMON & G.S. MOSS (eds.): Principles of transfusion medicine, pp. 91-93, Baltimore, Hong Kong, London, Munich, San Franciscio, Sydney, Tokyo: Williams & Wilkins.
6. SCHUSTER, K.-D., K.P. PFLUG, H. FÖRSTEL & J.P. PICHOTKA (1979): Adaptation of respiratory mass spectrometry to continuous recording of abundance ratios of stable oxygen isotopes. In: A. FRIGERIO (ed): Recent developments in mass spectrometry in biochemistry and medicine, Vol. 2, pp. 451-462, New York: Plenum Publishing Corp.
7. SCHUSTER, K.-D. (1985): Kinetics of pulmonary CO_2 transfer studied by using labeled carbon dioxide $C^{16}O^{18}O$. Respir. Physiol. 60, 21-37.

8. SCHUSTER, K.-D. & K.P. PFLUG (1989): The overall fractionation effect of isotopic oxygen molecules during oxygen transport and utilization in humans. Adv. Exp. Med. Biol. 248, 151-156.
9. SIMON, T.L. (1991): Red cell transfusion. In: ROSSI, E.C., T.L. SIMON & G.S. MOSS (eds.): Principles of transfusion medicine, pp. 95-98, Baltimore, Hong Kong, London, Munich, San Franciscio, Sydney, Tokyo: Williams & Wilkins.

Power spectral analysis of the heart period duration under conditions of rest and load

E. Schubert, W. Laube* and A. Patzak

Institute of Physiology, Humboldt-University of Berlin and
*Klinik Bavaria, Kreischa

Introduction

The cardiovascular system adapts its performance to O_2-demands in man mainly by setting the heart rate via vagal and sympathetic efferents [20]. Influences of age, load, training conditions and diseases have been well investigated and make a distinction between vagal effects upon sinus arrhythmia and sympathetic drive mainly on the heart rate [6, 23, 24]. The analyses do not allow to discriminate diverse origins of regulatory effects or changes in the information processing of the vegetative cardiovascular centres, especially under the influence of "higher control" called central command. This mechanism is most likely to be responsible for the setting of cardiac action under physical load. An exact adjustment of respiration and circulation to the requirements of the tissues is only possible with afferent inputs from peripheral receptors reflecting the metabolic situation of supply and export. In this respect, the phenomenon of the respiratory sinus arrhythmia (RSA) hints at influences of respiration on the heart either by means of central co-activation and interaction of both regulatory centres, respectively, or by afferent pathways from baro- or stretch receptors in the thorax. Hitherto, other inputs may participate in the efferent vago-sympathetic control of the cardiac rhythm [11].

Via power spectral analysis one may gain further insight into the vago-sympathetic influences on the heart rhythm. It is known that the power spectrum of the heart period variability in adult men shows three peaks: A high-frequency band (HF) is centred at the respiratory frequency and its amplitude reflects quantitatively the respiratory arrhythmia. This component is mainly mediated by the vagus [2]. The mid-frequency part (MF) around 0.1 Hz corresponds to the blood pressure rhythm, visible in the Hering-Traube-Mayer waves. In the range between 0.01 and 0.05 Hz, a low frequency (LF) peak becomes evident, which is assumed to be of vasomotor origin. These MF- and LF-bands are attributed both to the sympathetic and parasympathetic activity [2]. However, a contradictory discussion about the results exists [1].

Changes of heart rate during exercise are produced by a reduction of vagal activity and simultaneous amplification of the sympathetic drive up to a rate of 120 bpm. Beyond that, the control is realised only by the sympathetic system [19, 23]. Our aim is to find out in which way spectral analysis can reveal origins of the different components of heart rate control during exercise.

Methods

The experimental group consisted of 16 adult and physically active men (age 25 years, SE ± 5.8 years). They were prepared for the experiment and gave their informed consent. The subjects performed a cycle ergometer program, which included an increase of load starting at 0.5 up to 3.0 W/kg body mass in steps of 0.5 W. Each phase of load lasted 5 min and was followed by recovery periods of 6 min. The rotation speed of the cycle ergometer was 75 cpm. The registration of the ECG began when the subjects mounted on the ergometer. After a resting period of 5 min the load-recovery cycles started. Heart period duration (HPD) was evaluated by measuring the interval length between successive R-waves in ms. A half-open system was used for the investigation of ventilation. The subjects breathed through a mask. Respiratory frequency and tidal volume were recorded continuously using a computer aided system. Changes in the metabolic milieu were surveyed by analysing lactic acid from capillary blood samples at rest, and in each phase of load and recovery.

Off-line analysis was performed on a digital computer. At first, the data of each experimental phase underwent a test of errors. After automatic correction, the data were linearly interpolated with a sampling frequency of 5 Hz. Trends were eliminated by high-pass filtering with a Bessel filter of 2nd order, limiting frequency 0.03 Hz. A fast Fourier transform based algorithm served for the calculation of the power spectrum in the range from 0 to 1 Hz. A Hanning-window was used for the estimation of the spectrum. Spectral terms for equidistant 256 data points were calculated, which corresponds to a period of 51,2 sec. The power spectra of load and recovery phases were expressed as the mean of 5 and 6 single spectra. As secondary parameters, we calculated: the total power as the sum of the power of all spectral terms and the relative power in percentage values in the ranges between 0.03 and 0.05 Hz (LF), 0.05 and 0.15 Hz (MF), and 0.15 and 0.5 Hz (HF).

Results

Fig. 1 represents the power spectra of a single subject of the experimental series for resting, loading and recovery phases. Despite poorly smoothed spectra and various smaller peaks, a mid- and high frequency peak can be seen. At rest, the HF-part consists of two peaks due to a change in the respiratory frequency. An LF-peak is absent. With increasing load the MF-peak remains stable. Beginning with a load of 1.5 W/kg b.m. an LF-peak becomes visible. The HF-part drastically decreases at 0.5 W/kg b.m. and now shows multiple peaks, whereby the central frequency of the main peak corresponds to the main frequency of the ventilation. Although the total power is drastically diminished at 2.5 and 3.0W/kg b.m., the spectra allow regularly a clear distinction between the low-, mid- and high-frequency region.

Resting conditions

The spectra of the heart period variability of the 16 volunteers regularly show two peaks, situated in the mid- and high-frequency range. Below 0.05 Hz (LF-region), a distinct peak is not always recognisable. The means of the absolute power of the LF-, MF-, and HF-regions are 856 ± 840 ms^2, 8552 ± 4377 ms^2, and 4379 ± 6628 ms^2, the relative parts of them lead to 6.8 ± 5.6 % (LF), 65.5 ± 14.4 % (MF), and 26.8 ± 15.0 % (HF). Respiration shows a mean frequency of 15.6 ± 3.8 breath/min and an average tidal volume of 819 ± 239 ml, corresponding to a total ventilatory rate of 13.1 ± 4.3 l/min. Lactic acid amounts to 1.45 ± 0.4 mmol/l.

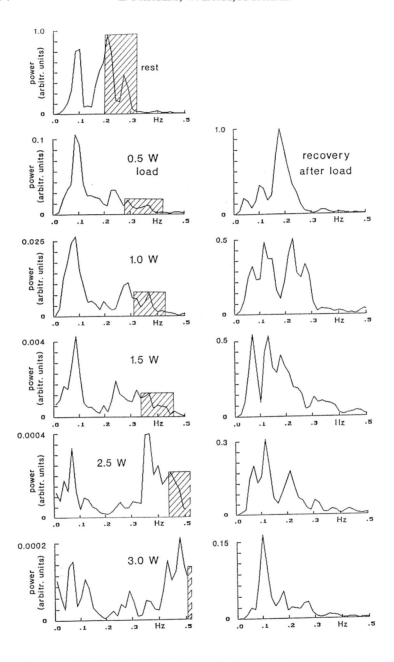

Fig. 1: Power spectra of the heart period variability from one subject for phases of load and recovery. The hatched regions mark the range of mean respiratory frequencies of all 16 subjects during phases of load.

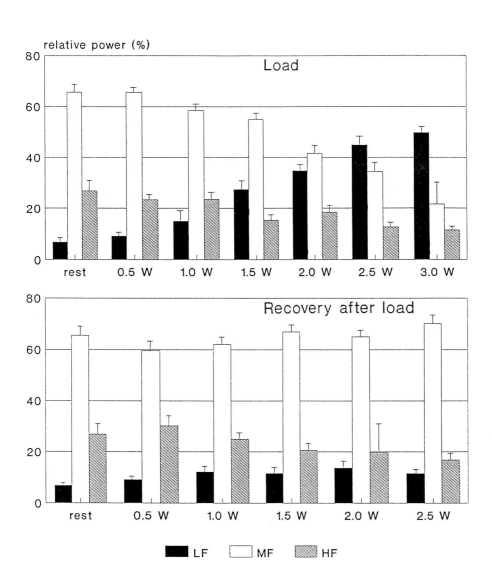

Fig. 2: Relative power of the LF-, MF-, and HF-frequency bands of the spectral density during load and in recovery.

Condition of load

Generally, during load, the total power of the heart period spectrum decreases by a factor of 10^3-10^4, starting from rest up to the level of the highest load. The power in the three defined ranges decreases in a different manner. The relative power of the LF-region increases from 6.8 ± 1.4 % up to 49.8 ± 2.6 %, that of the MF-region drops from 65.6 ± 3.6 % to 31.6 ± 3.7 %, and that of the HF-band decreases slightly from 26.8 ± 3.8 % to 11.5 ± 1.3 % (Fig. 2). The respiratory rate increases from 15.6 ± 3.8 /min at rest to 36.7 ± 6.4 /min (3 W/kg b.m.) and the tidal volume rises from 819 ± 239 ml to 2624 ± 378 ml. This corresponds to a total respiratory rate of 13.1 ± 4.3 l/min and $95.5 \pm 16,7$ l/min, respectively. The lactic acid reaches a maximum of 7.33 ± 1.9 mmol/l after the maximal load.

Recovery between phases of load

During recovery the total power remains nearly unaffected after a load of 0.5 W./kg b.m.. At loads greater than 1.5W/kg b.m., it is reduced by a factor up to 10^1, reflecting an incomplete recovery. The relations between the parts of the spectrum change in different ways: the LF-part increases from 6.8 ± 1.4 % at rest to 11.6 ± 1.3 % after load of 2.5 W/kg b.m., the HF-region decreases from 26.8 ± 3.8 % to 16.8 ± 3.2 %, and the MF-part depicts no clear fluctuation (65.6 ± 3.6 % and 70.2 ± 2.9 %, Fig. 2).

Discussion

Several authors were able to demonstrate power spectra of heart rate variability in man and mammalians containing three major components, which are characterised by more or less distinct peaks of power in a low-, middle-, and high-frequency range [2, 9, 17, 21, 22]. This is consistent with the results of our subjects in resting conditions. As Fig. 1 shows, the appearance of such spectra is variable. The variability of the patterns of the spectra depends on the individual characteristics of the investigated subjects and on the non-stationarity of biological rhythms. Changes in biological rhythm are observed, even during rest (12). However, one of the important requirements of spectral analysis is the stationarity of the signal. Therefore, spectral patterns with more than one peak in the high-frequency or mid-frequency range occur as demonstrated in the Fig. 1, particularly in the recovery periods. As for the contribution of trends to the low-frequency variability, a great portion of it is removed by the filtering procedure required because of the short interval of analysis. Thus, at rest, the mid-frequency peak dominates in the majority of the subjects (Fig. 2), a common finding in the orthostatic position [14, 17]. The MF/HF-relation is lower in supine position and reflects the changes in activity of the sympathetic system.

Studies of heart rate variability have elucidated the main role of the vagus [23]. In these studies the RSA as measured in the time domain variability was taken into account. Akselrod et al. [2, 3] demonstrated by spectral analysis that the high-frequency band of the spectrum corresponds to respiration and is mainly parasympathetically mediated. These authors [14, 18] proved LF and MF as jointly mediated by the parasympathetic and -sympathetic system.

During physical load the predominant phenomenon is the decrease of total power. This corresponds to the investigations of the overall heart rate variability (HRV). In our experiments, the logarithm of total power decreases linearly with increasing load from 0.5 to 3.0 W/kg b.m., reflecting the mathematical relation between HRV expressed in ms and the power measured in ms^2. Although HRV reaches values near the noise level of 1 ms during high load, the spectrum offers distinct peaks, which are related to all three frequency bands.

This raises the question of which mechanisms are involved in generating the different frequency bands. Until now, the generation of the respiratory rhythm is not quite clear. A central rhythm generator and afferent discharge from mechano- or pressoreceptors in the thorax are under discussion [11]. Since the respiratory component is assumed to be of vagal origin, a residual activity should be taken into consideration under condition of high load. On the other hand, studies in patients with heart transplantation hint at the possibility of an intrinsic ability to vary heart rate synchronously with respiration in consequence of myocardial stretch [5]. A respiratory drive under conditions of load moreover can result from central activation, chemo- and metaboreceptive afferents from the muscle and receptors in the vascular system [13, 25, 26].

The main frequency of the HF region shifts to higher frequencies with growing respiratory rate during stepwise increasing load. This is demonstrated also in voluntarily breathing subjects, when respiratory rate is changed [10, 15]. It is known that the respiratory sinus arrhythmia increases if the tidal volume is enhanced [7, 8]. Arai et al. [4], reflecting the frequency effect of respiration on heart rate, calculated an increasing effect of about 25 % for the high-frequency power. HF-power however drastically decreases during load. This agrees well with our study and suggests the maximal reduction of the vagal drive to the heart.

The mechanisms for the 0.1 Hz rhythm are very complex and include fluctuations in cardiovascular parameters as well as arterial and venous pressure and vascular volume. Akselrod et al. [2] assumed a combined sympathetic and vagal response below 0.1 Hz. At lower frequencies from 0.05 to 0.01 Hz, variabilities of the vasomotor activity are important, whereby the renin-angiotensin system is reported to have a damping effect [3]. Under these aspects the relation between high- and mid-/low-frequency power should reflect changes in the sympatho-vagal interaction of the heart rate control. In our study the relative power of the low frequency range increases, the mid-frequency part decreases and the power of the high-frequency range is slightly diminished. These results are in good agreement with measurements of Perini et al. [16] and point to a sympathetic influence on the low-frequency component during load. However, the low-frequency part contains an undefined portion, possibly due to a trend effect which increases under loading conditions.

In the recovery phases, the power decreases only slightly after a load of 1-2 W/kg b.m.. At 2.5 and 3 W/kg b.m. the decrease is clear. The factor of the decrease amounts to 10^1 and is smaller than at load. Interestingly, the beginning of the reduction in the total power at a load of 1 W/kg b.m. corresponds to a distinct increase in lactic acid to 1.9 ± 0.6 mmol/l. Possibly, this indicates a role of chemo-afferents from the muscle in the modulation of the vagal cardiac activity.

In summary, our results confirm the applicability of power spectral analysis for the estimation of rhythms in the heart rate variability at rest and load. In contrast to studies of the overall variability, power spectrum analysis gives an insight into various components of the heart rate regulation reflecting respiratory, vasomotor and possible chemosensitive influences. It remains unclear whether the spectrum reflects the vago-sympathetic balance under load, as the reduction of power across the entire spectrum is dominant. Indeed the increase of the normalised low-frequency power is associated with a prevalence of the sympathetic drive, but it cannot be distinguished from the trend effects.

References

1. ABEL, H.-H., D. KLÜSSENDORF, R. DROH & H.-P. KOEPCHEN (1991): Cardiorespiratory relations in human heart rate pattern. In: Cardiorespiratory and motor coordination. KOEPCHEN, H.-P. & T. HUOPANIEMI, pp. 307-318, Springer-Verlag, Berlin, Heidelberg, New York.
2. AKSELROD S., D. GORDON, F.A. UBEL, D.C. SHANNON, A.C. BARGER & R.J. COHEN (1981): Power spectrum analysis of heart rate fluctuation: A quantitative probe of beat-to-beat cardiovascular control. Science 231, 220-222.
3. AKSELROD, S., D. GORDON, J.B. MADWED, N.C. SNIDMAN, D.C. SHANNON & R.J. COHEN (1985): Hemodynamic regulation: investigation by spectral analysis. Am. J. Physiol. 249, H867-H875.
4. ARAI, Y., J.P. SAUL, P. ALBRECHT, L.H. HARTLEY, L.S. LILLY, R.J. COHEN & W.S. COLUCCI (1989): Modulation of cardiac autonomic activity during and immediately after exercise. Am. J. Physiol. 256, H132-141.
5. BERNARDI, L., F. KELLER, M. SANDERS, P.S. REDDY, B. GRIFFITH, F. MENO & M.R. PINSKY (1989): Respiratory sinus arrhythmia in the denervated human heart. J. Appl. Physiol. 67, 1447-1455.
6. ECKBERG, D.L. (1983): Human sinus arrhythmia as an index of vagal cardiac outflow. J.Appl. Physiol. 54, 961-966.
7. ECKOLDT, K. & E. SCHUBERT (1975): Zum Einfluß der Atemtiefe auf die Sinusarrhythmie des Herzens. Acta biol. med. germ. 43, 767-771.
8. HIRSCH, J.A. & B. BISHOP (1981): Respiratory sinus arrhythmia in humans: how breathing pattern modulates heart rate. Amer. J. Physiol. 241, H620-H629.
9. HYNDMAN, B.W. & J.R. GREGORY (1975): Spectral analysis of sinus arrhythmia during mental load. Ergonomics 18, 225-270.
10. KITNEY, R., D.A. LINKENS, A.C. SELMAN & A. MCDONALD (1982): The interaction between heart rate and respiration: part II - nonlinear analysis based on computer modelling. Automedica 4, 141-153.
11. KOEPCHEN, H.-P. (1982): Zentrale und reflektorische Steuerung der Herzfrequenz. In: Autonome Innervation des Herzens. BRISSE, B. & F. BINDER (eds), pp. 66-85, Steinkopf, Darmstadt.
12. KOEPCHEN, H.-P. (1991): Physiology of rhythms and control systems: An integrative approach. In: Rhythms in physiological systems; HAKEN, H. & H..-P. KOEPCHEN (eds.). pp. 3-20, Springer-Verlag, Berlin, Heidelberg.
13. KOIZUMI, K. & M. KOLLAI (1980): Differential sympathetic responses to stimulation of arterial chemoreceptors: The laterality of cardiac sympathetic nerve responses. In: Central interaction between respiratory and cardiovascular control system. KOEPCHEN, H.-P., S.M. HILTON & A. TRZEBSKI (eds), pp. 152-157, Springer Berlin, Heidelberg, New York.
14. PAGANI, M., F. LOMBARDI, S. GUZZETTI, O. RIMOLDI, R. FURLAM, P. PIZZINELLI, G. SANDRONE, G. MALFATTO, S. DELL'ORTO, E. PICCALUGA, M. TURIEL, G. BASELLI, S. CERUTTI & A. MALLIANI (1986): Power spectral analysis of heart rate and arterial pressure variabilities as a marker of sympatho-vagal interaction in man and conscious dog. Circ. Res. 59, 178-193.
15. PATZAK, A., C. JOHL, & J. EBNER (1991): Effect of breathing rate and amplitude on heart rate power spectra. J. Interdisc. Res. 22, 166-167.

16. PERINI, R., C. ORIZIO, G. BASELLI, S. CERUTTI & A. VEICSTEINAS (1990): The influence of exercise intensity on the power spectrum of heart rate variability. Eur. J. Appl. Physiol. 61, 143-148.
17. POMERANZ, B., R.J.B. MACAULAY, M.A. CAUDILL, I. KUTZ, D. ADAM, D. GORDON, K.M. KILBORN, A.C. BARGER, D.C. SHANNON, R.J. COHEN, & H. BENSON (1985): Assessment of autonomic function in humans by heart rate spectral analysis. Amer. J. Physiol. 248, H151-H153.
18. RAEDER, E.A., R. BERGER, R. KENET, J.P. KIELY, H. LEHNERT, R.J. COHEN & B. LOWN (1987): Assessment of autonomic cardiac control by power spectrum of the heart rate fluctuations. J. Appl. Cardiol. 2, 283-300.
19. ROBINSOHN, B.F., S.E. EBSTEIN, G.D. BEISER & E. BRAUNWALD (1966): Control of heart rate by the autonomic nervous system. Studies in man on the interrelation between baroreceptor mechanisms and exercise. Circ. Res. 19, 400-411.
20. RUSHMER, R.F. (1970): Cardiovascular dynamics. 3rd ed., Sounders Co, Philadelphia-London-Toronto.
21. SAUL, J.P., Y. ARAI, R. D. BERGER, L. LILLY, W.S. COLUCCI, & R.J. COHEN (1988): Assessment of autonomic regulation in chronic congestive heart failure by heart rate spectral analysis. Am. J. Cardiol. 61, 1292-1299.
22. SAYERS, B.M. (1973): Analysis of heart rate variability. Ergonomics, 16, 17-32.
23. Schubert, E. (1981): La détermination quantitative de l'activité du nerf vague et sa valeur pour la régulation du fonctionnement du coeur. Bull. et Mém. Acad. Roy. Méd. Belg. 136, 195-206.
24. SCHUBERT, E., K. ECKHOLDT & B. PFEIFER (1981): Normal ranges and deviations of the heart rhythm regulation in man. In: New frontiers in electrocardiology, F. DE PADUA, & P.W. MACFARLANE (eds.), pp. 409-413, Wiley, Chichester.
25. SCHUBERT, E., W. DINTER & W. RILKE (1991): Heart rate control and metabolic parameters after fatiguing exercise. In: Cardiorespiratory and motor coordination, KOEPCHEN, H.-P. & T. HUOPANIEMI (eds.), pp. 300-306, Springer-Verlag, Berlin, Heidelberg, New York.
26. TIBES, U. (1981): Kreislauf und Atmung bei Arbeit und Sport - Spiegel des Muskelstoffwechsels. Schriften der Deutschen Sporthochschule Köln, Bd. 6, Hans Richarz, Sankt Augustin.